Assessing Negative Response Bias in Competency to Stand Trial Evaluations

Assessing Negative Response Bias in Competency to Stand Trial Evaluations

STEVE RUBENZER

OXFORD
UNIVERSITY PRESS

OXFORD
UNIVERSITY PRESS

Oxford University Press is a department of the University of Oxford. It furthers the University's objective of excellence in research, scholarship, and education by publishing worldwide. Oxford is a registered trade mark of Oxford University Press in the UK and certain other countries.

Published in the United States of America by Oxford University Press
198 Madison Avenue, New York, NY 10016, United States of America.

CIP data is on file at the Library of Congress
ISBN 978-0-19-065316-3

CONTENTS

PREFACE

I've done a lot of competency evaluations: about 3,500 in Texas, on cases from trespassing to the highest-profile capital murder case, another 500-plus in New Hampshire, and about 100 in Alabama. I love the work. Many entering forensic work believe competency evaluations are pretty simple. And if you don't know what you're doing, they are. If you are knowledgeable about the law, psychological approaches to its definition and measurement, and assessment of response style, it is a topic of many subtleties.

My work at the Harris County Jail in Houston typically involved seeing two examinees each workday and performing a competency and sanity evaluation on each. On some days, I saw three or four defendants. It was possible to do fairly thorough evaluations because of several aspects of the Harris County system. Nearly all defendants were in custody at the jail, where my office was located. We had automatic access to the jail's medical chart and state psychiatric hospital records, as well as the offense report, rap sheet, and name and contact information for the defense attorney. If I needed observations from the jailers, I could call up to the pod and identify myself as a court-appointed examiner, and most of them would talk to me. Despite doing as many as 800 evaluations a year (counting competency and sanity evaluations separately), I typically testified only a couple times most years.

In 2002, I attended the first state-sponsored training program for competency examiners in Texas featuring Norm Poythress and Mary Alice Conroy. I also began pursuing my diplomate in forensic psychology and submitted work samples for CST and Mental State at the Time of the Offense exams. I successfully defended in 2004.

In 2010, I accepted a position with the Office of the Forensic Examiner in New Hampshire, providing court-appointed CST exams for defendants throughout New Hampshire. Things worked very differently in New Hampshire than in Texas. First of all, defendants were not presumed to be competent once the issue was raised. Most examinees were not in custody and came to the evaluation at our building in Concord. If medical or school records were available at all, they came through the defense attorney, often with missing pages or redactions. And attorneys, at least the public defenders, typically accompanied their clients to the evaluations and, prior to my arrival, had been permitted to stay during validity testing. Finally, a very substantial number of cases, perhaps one third, went to a formal hearing requiring testimony.

My introduction to malingering occurred in the 1980s when I saw eminent psychiatrist Phillip Resnick present in Houston. I began writing about negative response bias for legal audiences in 2004. In New Hampshire, I soon found that there were many defendants who had previously been found incompetent by the past chief examiner, a general (not forensic) psychiatrist. Many of these defendants failed validity tests in his evaluation: Some of these scored below chance on the Test of Memory Malingering or Competence Assessment for Standing Trial for Defendants with Mental Retardation, but the findings were soft-pedaled and rationalized.

Assessment of response style became the primary focus of my work. This included both exploring instruments for this purpose and identifying and contacting collateral sources—sometimes going well beyond the ones that are typically considered. This book attempts to summarize what I've learned, both from academic literature on response style and from nearly 15 years of full-time practice as an examiner. It is intended as a comprehensive summary and guide to assessing negative response bias in CST assessments. It does not address the full range of response style measures available in the neuropsychological literature, as tests like grip strength and finger-tapping are rarely used in CST exams, and there are already multiple books devoted to response style assessment in neuropsychological exams. Assessment of response style in CST examinations constitutes a specialized area of competence and requires some devotion to the field. Within 10 years, I believe that true competence in this area will be seen as indispensable by forensic professionals, prosecutors, and judges, and that CST examiners will neglect it at their peril.

ACKNOWLEDGMENTS

I would like to thank Hope Goldberg, Debbie Green, and Denis Zavodny for their input and feedback on earlier versions of this work. I would also like to thank Vicky Campagna and Eileen Kohutis for their feedback and suggestions on a considerably longer and revised version, and Michael Perlin for his assistance with legal citations. Finally, a number of forensic psychologists provided input and advice regarding the CST report checklist presented in Chapter 9. These included Thomas Schacht, Bruce Borkosky, Michael Thompson, Jill Durand, Kim Brown, Angela Torres, Vicky Campagna, Marla Domino, Tom Gray, and Terry Kukor.

ABOUT THE AUTHOR

Steve Rubenzer, PhD, ABPP, received his doctorate in clinical psychology at the University of Houston. He has worked in the field of forensic psychology since 1995, earned his board certification in forensic psychology in 2004 after completing work samples in competency and sanity assessment, and has authored multiple peer-reviewed papers on response style assessment in competency to stand trial and disability evaluations. He has performed approximately 4,000 competency exams in Texas, New Hampshire, and Alabama on cases ranging from trespassing to the highest-profile capital murder.

1

Introduction

There may be great fraud in this matter . . . [the judge] may do well to inquire . . . whether it (incompetence) be real or counterfeit. (Hale, 1736)

A defendant in a criminal case has a constitutional right to be able to understand the charges and proceedings against him or her. The seminal case, *Dusky v. United States* (1960), set out for the first time in the United States what would become the guiding language for the competency standard in nearly all jurisdictions: "Whether the defendant has sufficient present ability to consult with his lawyer with a reasonable degree of rational understanding and whether he has a rational as well as factual understanding of the proceedings against him" (p. 402). Although it is not explicitly stated, most jurisdictions require a mental condition or defect as the cause of any such deficits (Zapf & Roesch, 2009).

Evaluations of a defendant's competence to stand trial (CST) are probably the most frequently performed forensic evaluations (Melton, Petrila, Poythress, & Slobogin, 2007). Bonnie and Grisso (2000) estimated 60,000 CST evaluations are conducted annually in the United States. Vitacco, Rogers, and Gabel (2009) considered the number of defendants nationwide and that attorneys have reported concern about competency in 10% to 15% of their clients. They estimated at least 700,000 defendants *should* be evaluated for CST annually. Several excellent books (Grisso, 1988; Zapf & Roesch, 2009) and book chapters (Grisso, 2003; Melton et al., 2007) have provided overviews of this topic and general parameters for assessment, and this book will assume the reader has an understanding of CST assessment from works such as these. All of them emphasize the need to assess for possible feigning or malingering. Yet there are accounts that indicate CST examiners often do not assess for feigning (Lander & Heilbrun, 2009; McDermott, Dualan, & Scott, 2013; *United States v. Tucker*, 2010) and fail to identify a considerable number of examinees who feign (D. Green, Rosenfeld, Belfi, Rohlehr, & Pierson, 2012; McDermott et al., 2013; Zavodny, 2016).

Malingering is the intentional production of false or grossly exaggerated physical or psychiatric symptoms, motivated by external incentives (American

Psychiatric Association, 2013). *Feigning* is a more general term that applies to the deliberate fabrication or exaggeration of symptoms without assumptions about its goal(s) (Rogers, 2008a), and does not require *gross exaggeration*. I will generally use the latter term because it is broader and less inferential. However, not all invalid responding is due to a deliberate intention to bias our instruments or impressions. Some examinees are not fully cooperative and do not put forth full effort on tests requiring effort. Others, such as those with a somatoform disorder or hysterical traits, may over-report on tests such as the Minnesota Multiphasic Personality Inventory-2 (MMPI-2) without intent to deceive.[1] All response styles that lead to an overestimate of psychiatric or cognitive impairment, or ignorance of the court system, can be referred to as *negative response bias*. This chapter will discuss rates and types of invalid responding in CST exams and report relevant case law.

RATES OF NEGATIVE RESPONSE BIAS

The rate of feigning or negative response bias in CST evaluations is not known with certainty. Rogers, Salekin, Sewell, Goldstein, and Leonard (1998) surveyed forensic practitioners, who reported an average *base rate* (percentage of the sample with the condition of interest) of 17.4% across different forensic settings. Several studies reported rates of apparent feigning in specialized referral groups. McDermott et al. (2013) reported that 17.5% of defendants who were previously assessed, found incompetent, and admitted for competency restoration were judged to be *possibly* or *likely* malingering. D. Green et al. (2012) reported psychiatrists suspected feigning in 21.2% of defendants in a similar sample that had previously been assessed by *two* CST examiners. L. Colwell and K. Colwell (2011) reported 17.1% of competency restoration patients were identified as feigning by the treatment team. Mittenberg, Patton, Canyock, and Condit (2002) reported a survey of clinical neuropsychologists, who estimated the base rate of exaggeration or malingering in criminal justice examinees at 19.3%, which the authors adjusted to 22.8% when the effect of referral source was removed. Ardolf, Denney, and Houston (2007) reported that 54.3% of defendants referred for neuropsychological evaluations met criteria for *probable* or *definite* malingering of neurocognitive dysfunction (Slick, Sherman, & Iverson, 1999). Others have reported probable feigning in more representative CST samples ranging from 8% (Cornell & Hawk, 1989) to 35% (Gierok, Dickson, & Cole, 2005; Table 1.1).[2] This author (Chapter 10, this volume) surveyed CST examiners across the country and found an average estimated rate of feigning of 24.1%, with a median figure of 20%. All these figures may be conservative given that some feigners likely went undetected because most instruments and practice recommendations emphasize specificity (avoiding false positives) at the expense of sensitivity (correctly identifying those who are feigning).

The rate of feigning in a competency assessment setting is likely affected by the following factors, real or perceived: (a) the advantages of being found incompetent

Table 1.1 BASE RATES OF FEIGNING FOR CST EXAMINEES

Source	Sample	Criterion	Base Rate
Steadman (1979)	CST examinees	Psychiatrist's judgment	5–15%
Cornell & Hawk (1989)	CST and MSO pretrial defendants	Clinician judgment	8%
Frederick (2000a)	Pretrial examinees	Clinician estimates	15.5%
Frederick, Crosby, & Wynkoop (2000)	Pretrial defendants	VIP NV Invalid VIP NV Malinger	43.7% 1.1%
Frederick (2000b)	Defendants	Normative floor Personal floor	16.9% 15.6%
Heinze & Purisch (2001)	CST restoration	Clinical team	13%
Cochrane, Grisso, & Frederick (2001)	CST and MSO examinees	Clinical opinion	10.9%
Lewis, Simcox, & Berry (2002)	CST mostly	SIRS	31.4%[a]
Weinborn, Orr, Woods, Conover, & Feix (2003)	CST & MSO neuropsychological referrals	TOMM	41%
Rogers, Jackson, Sewell, & Harrison (2004)	CST (restoration)	SIRS	14.8%
H. A. Miller (2004)	CST (restoration)	SIRS[b]	28%
Gierok, Dickson, & Cole (2005)	CST	TOMM	30–35%
Boccaccini, Murrie, & Duncan (2006)	Pretrial federal prisoners	SIRS	29%
Kucharski, Toomey, Fila, & Duncan (2007)	Pretrial prisoners	SIRS	26.7%
Vitacco, Rogers, & Gabel (2007)	CST examinees, "quasi-random"	SIRS	21%
Barber-Rioja, Zottoli, Kucharski, & Duncan (2009)	Pretrial defendants	SIRS	22.9%
Toomey, Kucharski, & Duncan (2009)	CST or MSO examinees	SIRS	23%
L. Colwell & K. Colwell (2011)	CST examinees	TOMM/ Clinical team	14.3%/ 18.2%
D. Green, Rosenfeld, Belfi, Rohlehr, & Pierson (2012)	Felony defendants, CST restoration	Psychiatrist's judgment	21.9%

NOTE: MSO = mental state at the time of offense; VIP NV Invalid = Validity Indicator Profile (Frederick, 1997) nonverbal subtest *invalid* classification of the profile; VIP Malinger = nonverbal subtest *malingering* classification of the profile; TOMM = Test of Memory Malingering (Tombaugh, 1996); SIRS = Structured Inventory of Reported Symptoms (Rogers, Bagby & Dickens, 1992); normative floor = a low score established by the range of scores of other examinees; personal floor = examinee's own level of performance on easy items.

[a] This sample consisted of 52 consecutive referrals, plus 12 from another facility who were *all* suspected of malingering.

[b] Failure of SIRS was defined by two scales in the *probable* feigning range; the standard rule is three scales in the *probable* range or one in the *definite* feigning range.

or insane at the time of the offense; (b) the seriousness of the defendant's predicament;[3] (c) the disposition of those found incompetent or insane (e.g., mandatory inpatient vs. community treatment); (d) the probability of successfully feigning; and (e) the cost of getting caught. Although there have been several federal cases in which feigning has brought obstruction of justice charges and a sentencing enhancement (*United States v. Greer*, 1998; *United States v. Binion*, 2005; *United States v. Batista*, 2007), in many settings there may be no tangible cost to a defendant who attempts to feign and is caught. Possible motivations for malingering in pretrial defendants include the following:

- Securing transfer to a psychiatric unit and doing easier time in jail,
- escaping a dangerous or undesirable situation in one's current setting,
- access to psychiatric drugs for recreation or barter,
- securing better treatment within the court system or transfer to a mental health court,
- being found incompetent and having charges dropped,
- better access to family and friends,
- to frustrate and annoy the prosecution,
- better opportunities for escape, sex, or criminal activity,
- delaying the case to allow time for witnesses to disappear or be compromised,
- setting up a disability claim,
- gaining a strategic advantage at trial (*Maggio v. Fulford*, 1983),
- keeping hope alive in one's case,
- better access to staff members of the opposite sex.

The defendant in *United States v. Binion* denied that he malingered to obstruct justice and said he feigned mental illness simply to amuse himself.

One of the factors that will likely affect the base rate of feigning is the perception of how capable CST examiners are at detecting it. Defendants may believe that mental health professionals are easy to fool because of their benevolent ethos, or they may know of other defendants who have done so successfully. Hickling, Blanchard, Mundy, and Galovski (2002) researched their own clinicians' ability to detect actors trained as post-traumatic stress disorder (PTSD) simulators and found troubling results. Despite having access to various self-report scales (but not ones with validity scales) and psychophysiological data, clinicians described as "highly experienced with a trauma population" failed to identify *any* of the six actors. When told the nature of the study, clinicians identified three of the six actors but also misidentified three patients. H. A. Miller (2005) reported that scores on the Miller Forensic Assessment of Symptoms Test (M-FAST; H. A. Miller, 2001) were modestly related to psychiatrists' (AUC = .65) and moderately related to psychologists' (AUC = .73) dichotomous judgments of malingering. McDermott and Sokolov (2009) reported that written suspicions of malingering in the jail medical chart bore no relation to classification on the Structured Interview of Reported Symptoms (SIRS; Rogers, Bagby, & Dickens, 1992). Martin, Schroeder, and Odland (2015) reported the neuropsychologists they surveyed overwhelmingly (88.9%) believed validity tests (tests designed to detect feigning or poor effort) were more accurate than clinical impressions of credibility. On the other hand, Bourg, Connor, and Landis (1995) reported forensic clinicians were quite accurate in classifying four case reports regarding malingering and insanity claims. Frederick and Bowden (2009a) reported that clinician estimates of the probability that a given defendant would feign cognitive or memory impairment strongly predicted subsequent performance on the Rey 15 Item Test (FIT; Rey, 1958). D. Green et al. (2012) reported that of 23 forensic patients suspected of feigning, all but 4 failed at least one validity test, suggesting good specificity (19/23 = 82.6%) for the psychiatrists' judgments. Nonetheless, the uncertain validity of clinical judgments, unaided by testing or collateral information, has important implications for the assessment of feigning, which I address later.

Numerous authors have emphasized the importance of response style assessment in forensic evaluations (Heilbrun, 2001; Melton et al., 2007), and specifically in CST evaluations (C. L. Ray, 2009; White, Batchelor, Pulman, & Howard, 2015; Zapf & Roesch, 2009). This task has become much more challenging in the past two decades, as CST assessments have largely moved from state hospitals to community or jail settings. Whereas examiners in the past might have had 60 to 90 days of inpatient, around-the-clock observations to draw upon, a community examiner may have little more than the defendant's presentation during a brief examination to consider.

This book takes the position that response style assessment is the primary differential diagnostic and assessment skill of the CST examiner. As such, careful attention should be paid to every phase in which errors might arise. Some sources suggest malingering in CST evaluations should be assessed whenever *suspected.* Soliman and Resnick (2010) specified the following indicators to trigger an assessment of response bias:

1. presence of atypical symptoms,
2. inconsistencies in history,
3. history of prior adjudicative competence,
4. uncooperativeness, and
5. claimed ignorance of very common information.

Although not explicit, it appears the presence of any one criterion would trigger further examination. In contrast, Grisso (1988) wrote, "Malingering must be considered whenever a pre-trial competency evaluation produces signs of psychotic

---

Box 1.1

Area under the curve (AUC): A measure of the relationship between a dichotomous (yes or no; faking or not) variable and another variable such as scores on a test. An AUC of .50 (50%) indicates no relationship between the variables (correlation = .00), whereas an AUC of 1.00 (100%) is the maximum obtainable. It takes into account all possible cutoff scores. See Appendix A for a more thorough explanation.

---

or organic disorders, mental retardation, deficits in competency abilities, or special states like amnesia" (p. 35). While Soliman and Resnick's criteria may be valid indicators of feigning, not all feigners will display any or all of them. For example, suppose a defendant, with no prior convictions, claims to hear voices that tell him his attorney is an agent for the prosecutor. The defendant is superficially cooperative and does not present as ignorant of the court system. Such a defendant passes Soliman and Resnick's criteria and would receive no further evaluation of response validity. So would a defendant with mild intellectual disability who answers honestly to most questions but intentionally fails some questions about the court system. It is crucial not to exclude the possibility of malingering prematurely, which may well happen if the initial hurdle is the examiner's suspicion. A low bar for suspicion is necessary because even defendants with schizophrenia (Raffard, Capdevielle, Boulenger, Gely-Nargeot, & Bayard, 2014), serious head injury (Bianchini, Greve, & Love, 2003; Sweet & Guiffre Meyer, 2011), or intellectual disability (Everington, Notario-Smull, & Horton, 2007) may exaggerate their disabilities. Thus, I endorse a variation of Grisso's recommendation: that any defendant presenting with deficits sufficient to warrant a finding of incompetence (or serious doubt about competency) be assessed for negative response bias. An exception can be made if there is compelling evidence of serious psychopathology or cognitive limitations *and* evidence that this is not being manipulated. For example, a defendant who has been screaming irrationally in the holding cell for six days and is being held on trespassing charges probably can be taken at face value. On the other hand, one should not underestimate the lengths that defendants facing dire circumstances will go to demonstrate they are incompetent.

TYPES OF NEGATIVE RESPONSE BIAS

There is a wide range of possible strategies for defendants who want to feign. Although malingering has received much more attention, *lack of cooperation*, illness, and distraction from the environment or personal problems also present a serious challenge to valid assessment. This is particularly so for assessment of cognitive abilities, which requires examinees to consistently perform to the best of their abilities. Similarly, defendants who put no effort into articulating their best answer to questions about the court system, or who are reluctant to discuss their thinking regarding their possible trial strategies, may not provide reliable data.

Heinze and Purisch (2001) described six varieties of feigned incompetence. This writer (Chapter 10, this volume) surveyed experienced CST examiners and queried them about the frequencies of invalid presentations they have encountered. The most frequently reported modalities were ignorance of the court system, amnesia for the crime, memory problems, and auditory hallucinations, but about a dozen more were reported. Table 1.2 lists the perceived prevalence of each feigned presentation, as well as other types of negative response bias, such as factitious disorder and lack of cooperation.

Table 1.2 Types of Invalid Responding in CST Evaluations

Invalid Presentation	Mean	Median	*SD*
Feigned ignorance of the court system	17.2%	15%	16.2
Feigned amnesia for offense	14.6%	10%	12.7
Feigned or exaggerated intellectual limitations	14.5%	10%	15.7
Feigned memory problems (*not* amnesia for offense)	12.8%	10%	11.8
Feigned hallucinations	10.5%	8%	10.2
Feigned depression	10.2%	5%	10.8
Feigned anxiety or PTSD	8.2%	5%	8.7
Feigned demeanor[a]	7.5%	5%	13.9
Feigned paranoia	6.7%	5%	6.1
Feigned/exaggerated medical issues[b]	4.3%	2%	5.2
Feigned agitation/mania	2.3%	1%	3.2
Feigned disorganized speech	1.7%	1%	2.4
Other feigned presentation (not listed above)	1.6%	0%	3.6
Any kind of feigning (all previous styles)	24.1%	20%	19.4
Factitious disorder	1.2%	1%	2.0
Somatoform or conversion disorder	1.9%	1%	4.2
Lack of cooperation *without* malingering, factitious or somatoform disorder	8.7%	5%	8.6

NOTE: Median values are reported in addition to the means because the median value can be a better index of representativeness when the distribution of scores is skewed, as many were in this study.

[a]E.g., helplessness, vulnerability, childlike demeanor, speech impediment.

[b]E.g., unneeded cane, wheelchair, oxygen tank.

IMPLICATIONS OF WIDESPREAD NEGATIVE RESPONSE BIAS

The preceding figures can be compared with those of Pirelli, Gottdiener, and Zapf (2011), who reported that across 59 samples, an average of 27.5% (*Mdn* = 25.3%) of CST examinees are found *incompetent*. Given that rates of malingering were not reported in many studies, it is likely that some of those found incompetent were in fact feigning or not providing valid data. If so, *the base rate of negative response bias might equal, or even exceed, that of defendants who are actually incompetent.* This is of great import: Prior to beginning the assessment, it may be as statistically likely that an examinee who presents as impaired is feigning as that he or she is incompetent. Thus, consideration of negative response bias is appropriate as soon as one receives a referral, and certainly once the defendant displays CST-related deficits. This observation has weighty implications for testing and interpretation of results, as it directly affects the likelihood that an examinee who obtains a given score is not responding validly.

POSITIVE RESPONSE BIAS

Although this book focuses on negative response bias, a few legitimate mentally ill examinees will underreport or deny psychiatric problems. Sometimes these persons have serious conditions, like paranoid schizophrenia, which may legitimately compromise their competence to be adjudicated. Such persons may perform adequately on instruments like the Evaluation for Competency to Stand Trial-Revised (Rogers, Tillbrook, & Sewell, 2004), and thus it would seem that their mental illness does not impair their competence. Certainly, a person can be schizophrenic, even currently psychotic, and yet be competent. However, a CST exam typically occurs on a single occasion and thus represents a small sample of observations, limited to a single setting and time, and a situation that is somewhat removed from the criminal prosecution. Examiners do not typically try to create stressful situations, yet court can be very stressful. In other words, the examinee may present quite differently in another setting under different circumstances, and examiners should remember the perils of generalization based on small, biased samples of observation.

A number of instruments, like the Structured Interview of Reported Symptoms-2 (SIRS-2; Rogers, Sewell, & Gilliard, 2010), MMPI-2 (Butcher et al., 1991), MMPI-2-Revised Form (RF; Ben-Porath & Tellegen, 2008), and Personality Assessment Inventory (PAI; Morey, 1991), have scales or indices designed to detect defensiveness or denial of psychiatric symptoms. However, this is different than detecting an underlying serious mental illness: Someone can be defensive on a test and yet be free of psychiatric illness.

Performance tests like the Rorschach have been touted as being able to detect hidden pathology, and proponents argue that although feigners are probably able to suppress giving responses with morbid or aggressive content, they are unable to greatly affect several perceptual variables such as the form quality of the responses. Several studies appear to support this claim (Hartmann & Hartmann, 2014; Nørbech, Fodstad, Kuisma, Lunde, & Hartmann, 2016; Wasyliw, Benn, Grossman, & Haywood, 1998). However, the studies by Nørbech et al. (2016) and Hartmann and Hartmann (2014) have significant methodological limitations, in that there was no incentive offered for successful feigning, no manipulation checks, and no assessment of possible feigning in those in the "standard administration" condition. Indeed, the mean F score of offenders in the presumed honest responding group of Nørbech et al. was 92. Further, both groups of authors reported limited engagement by subjects, with Hartmann and Hartmann writing:

> During the interviews at the end of the assessments, most of the faking patients reported that they, for various reasons, had either given up or forgotten to try to simulate being well-adjusted on the Rorschach. Either they had no strategy for how to fake good on this test or they got so absorbed by the images that they failed to remember to fake responses. Therefore, only a few had been able to hold back some aggressive, sexual, and other provocative

> images and they did not otherwise know how they could have altered their manner of responding. (p. 440)

Hartmann and Hartmann's work is the only study since Ganellen's (2008) review that addressed examinees with schizophrenia or psychotic-spectrum illness. Ganellen concluded that the Rorschach, as a stand-alone measure, has not been demonstrated to be useful in detecting either defensiveness or feigning.

The MMPI-2, MMPI-2-RF, and PAI all have scales and indices to detect defensiveness. Greene (2008) reviewed data for a variety of indices on the MMPI-2, including L, K, F-K, Obvious-Subtle, the Superlative scale, Positive Malingering (Mp), and Social Desirability (Sd), and noted that a prior meta-analysis (Baer, Wetter, & Berry, 1992) found the latter two indices to have higher average effect sizes ($d = 1.5$) than the traditional L and K indices, both of which averaged about 1.0. Several issues should be considered. First, there is a substantial chance that defensiveness may not be detected given the modest effect sizes and the recommended cutoff scores. Second, even if defensiveness is detected, it is likely that the rest of the clinical scales will be suppressed and provide little, if any, useful clinical information (Nørbech et al., 2016). Lastly, defensiveness on the MMPI (or PAI) is a general concept that does not distinguish denial of psychosis, which is relevant to CST, from denial of other problems that are not. Thus, the total yield from such a protocol may be that the examinee was defensive, with no information about whether mental illness is present.

In sum, testing can provide evidence of generalized defensiveness, but its value in assessing for hidden pathology is limited and unproven. Collateral data, particularly from family, the defense attorney, and jail staff, are likely to be the best means for detecting serious pathology that is not acknowledged by the examinee.

Defendants may present invalidly for many reasons, and in many different ways. Recent estimates of feigning in CST exams run over 20%, with feigned ignorance of the court system, amnesia for the offense, intellectual limitations, and memory problems being the most commonly reported approaches. Even putting aside *lack of cooperation* and other forms of negative response bias, the base rate of feigning is close to the base rate of defendants found incompetent. With rare exceptions, examiners should assess for negative response bias whenever a defendant presents with significant CST-related impairment. Some mentally ill defendants may deny their symptoms, although this is probably much less common than negative response bias. For both types of defendants, collateral data may be crucial.

LEGAL PERSPECTIVES

CST evaluations, like other forensic exams, take place within a legal framework (Melton et al., 2007). No Supreme Court cases were found regarding malingering within a CST exam, so the reader should be mindful that the cases cited are directly applicable and binding only within their respective jurisdictions. However, published opinions in other jurisdictions are often cited by courts elsewhere if the issue has not been addressed in local case law, and they may be relied upon to decide the issue. This section will review the limited legal literature that addresses feigning in the context of a CST evaluation or hearing.[4] Readers interested in a review of cases pertaining to CST in general are referred to *Examinations of Competency to Stand Trial: Foundations in Case Law* by Frederick, DeMier, and Smith (2014).

In a law review article, Friedland (1998) noted that traditionally the judge or jury was entrusted with assessing the credibility of the defendant and witnesses, including on issues of malingering. Doing so was deemed to be within the purview of common sense and observation, as the judge or jury not only could listen to the witness's or defendant's words but also could observe his or her body language, expressions, and telltale errors of speech. Courts have at times jealously guarded this prerogative, as with testimony about eyewitness accuracy factors, and been skeptical about whether experts provide information that is beyond lay knowledge. Further, judges' rulings have sometimes been reversed for taking this matter out of the hands of a jury. In *United States v. Denny-Shaffer* (1993), the defense presented testimony that the defendant experienced a dissociative disorder. The judge was apparently unimpressed, concluded the defendant was malingering, and did not allow presentation of the defense to the jury. The defendant was convicted but appealed the exclusion and won.

Yet, Friedland provided examples of professionals testifying on the topic of malingering dating back more than a hundred years (*Ney v. City of Troy*, 1888; *Hickenbottom v. Delaware, L. & W. R. Co.*, 1890). He also noted that in *United States v. Kokoski* (1994), psychologist Richard Rogers was approved to assess a defendant and to testify as an expert on malingering in a federal court CST hearing. Friedland noted that the courts have occasionally refused to admit expert testimony of malingering based on psychological testing or scientific principles for fear that it will overawe and unfairly prejudice the jury, that the jury will mistakenly infer the expert is unbiased, or that testimony will be too general or abstract to address the case at hand. Testimony that is based on simple observations of changes in demeanor or impressions of evasiveness may be judged simple common sense, duplicative, and thus a waste of the court's time. This argument assumes that the jury either has access to the same set of observations, perhaps from the examiner's report, or can make a set of parallel observations of the defendant in the courtroom.

In *State of Louisiana v. Brooks* (1995), a defendant claimed that he was retarded or brain damaged and not competent to waive his Miranda rights. However, the Louisiana Supreme Court took note of highly discrepant IQ scores on different occasions, which were apparently attributed to malingering. The court stated,

> This picture of Brooks as a man capable of selectively exercising discernment when it suited his purposes accords with the consistent and uncontroverted testimony of Detective Reynolds concerning Brooks' apparent frankness and coherence during the course of his confession. (p. 374)

A high profile, contested competency case involved mob boss Vincent Gigante, who claimed to be incompetent due to dementia (*United States v. Gigante* (1997)). A battle of multiple experts ensued, but observations by a corrections officer and nurse were apparently more credible to the judge than some very respected professionals' opinions. The corrections officer and nurse reported that Mr. Gigante conversed normally when, for example, on the phone to family members, and showed above average capability in handling assigned jobs.

In *Lewis v. State of Alabama* (2003), the defendant was assessed by three CST examiners, all of whom expressed the opinion that he was malingering. Lewis objected that his CST jury was prejudiced by the state's disclosing facts of the crime (and the defendant's other crimes), his level of cooperation with investigators, and his confession. The Alabama Criminal Court of Appeals concluded:

> If a jury is to determine a defendant's competency to stand trial and a part of the test for competency is an understanding of the facts and nature of the charged crimes so that he may assist in his defense, such facts are not irrelevant and it is not error for the State to present to the jury evidence regarding those facts. (p. 34)

In a civil case (*Bonds v. Padlock* et al., 2008), a family physician's testimony regarding the plaintiff's malingering pain from a 2002 accident prior to the claimed injury in 2005 was rejected. The plaintiff asserted the physician (Dr. Kulick) did not use any tests or validated procedures and relied on chart notes from a colleague. Although the US District Court of the Eastern District of Louisiana ruled Dr. Kulick was competent to render such an opinion in his role as a physician and did not object to reliance on medical records, it concluded:

> (Dr.) Kulick's deposition testimony suggesting that Bonds malingered as to her injuries from the 2002 accident [*12] should be excluded under Rule 402 because it is not relevant to any fact in issue in the present case. In addition, to the extent that Kulick's malingering testimony is at all relevant to Bonds's claims in the instant matter, that testimony should nonetheless be excluded under Rule 403 because any marginal relevancy would be substantially outweighed by the danger of unfair prejudice and confusion of the issues. (p. 5)

In *State v. Demesmin* (2010), the New Hampshire Supreme Court ruled that the trial court may order a second CST evaluation if there was evidence of malingering in the first evaluation. In *United States v. Tucker* (2010), an expert's failure to consider malingering was deemed "problematic."

In *United States v. Rothman* (2010), the defense argued that the defendant suffered from dementia and was thus unable to assist in his defense. The government contended that even though the defendant likely suffered from dementia, the defense experts' reports did not directly assess his cognitive deficits or their effect on his ability to assist in his defense. The US District Court of Southern

Florida found the defendant incompetent, apparently putting great weight on the physicians' diagnoses of dementia and the implication that dementia would cause deficits sufficient to impair competence. The defense experts did state that the defendant's condition would impair specific CST capacities, but it is unclear from the court's opinion whether the physicians directly assessed impairments or if they were simply inferred from the dementia diagnosis.

In *United States v. Merriweather* (2011), the defendant was examined by multiple state and defense experts who came to widely differing opinions. The time involvement and methodologies employed by the experts also varied, with one expert spending only an hour and a half and another having had daily interaction over the course of more than a year while the defendant was incarcerated at the Bureau of Prisons. In attempting to resolve the differences, the the following text was presented by the court:

> Because of the particular set of facts in this case, there was one measurement that effectively encapsulated all of these criteria: the duration of continuous interaction between the expert and Merriweather. The validity of using the amount of time spent with Merriweather in evaluating an expert witness' credibility is undisputed between the parties. Indeed, the Defense has suggested that the court should completely discredit the evaluations conducted by Dr. Gualtieri because "[h]is exposure to Merriweather was limited."

Philipsborn (2015) cautioned that experts may be questioned if they spent sufficient "*Merriweather* time" to produce reliable conclusions from their examination. However, the court continued:

> The court is quick to note that the amount of time spent with Merriweather is but one of the factors the court has considered in crediting the testimony of Drs. Pietz and Berger. Indeed, the court was impressed with the testimony of Drs. Pietz and Berger, particularly the latter. Of all the experts called to testify, Dr. Berger appeared to be the most balanced and careful. He was not an "advocate" in any sense. (156 at 42).

In *Dorgan v. O'Connor* (2011), the plaintiff in a civil case claimed a traumatic brain injury in a personal injury claim and was assessed twice, the second time by a physician who used the SIRS. The plaintiff objected to testimony derived from the SIRS, and a *Daubert* hearing was held. The Appeals Court of Massachusetts noted that the trial court judge held extensive hearings regarding the SIRS and the evidence regarding its validity, and upheld the lower court's decision allowing SIRS-based testimony.

In *Washington v. State of Florida* (2015), the defendant was examined by five mental health professionals, three who concluded he was incompetent and two who concluded he was malingering. The latter two experts did not offer an opinion on competency, noting it was possible that the defendant was both malingering and incompetent. The case was appealed and the judge's decision overturned. The District Court of Appeal of Florida, Fourth District, noted that there was no testimony on which to support the judge's finding of competence; citing earlier Florida cases, it concluded that a prior evaluation from 2011 was "stale" and thus not "competent, substantial" evidence of competency. One of these earlier cases (*Brockman v. State*, 2003) made a similar ruling regarding a competency exam completed only 4 months prior.

In *United States v. Deruiter* (2015), two neuropsychologists evaluated a defendant and came to opposing conclusions about malingering, forcing the court to weigh the relative credibility of each assessment. The first expert (Dr. Ouaou) administered many neuropsychological tests, the Test of Memory Malingering (TOMM), and three other unidentified performance validity tests (PVTs). The second expert (Dr. Buigas) administered the MMPI-2-RF, SIRS-2, Validity Indicator Profile (VIP), and Inventory of Legal Knoweldge (ILK). The court[5] concluded:

> In this case, however, the Court gives Dr. Ouaou's opinion less weight than Dr. Buigas' opinion because Dr. Ouaou evaluated the Defendant over a shorter period of time. Dr. Buigas and his staff evaluated the Defendant over the course of several weeks and administered tests for roughly 10 hours and 15 minutes. (p. 15)

In *Kentucky v. McGorman* (2016), a defendant was referred for a CST assessment and was found competent. In the courtroom, he exhibited rocking motions. His attorney, fearing the jury would perceive the rocking as malingering, waived the defendant's right to be present during the trial and did not seek a second CST evaluation. The Kentucky Supreme Court held this decision did not constitute ineffective assistance of counsel.

This section has provided an overview of topics and options addressed in appeals courts across the United States, including both federal and state jurisdictions. No cases were located in which an expert was barred from testifying on malingering. One court explicitly endorsed the inclusion of details from the crime if relevant to the issue of competency when malingering was strongly suspected, but it did not limit its opinion to cases involving feigning. Although Friedland (1998) suggested that simple behavioral observations regarding malingering could be excluded, no examples of this occurring were located. The one case in which a test was subjected to a *Daubert* challenge, the judge's ruling to admit was upheld.

In cases where a disagreement among examiners about malingering was present, it appears examiners differed largely because of the validity test results. In some cases, experts made no assessment of feigning or else used a single, relatively insensitive test. With the exception of the judge in the *Gigante* case, judicial opinions often make little reference to the use of collateral sources, implying examiners did not utilize them and relied primarily on testing to assess validity of presentation.

Box 1.2

False positive rate (FPR): The percentage of genuine examinees who are incorrectly identified as feigners. The FPR ranges from 0% to 100% (also written as .00–1.00), although very high values are rare and undesirable.

Sensitivity: The percentage of fakers who are "caught" by the test; also the accuracy rate for feigners. It ranges from 0% to 100% (also written as .00–1.00).

A GLANCE AHEAD

In the chapters to follow, I will discuss assessment practices, review validity tests, and introduce readers to aspects of the vibrant neuropsychological response style literature, which many forensic psychologists appear to have overlooked. I will discuss ways of combining data from different tests and observations, report writing, and testimony and will consider some research and policy issues pertinent to CST assessment. I do not provide extensive descriptions of the tests reviewed because doing so could compromise test security. In addition to CST examiners, this book may be read by attorneys and even examinees.

The majority of the material presented in this book is based on studies and professional literature for adult CST referrals, not juveniles. At present, there are very few studies on response style in juvenile CST examinees. The available data suggest that PVTs like the TOMM can be used confidently with adolescent subjects (DeRight & Carone, 2015), provided minimal reading levels are met for verbal tests. The limited data on this topic is reviewed in Chapter 8.

The following chapters will review quite a few tests, and it is desirable to have a rubric to help make meaningful comparisons between them. In the past, many researchers sought to identify cutoff scores that would yield the highest overall classification rate. In contrast, Greve and Bianchini (2004) argued that to compare validity tests, one should set the cutoff score to achieve a false positive rate of 10% or less, and let the resultant sensitivity "fall where it may." I have followed this convention in reporting cutoff scores and diagnostic statistics throughout the book. Because it may be useful to have the figures for different tests in one place, a master table is presented in Appendix B.

NOTES

1. Jean Martin Charcot, the most prominent author writing on hysteria at the time, reportedly stated, "Malingering is to be found in every phase of hysteria" (Merskey, 1979; cited by Maldonado & Spiegel, 2001). See also Merten and Merckelbach (2013).
2. I do not cite some studies with higher estimates because they either preselected subjects for suspicion of feigning or included those who were classified as showing poor effort (but were not necessarily feigning).

3. The seriousness of the charges is only one factor. New charges may violate probation or bail conditions. Some convictions may have devastating consequences for some professions, such as a DUI for an airline pilot. Although a 30-day jail sentence may be little more than an inconvenience to someone in their early 20s with an unsettled lifestyle, readers might consider how this would impact their own life.
4. I used combinations of the following terms to search Lexis-Nexis: competency to stand trial, CST, competency, malingering, evidence of malingering, exclusion, exclusion of evidence, and exclusion of testimony.
5. US District Court for the Middle District of Florida, Fort Myers Division.

2

The Evaluation

Data Gathering and Interview Strategy

This chapter considers evaluation strategies beginning from receipt of the referral to the conclusion of the interview. Most of what follows is based on my personal experience, so I will occasionally use the first-person pronoun. Before delving into ways of gathering observational and collateral data, it is important to consider the goals and caveats involved.

While there is a wide range of data that may be relevant to a competency exam, there are only a few broad themes that are important in most cases: Does the defendant have a psychiatric or cognitive condition? If so, to what extent is it impairing? Is the defendant's presentation in the CST exam a valid representation of his/her typical performance and demeanor?

There is evidence of considerable unreliability in the conclusions of competency examiners. Guarnera and Murrie (2017) reported on a meta-analysis of competency evaluations by two or more examiners. They reported a kappa of .45, which fell in the *moderate agreement* range. Murrie, Boccaccini, Zapf, Warren, and Henderson (2008) reported that different CST examiners varied widely in the proportion of examinees they deemed incompetent, from 0 to 62%.

A few suggestions have been advanced for how forensic clinicians might reduce bias, such as actively generating alternative conclusions, identifying and using relevant base rates, minimizing the role of memory, and identifying and weighing the most valid sources of data (Arkes, 1981; Borum, Otto, & Golding, 1993). Interest in forensic science decision-making has only grown following the report by the National Research Council (2009), which found most of the traditional disciplines (fingerprints, ballistics, arson investigation) were not based on scientific methodology or data. While forensic psychology and psychiatry were not addressed in this report, surveys indicate legal professionals perceive medical and other professionals as quite subject to bias (Krafka, Dunn, Johnson, Cecil, & Miletich, 2002; Shuman, Whitaker, & Champagne, 1994).

Dror (2016) distinguished between two basic properties of decision making, *reliability* and *biasability:* Reliability refers to the consistency or, reproducibility of decisions. For example, would different forensic evaluators reach the same conclusions? *Biasability* refers to the potential effects of irrelevant contextual information and other biases (e.g., leniency) that may impact the decision. For example, would a criminal defendant's race or religion influence the forensic evaluator's decisions? A full discussion of these issues is beyond the scope of this chapter, and the reader is referred to Borum, Otto, and Golding (1993) and recently published works (Dror & Murrie, 2017; Guarnera, Murrie, & Boccaccini, 2017; Lockhart & Satya-Murti, 2017; Neal, 2016; Neal & Grisso, 2014; Zapf & Dror, 2017) that provide recommendations for examiners. However, a brief primer is presented here.

Dror (2016) presented an eight-level taxonomy of judgments for forensic psychological exam based on three variables: stage of process (observation vs. decision), type of reliability examined (intra vs. inter-rater), and type of potential error (unreliability vs. biasability). The most basic type of reliability that must be demonstrated, for a court to trust data from a given field, is that a particular expert in that field can provide reliable observations (for example, regarding a fingerprint pattern) on different occasions. The most rigorous demonstration would be that *different* experts can *avoid bias* when rendering *conclusions*.

Zapf and Dror (2017) applied a different seven-level schema that identified possible origins of bias, ranging from cognitive architecture (e.g., short term memory limitations; top-down processing) to case evidence. Zapf and Dror noted that just as criminologists must take steps to avoid contamination of physical evidence, such as blood samples, forensic psychologists must strive to avoid cognitive contamination from irrelevant or biasing information. They provided two prominent examples. Collateral sources may communicate inaccurate or emotionally biased information that could be unconsciously credited by the examiner. Offense reports, and medical records, may also contain much information that is not directly relevant to the issue of competency, but could be quite prejudicial. For example, in a murder case, the prosecutor may include crime scene photos in the materials sent to the forensic examiner. Medical records may include information about substance abuse or sexually-transmitted diseases, and the offense report often paints the defendant in a negative light. Zapf and Dror suggest that a third neutral party review such data and extract that which is relevant to forward to the examiner. In that way, the examiner is shielded (or *blinded*) from irrelevant or potentially biasing information.

Two groups of authors have surveyed forensic practitioners about their knowledge and beliefs about dealing with bias (Kukucka, Kassin, Zapf, & Dror, in press; Neal & Brodsky, 2017; Zapf, Kukucka, Kassin, & Dror, in press). Neal and Broskey reported their respondents endorsed some empirically-supported debiasing strategies, such as training, slowing down (taking time to review and question one's assessment), structured evaluation methods (use of checklists or actuarial instruments), and considering the opposite point of view. However, the authors noted that effective *training* needed to be focused on debiasing techniques, and that *considering the opposite point of view* required true consideration of the opposing perspective rather than attempting to defeat a straw man. No survey respondents cited *blinding*, one of the best empirically-supported strategies, and most endorsed *introspection*, which has been shown to be ineffective. A potentially useful strategy was (realistically) taking professional pride in one's objectivity. Survey respondents were more likely to perceive bias in colleagues and opposing experts than themselves, and years of experience was negatively related to concern about bias (Zapf et al., 2017). The examiner's personality may also be relevant: Miller, Rufino, Boccaccini, Jackson, and Murrie (2011) reported raters scoring high on some Agreeableness subscales assigned lower Psychopathy Checklist *Interpersonal* facet scores than low scorers.

Examiners may want to consciously order their review of collateral data. In order to prevent premature conclusions and maintain an open mind, sources that are likely to be prosecution or defense-friendly might be staggered. Because examiners appointed by one side might be biased by allegiance (Murrie, Boccaccini, Guarnera, & Rufino, 2013), they might intentionally begin and end their analysis with sources likely to favor the other side, since information that is considered first and last tends to have the most impact on judgments (Kahneman, 2011). Thus, if one is defense-appointed, one might start by reviewing the Offense Report; if prosecution or court-appointed, with the defense attorney's motion. Table 2.1 provides a summary of steps an examiner can use to mitigate the influence of bias during the assessment process.

COLLECTING DATA

Court-appointed examiners will typically receive the order authorizing the examination, whereas those in private practice may receive a phone call from a defense

Table 2.1 Means of Reducing Bias During the Evaluation Stage

- Avoid exposure to irrelevant, prejudicial information
- Consider beginning and ending review of collateral data with material likely to favor the non-referring party, and staggering the review of defense- and prosecution-friendly sources
- Use structured evaluation methods (checklists or standardized instruments) when available and appropriate
- Minimize the role of memory (record interviews and score or summarize material ASAP)
- Actively generate alternative hypotheses; consider the opposite point of view
- Identify and obtain the most valid sources of data
- Seek out information that would disprove one's hypothesis rather than corroborate it
- Strive for objectivity in formulating questions, recording answers, and in one's attitude and demeanor towards all sources

attorney to initiate the referral. I find it advantageous to obtain considerable information before the evaluation, particularly the police report, as well as the indictment, input from the defense attorney, school and/or psychiatric records, and, if available, recordings or transcripts of police interviews. This will permit early identification of issues that are relevant to the defendant's specific case(s) to be addressed in the interview.

Any contact with the defendant, such as a phone call confirming the appointment time, can potentially yield useful data: Does the defendant make the call personally or have someone else do so? If the defendant calls, how does he or she sound? Even better, if the defendant is called and doesn't answer, is there a recorded message? What does this message convey in terms of the defendant's personal style and ability to communicate? Perhaps most important, how does the persona in the message compare with the one on display in the evaluation? By comparison, during the interview, the defendant may present as having a speech impediment, as intellectually disabled, or as too depressed or psychotic to stand trial.

The examiner should plan, to the extent possible given one's office layout, to covertly observe the defendant before, during, and after the interview. Changes in demeanor in the first second or two when the defendant meets the examiner can be quite telling, as can changes as he or she leaves the building. Defendants may swagger and have a very intact "street" demeanor before and after the evaluation, or during cigarette breaks, but adopt a vulnerable, dependent, or sympathetic persona for the interview. Many times, I have seen a defendant swagger into our building only to adopt a dependent, wide-eyed sincerity in the evaluation that was quickly shed at the front door on the way out. One defendant was observed talking and joking with a group of cellmates, but when called for the evaluation, he crossed his eyes and walked past me as if he were blind. It may be desirable to plan on at least one break during the evaluation that will allow the defendant to transition to a different setting, such as getting snacks or simply taking some time to unwind. If the defendant traveled to the exam, the examiner might ask if he or she came alone, drove, and/or had any trouble finding the building or office.

The examinee will need to be informed of the purpose of the evaluation, the examiner's role, and, in general terms, the exam's parameters. He or she should *not* be warned about the use of validity tests, as such warnings tend to lower these tests' sensitivity and probably do not deter feigning. However, examinees can be informed of the importance of complete honesty and putting forth their best effort at all times (Boone, 2007a). After providing the notification of the examination's parameters, I recommend testing the examinee's retention of the material. Defendants may not treat this as part of the competency evaluation and may perform much better than when asked about the court system later in the evaluation. These and other observations regarding possible exaggeration should be recorded in real time.

For the psychosocial interview, a focus on education, job history, and criminal history is important for context if the person presents as limited either cognitively or in knowledge of the court system. Defendants should be asked about psychiatric and medical conditions, particularly conditions (e.g., head injuries, stroke, and dementia for the elderly) or medications that can affect mental functioning. Many defendants will report head injuries, and examiners need to know how to assess head injury severity (see Ruff, Iverson, Barth, Bush, & Broshek, 2009). Defendants should be asked what happened, if they lost consciousness and for how long, what led up to the injury, if and where they were treated, and about any complications in their recovery or long-term effects. Intact memory for the injury and the event immediately preceding it indicates a mild injury. Although there has recently been much attention paid to concussions, research has repeatedly shown that the typical course for a single mild traumatic brain injury (mTBI; 30 minutes or less of unconsciousness, no abnormality on CT scan) is recovery of baseline cognitive functioning within 3 months of the injury (Karr, Areshenkoff, & Garcia-Barrera, 2014).

During the interview, the examiner can pursue multiple tasks simultaneously. In addition to obtaining standard background information, the examiner should listen carefully for collateral sources to corroborate or disconfirm what the defendant says. Thus, it can be important to ask which school he or she last attended, and to identify treatment providers or family members with whom the defendant is in contact—and their phone numbers. I am interested not only in the phone number but also in how it is provided. Does the examinee recall it from memory or pull out the latest smartphone and quickly retrieve the requested information? Similarly, I might ask to see a picture identification. This is crucial to confirm that the person you are evaluating is the defendant referred for the evaluation, but it has another purpose as well. When the examinee opens a wallet or purse, is it stuffed full of old papers and tissues, or is it neatly organized with multiple credit cards and other indications of lifestyle? One might also compare the persona of the person in the identification photo, and the signature, with those presented in the evaluation.

A cognitive mini-mental state examination (MMSE) can provide some information about overall cognitive functioning and, potentially, cognitive feigning. The original MMSE (Folstein, Folstein, & McHugh, 1975) has several supportive publications examining its use as a validity measure (Gierok, Dickson, & Cole, 2005; Myers, Hall, & Tolou-Shams, 2013; Myers, 1987), and it outperformed the Rey 15 Item Test in a small sample of homicide cases (Myers et al., 2013). Myers (1987) examined the MMSE among intellectually disabled (ID) persons and concluded, “In the absence of a psychiatric disorder, it takes moderate intellectual disability (IQ less than 55) or severe reading disability with IQ less than 70 to produce an MMSE score of less than 24” (p. 85). Rienstra et al. (2013) reported that memory-disordered patients with MMSE scores of 24 or greater were able to pass the TOMM. Finally, because the MMSE is widely used in psychiatric settings, it may be possible to directly compare scores the defendant has produced in different settings with those produced during the competency evaluation. However, a good score on the MMSE should not be taken as evidence that no cognitive impairment exists.

When querying psychiatric symptoms, several authors (Drob & Berger, 1987; Soliman & Resnick, 2010) suggest beginning with a very general inquiry, such as,

"Are you having any emotional or psychiatric problems? What are they?" One can always follow up with more specific questions, but these answers should be interpreted in context. Some defendants may be stumped by open-ended questions about symptoms but agree to leading questions like "Are you hearing voices?"

Although there are studies of the phenomenology of actual psychotic patients (e.g., Goodwin & Rosenthal, 1971) that may have guided item development for the SIRS, Structured Inventory of Malingered Symptomatology (SIMS; Widows & Smith, 2005), and M-FAST (H. A. Miller, 2001), the results among these and later studies (Larøi et al., 2012; McCarthy-Jones & Resnick, 2014; McCarthy-Jones, Trauer, Mackinnon, Sims, Thomas, & Copolov, 2014; Nayani & David, 1996; Pollock, 1998) are not entirely consistent. Rather, the examiner might focus on whether the defendant's descriptions are congruent with other sources or the typical course of the disorder. A defendant may report hearing voices "all my life" despite not reporting such symptoms to jail staff over the last 3 months. Voices heard only at night would not seem to affect court proceedings during the day. Assessment with the M-FAST, SIRS/SIRS-2, MMPI-2, and/or MMPI-2-RF should also be considered.

Examiners should also pay attention to variation in the defendant's clarity, manner, and memory as the interview broaches different topics. Defendants who are feigning sometimes will convey positive information (job history, anecdotes suggesting responsibility or good character) or accounts of psychiatric treatment with great clarity but be foggy or evasive when asked questions about previous arrests or drugs used or questions that could lead to unfriendly sources, like past and present probation officers.

FACT PATTERNS AND BEHAVIORAL INDICATORS

Lists of behaviors and observations suggestive of malingering have been proposed by Resnick (1984) and Rogers (1984). These include items such as poor cooperation, calling attention to symptoms, atypical reports of hallucinations, *Ganser*-type answers (answers that are wrong but close: e.g., an octopus has seven arms), and symptoms that do not conform to known psychiatric symptoms. These indicators were proposed based on case reports or a rational basis, and little or no empirical justification was presented (Rogers & Correa, 2008).

There have been several attempts to create formal rating scales based on such items. The Tehachapi Malingering Scale (Haskett, 1995) was developed in the California prison system and has gone through several revisions, but no peer-reviewed research has been published. The Barkemeyer-Callon-Jones Malingering Detection Scale (Barkemeyer & Callon, 1989) was examined in two studies by the authors (Barkemeyer, Wymer, Jones, & Callon, 2003; Wymer, Barkemeyer, Jones, & Callon, 2006). Excellent sensitivity and specificity were reported in classifying *neurology* patients determined otherwise to be genuine or malingering, with a Cohen's *d* of 3.09. However, Smith (2008) noted that studies demonstrating generalization to other settings and in simulating samples are needed.

Box 2.1

Specificity: The accuracy of a test in classifying persons who do not have the condition of interest, such as faking. Thus, specificity is the accuracy of a malingering test in classifying *honest* respondents and ranges from 0% to 100%. Specificity also equals 100%–the false positive rate.

Cornell and Hawk (1989) distilled 24 observations relevant to malingering among CST examinees from an original list of about 100 such descriptors. They then examined the correlation of indicators, coded by independent raters, from the clinical reports and conclusions of the examiners. Thus, although examiners coded the indicative behaviors and malingering status, the transformation of data into ratings on the behavioral indicators was made by separate raters. Cornell and Hawk found significant differences on 14 of the items. Pretrial defendants judged to have legitimate psychiatric problems were more likely to show verbosity, neologisms, incoherent speech, concrete thinking, delusions and ideas of reference, poor hygiene, concentration problems, and disturbed affect. Malingerers were more likely to show exaggerated behavior and to report visual hallucinations, to report unusual groupings of symptoms, to endorse bogus symptoms, and to report suicidal ideation. Interestingly, guardedness and claimed memory problems did not distinguish the groups. It should be noted that some malingerers presented with symptoms that are often regarded as unusual or hard to feign, such as neologisms and incoherent speech.

Kucharski, Ryan, Vogt, and Goodloe (1998) had two experienced forensic psychologists review the mental status portion of psychological reports of 60 CST or not guilty by reason of insanity examinees, all charged with felonies. The examinees divided into two groups: those who had previous, documented history of psychiatric treatment and those that did not. The former were believed to be at low risk of malingering, while the latter were deemed high-risk. Raters coded each mental status narrative through ratings on six items, each on a 5-point Likert scale. These included common versus unusual symptom presentations and combinations, presentation consistent with the global assessment of functioning rating or not, concordant versus discordant affective presentation, and thought disorganization. Raters showed very high inter-rater agreement (interclass correlation coefficients [ICCs] = .92 to .97) on individual items and the total score of the six items (ICC = .98). Stepwise discriminate analysis found that three items (*presentation inconsistent with GAF, common/unusual hallucinations, common/unusual symptom presentation*) performed as well as the six items and produced 90% accuracy in assigning defendants to criterion (honest vs. malingering) groups. Summarizing, the authors reported that the results provide support for a "clinical" approach to validity assessment. No subject attempted to feign mania, and among identified malingerers, thought disorder was "often absent."

A few studies have produced empirical support for individual behavior rating items. Webb, Batchelor, Meares, Taylor, and Marsh (2012) reported that the item "exaggerated displays of behavior" predicted cognitive validity test failure (odds ratio = 5.84) in an archival sample of 555 adults with traumatic brain injury (TBI). Chafetz, Abrahams, and Kohlmaier (2007) sought to develop a validity scale for Social Security disability applicants that required little additional testing beyond the Wechsler Adult Intelligence Scale-III (Wechsler, 1997). They observed that a variety of floor effect items (e.g., presented inability to state one's age or date of birth or to name the current president, highly improbable answers, two or more Ganser responses, inability to complete simple numerical sequences, WAIS coding errors) were strongly related to failure on the Medical Symptom Validity Test (MSVT; P. Green, 2004) and TOMM (Tombaugh, 1996), as were reports of improbable psychiatric symptoms. Denning (2014) reported that a tendency to respond by pointing and naming TOMM responses was moderately associated with PVT failure. J. M. Williams (2011) noted that among the major forms of dissimulation in neuropsychological testing identified by Meyers (2007; *intentionally answering incorrectly, performing slowly, being inattentive*, and *responding haphazardly*), *performing slowly* is both common and underassessed. No major PVT reviewed in this work incorporates time to respond as a variable, and this could be easily incorporated in computer-administered PVTs like the Word Memory Test.

Akehurst, Easton, Fuller, Drane, Kuzmin, and Litchfield (2015) developed a 28-item checklist of malingering behaviors in a medico-legal context, drawing items from the separate literatures on malingering and assessment of credibility. Raters who used the checklist classified experimental malingerers better than chance and raters who did not use the checklist, and obtained an overall accuracy rate of 70%. A discriminate analysis classified 81% of subjects, with a $d = 1.08$. Nine items were identified as the best discriminators. However, an abbreviated checklist based on the 9 items was not found valid in a follow-up study (Easton, Akehurst, Satchell, & Turtle, 2017), whereas the full 28-item checklist showed better accuracy (86%) than in the original study. The researchers also identified 5 items that were particularly discriminating, although these were different than the 9 items from the prior study. Although sensitivity and specificity are reported for discriminate analysis function, no raw cutoff score or associated diagnostic statistics were reported.

Keesler, McClung, Meredith-Duliba, Williams, and Swirsky-Sacchetti (2017) reported on mTBI plaintiffs undergoing neuropsychological examination. The examinees were asked the date of their injury and about how long, if at all, they were unconscious. Their answers were compared with medical records from the

---

Box 2.2

Odds ratio: The relative likelihood that a subject with a risk factor (e.g., exaggerated behavior) will show the condition of interest (feigning) relative to someone who does not display that risk factor: percent positive with risk factor ÷ percent positive without risk factor.

---

accident date. Inaccurate reporting of the period of unconsciousness was predictive of failure on cognitive validity tests.

The data in this section support the clinical signs identified by early case studies of individual malingerers, but studies were often not strong in methodology. Only a handful of indicators are supported by two or more studies (Table 2.2). It should be remembered that these examples are all generated by feigners who were caught: Those who escaped detection are not represented.

Examiners should also consider that various aspects of an examinee's presentation may not be what they seem. About twenty years ago, I shared an elevator at a mental health clinic with a patient (not mine) and her friend. The patient told her friend she had a Social Security disability examination coming up, so she planned not to shower for a week before it. In a CST exam, an elderly man showed up 3 hours early for his appointment, seemingly confused. Collateral sources portrayed him as quite competent in remembering the dates and times of community events, birthdays of ladies in his area, and so forth. Such affectations may mislead an unwary examiner who does not question the validity of nonverbal behavior as well as accounts from the defendant.

As important as identifying atypical symptoms to identify feigners is knowing the true diagnostic information provided by a given presentation. It has often been asserted that disorganized speech is difficult to fake. However, there have been no studies in which, for example, aspiring actors are given tutoring, 10 hours to prepare, and a high incentive to deceive forensic examiners. Although many defendants seem to devote little time to preparing for an evaluation, those

Table 2.2 Behavioral Indicators of Feigning

Indicators of Feigning	Indicators of Genuine Psychopathology
• Endorses bogus/unusual symptoms[a]	• Incoherent speech/thought disorganization[a]
• Positive but no negative symptoms[a]	• Disturbed affect[a]
• Unusual groupings of symptoms[a]	• Verbosity
• Very slow performance[a]	• Neologisms
• Inconsistent performance on similar tasks[a]	• Concrete thinking
• Exaggerated behavior[a]	• Delusions and ideas of reference
• Fails floor effect items[a]	• Poor hygiene
• Gives improbable answers[a]	• Concentration problems
• Reports visual hallucinations	
• Reports suicide ideation	
• Affect discordant with topic	
• Presentation incongruent with GAF	

NOTE: Items in this table have been empirically evaluated and supported in at least one study.

[a] Supported in two independent studies. Indicators of genuine psychopathology are from Cornell and Hawk (1989).

facing a long prison sentence, the death penalty, or a career-ending conviction (e.g., a DUI for an airline pilot) may do so. Conversely, spending time on preparation might have much to do with having time available to do so (e.g., because of unemployment or incarceration). Examiners should be alert to circumstances and personal attributes of the defendant (e.g., intelligence, persistence, ingenuity, skill in manipulation, self-control, history of fraud, access to professional materials or family members with mental illness) that might enable successful portrayal of mental illness, including disorganized speech. One infamous multiple murderer, Ángel Maturino Reséndiz (known as the Railway Killer) worked in a prison library, where he researched professionals' strategies of malingering assessment and coached other prisoners.[1]

Some early sources listed *lack of cooperation* as an indication of malingering. My impression is that feigners/malingerers now are more likely to adopt a sincere, sympathetic demeanor and to appear to put forth good effort on assessment tasks—although a few will still be surly. Faced with an overtly uncooperative defendant, it may be worthwhile to ask why he or she appears unhappy.

Predictors of feigning have been examined in several studies. Despite being listed as one of four criteria for suspected malingering in the fifth edition of the *Diagnostic and Statistical Manual of Mental Disorders* (*DSM-5*; American Psychiatric Association, 2013), antisocial characteristics are not reliably related to malingering (Niesten, Nentjes, Merckelbach, & Bernstein, 2015).[2] Two sets of authors (McDermott et al., 2013; Weinborn, Orr, Woods, Conover, & Feix, 2003) reported that defendants facing more serious crimes were much more likely to malinger, but three other publications (Cochran, Grisso, & Frederick, 2001; McDermott & Sokolov, 2009; Vitacco et al., 2007) reported otherwise. Lower levels of education have been found to be associated with feigning in some samples (Duncan & Ausborn, 2002; Heinze, 2003; McDermott & Sokolov, 2009; Norris & May, 1998) but not in others (Gothard, Viglione, Meloy, & Sherman, 1995). African Americans had higher rates of feigning in two studies (Cornell & Hawk, 1989; Vitacco et al., 2007).

While the preceding indicators have received some empirical evaluation, they generally should not replace validity tests and collateral data. Indeed, many of the behavioral indicators are much more potent if behavior in the interview contrasts with behavior described by collateral sources. More unusual or bizarre behavior or representations should certainly raise suspicion of feigning, but they also are valuable in another way: If legitimate, they are likely to be observed and remembered by collateral sources, even those who have casual contact with the defendant. For example, I once evaluated a defendant whose gait was truly bizarre—something you might have seen, if you are old enough, in the Monty Python skit "Ministry of Silly Walks" (available on YouTube). A quick check with the deputies revealed he walked that way all the time. Given the effort this walk appeared to take, it is unlikely it was feigned. Another defendant was described as speaking in word salad (gibberish) throughout a 3-hour CST interview. Yet, phone recordings from the jail revealed him speaking completely coherently to a family member in lengthy conversations the week before and the week after the defense examination.

TESTING

Any standardized tests should be administered according to their instructions unless an accommodation is required to collect valid data. This can occur if, for example, an examinee has trouble operating a mouse for computer-administered tests. One aspect of standardization is that the test administration is conducted with only the examiner and examinee present. If a family member or the defense attorney has accompanied the defendant to the evaluation, he or she should be excused before starting the testing. In addition to standardization, psychologists are ethically obligated to maintain test security (American Psychological Association, 2013). Allowing observers, unless required by statute or court order, violates this prescription.

COLLATERAL DATA

Collateral information is vital to forensic assessment (Heilbrun, 1991; Melton et al., 2007; Otto, Slobogin, & Greenberg, 2007; Zapf & Roesch, 2009). Stredny, Torres, and Wolber (2009) described how collateral sources can provide a "parallel assessment" of the cognitive abilities (e.g., attention, receptive and expressive language, memory) required for CST, which is particularly useful if the defendant does not present validly during the evaluation interview.

Although psychiatric treatment records can be highly informative, examiners should be aware of their limitations. Few clinicians critically examine or seek to verify information that their patients tell them. I evaluated a defendant with perhaps 20 drug-related arrests. The defendant's treating psychiatrist of 5 years, when interviewed, denied the patient had a substance abuse issue, although he did say she tended to beg for free samples from his drug company representatives. Such defendants may carry on a long-term relationship with a treatment provider to obtain desired medications, for either personal use or sale, to support disability claims, or to evade criminal prosecution. Van Egmond and colleagues (Van Egmond & Kummeling, 2002; Van Egmond, Kummeling, & Balkom, 2005) reported that 10% to 42% of psychiatric patients in treatment had agendas that they had not disclosed to their therapist or psychiatrist. Psychiatric admissions or emergency room evaluations may also be driven by external incentives, such as obtaining shelter during winter months (Brady, Scher, & Newman, 2013).

Cognitive test scores have traditionally been interpreted without concern about effort or external motivation. Although the National Academy of Neuropsychologists (Bush et al., 2005; see also Bush, Heilbronner, & Ruff, 2014) declared assessments of response validity as medically necessary for *all* neuropsychological evaluations, substantial numbers of practitioners do not use them. Such evaluations risk "validating" feigned cognitive impairment. And although many might assume that cognitive assessments carried out when a defendant was in school would be valid, Kirkwood and colleagues (Kirkwood &

Kirk, 2010; Kirkwood, Kirk, Blaha & Wilson, 2010) found that not all children put forth good effort on cognitive testing.

Collateral information is most useful when it is not subject to manipulation or impression management, or is obtained in a different motivational context (e.g., bail applications or in a contested custody case). In these situations, or when seeking a job within the jail (e.g., trustee or in the kitchen), the defendant is motivated to appear normal and functional. If the examiner works as part of a unit or with security staff, an attractive member of the opposite sex of the defendant, if not identified as associated with the CST exam, can sometimes elicit a very different demeanor than is presented during the evaluation interview.

Usefulness of collateral data is maximized when legal knowledge and decision-making are involved. Police reports should be always be provided for CST examiners. In small towns or cities with neighborhood stations, police officers may have had dozens of contacts with a defendant, sometimes also as a complainant or witness in another crime. Sometimes former lawyers can be identified and asked about their experiences interacting with a defendant. If topics are limited to the defendant's ability to understand and assist them, not the content of their disclosure, attorney-client privilege is preserved.

If the defendant is in custody or in a state hospital, there often will be considerable data from the facility bearing on competence. These may include medical and psychiatric records, although they may require a release or a separate court order. Examiners should be aware that malingering appears even more common in jail treatment settings than in CST referrals (McDermott et al., 2013, reported 66%; Norris & May, 1998 reported 45.3%) and may not be detected by treatment staff. Examiners may be tempted to speak to mental health professionals, but a defendant who makes any effort to keep up an act outside of the CST exam will likely also feign to the unit psychiatrist and psychologist. For this reason, I am often more interested in what the auxiliary staff (psychiatric technicians, nursing assistants, correction officers, and housekeeping staff) can tell me. They see things that may never be passed on to the treatment professionals.

Observations by jail staff are usually available as public information, subject to the approval of the jail superintendent or lead security officer. For this reason, it is desirable for examiners to develop a cooperative relationship with the facility leadership. Jail disciplinary hearings are an analogue of the trial process and may lead to telling accounts of the defendant's ability to defend him- or herself and convey relevant information. However, often the best evidence to be had comes from recordings of inmate phone calls. Defendants are advised that calls are recorded, and a few do display some guardedness, but the value of phone recordings in some cases cannot be overestimated.

Family members and friends can be important sources, despite loyalty to the defendant. They should, with very few exceptions, be interviewed separately from the defendant and each other to allow each source to be heard independently, and to avoid efforts to present a unified but misleading front. Apparent discrepancies should be queried.

The defendant's treatment providers, attorney, family members, and friends are what I call *friendly sources*. Because of their emotional ties, professional obligations, shared interests, or perceptual biases, they may portray the defendant as more sympathetic and less substance-abusing and criminally inclined than other sources would suggest. This is not always true: Some parents are fed up with a defendant's lifelong antisocial behavior and take the opportunity to air their suffering; ex-spouses and ex-lovers are more likely to be forthcoming with information suggestive of feigning than current ones. Probation or parole officers can be excellent sources and, unless the defendant is or was a juvenile during the period of supervision, are free to talk to the examiner without a release or court order. In some cases, I have contacted others who have had more incidental contact with the defendant, including convenience store or laundry employees, or the cab driver who drove the defendant to the exam. Finding a balance between friendly and unfriendly collateral sources is needed when trustworthy, neutral sources are unavailable or provide insufficient information.

The examiner should ask about the collateral's relationship with the defendant. You do not want to learn that the defendant stole that person's car or girlfriend for the first time when you are on the stand. In *United States v. Tucker* (2010), an expert interviewed the defendant's mother and girlfriend and relied on their input. In cross-examination, the expert admitted he was not aware that the girlfriend had been convicted of perjury for lying to protect the defendant in a previous case. The examiner might ask if there is anything in their relationship that the attorneys might point to as evidence of bias, with the goal of drawing out any such issues.

Occasionally, a collateral will provide information that pulls everything together in the case. I once had a police officer tell me that a defendant had hundreds of prior arrests, including several in similar circumstances to the current charge. I accurately quoted him in my report. On the stand, I was asked if I would be surprised to learn that the defendant had been arrested only 39 times. Every source is fallible, and it is a mistake to rely on information that, upon reflection, may be an exaggeration.

Sometimes the complainant knows the defendant and will have some very telling observations or reports about his or her capabilities and lifestyle. Of course, such witnesses may be biased (as may any other witness), and particular care should be exercised to corroborate such accounts. In addition, the examiner should seek guidance from the prosecutor or retaining attorney before contacting a witness in the case in chief.

Results from disability evaluations should be viewed skeptically because, by definition, there is an external incentive for presenting as impaired. People applying for Social Security disability status must be determined to be unable to work in any capacity to qualify for benefits, which means even many people with legitimate disabilities will have to exaggerate to qualify. Further, the Social Security Administration has resisted the use of validity measures, does not pay for examiners to administer them,[3] and has described their use "not programmatically useful" (Chafetz, 2008; Dunlop, 2005; Social Security Administration, 2013; see also Chafetz, 2015, for a history of this issue through 2013). Even administrative law judges have reported feeling pressured to approve claims (Ohlemacher, 2013). Similarly, pressures that discourage response style assessment have been reported within the Veterans Administration (*Hodge v. West*, 1998; Poyner, 2010; Russo, 2014; Worthen & Moering, 2011), despite high failure rates on validity tests and evidence of malingering within these populations (Armistead-Jehle, 2010; Burkett & Whitley, 1998; Chafetz, 2008; Chafetz & Underhill, 2013; Freeman, Powell, & Kimbrell, 2008). Although many Veterans Administration disability examiners do use response style measures, Congress recently allocated $5.8 billion to private evaluation companies. I have never seen a report from one of the private vendors address response style or the possibility of malingering. Thus, even a verified claim of disability status should be taken with a very large grain of salt.

Treatment providers may also experience strong disincentives from diagnosing malingering, even if they suspect it (P. Green & Merten, 2013; Resnick & Knoll, 2008): Such a diagnosis may lead to a board complaint, threats of violence, a lawsuit, or simply loss of the patient. Even if prior examiners or treatment providers addressed response style, the thoroughness and competence of this effort should be carefully considered and not assumed: Outside of neuropsychology, few mental health clinicians are expert in this area.

Otto et al. (2007) provided a review of legal and ethical issues in using collateral sources. They distinguished between court-appointed examiners and those retained by either the defense or the prosecution. Court-appointed examiners have the most freedom of operation and may contact collaterals without obtaining permission from the parties under the aegis of the court order appointing them. Examiners appointed by the defense are much more restricted and, according to the authors, should not contact any collateral without first seeking permission from the attorney who retained them. Failure to do so could inadvertently spoil witnesses, disclose defense strategy, and waive privilege. The authors recommend that an examiner employed by the state notify the defense attorney before contacting collaterals.

Otto et al. (2007) recommended that examiners assess the credibility of collateral sources and justify why they relied on a particular source as opposed to others. They suggested that examiners' collateral sources be given a notification to include the following:

- The examiner's role, and who he or she is working for;
- That his or her participation is voluntary;
- That the examiner is independent and interested in data that would help either side; and
- That the interview is not confidential, and the collateral may be questioned by others in the future.

Interestingly, they do not include the possibility that the collateral sources could be called to testify, a point they made earlier in their chapter in discussing *Crawford v. Washington* (2004). The authors also suggested questions that should be posed:

- Have they spoken with the defendant or attorneys regarding the case?
- What is their relationship with the defendant and any other persons (e.g., witnesses, complainant) in the case?
- Have they been told not to discuss or mention any topics?

The authors also recommended inviting the collaterals to verbally review the examiner's notes for accuracy and to contact the examiner if there is any additional information they would like to share.

Near the end of a collateral interview, I sometimes ask if the source has an opinion about the defendant's ability to understand the court system and help the attorney, and if so, to justify that opinion. Of course, I am more interested in the reasons cited than the conclusion. Such discussions can not only bring forth helpful data on the issue of CST but also provide a sense of the bias of the source.

As a court-appointed examiner, I prefer to receive records directly from the relevant facility. If an attorney provides them, it is possible that "unhelpful" material may have been removed or redacted. Attorneys will probably be reluctant to lie to an examiner, but one should listen closely for evasive language (e.g., "These are all the records I have for you"). Examiners can include the expectation regarding full disclosure of records relevant to one's opinion in the retention agreement.

Examiners might consider doing an Internet search on the defendant and accessing social media pages. These may present the defendant in a quite different light than that portrayed during the evaluation. If the examiner is court-appointed or employed by the state, and the material reviewed is open to the public, there is no need for release. Defense experts should discuss this issue with the retaining attorney at the time of hire or in the retention agreement—and, if agreed upon, immediately do the search. Many defense attorneys will want to see it first and remove material that puts their client in a bad light. If relevant information is found, screenshots should be taken to preserve the evidence.

Pirelli, Otto, and Estoup (2016) examined the use of web-based information in forensic psychological exams. They wrote:

> Taken together, we can say with certainty that (a) neither ethical standards nor professional guidelines in forensic psychology directly speak to the appropriateness of searching for and using examinees' Internet-based data; (b) there is no empirical research or published professional commentary discussing the appropriateness of searching for and using Internet data when conducting forensic psychological evaluations; and (c) forensic psychiatric practice guidelines and literature surrounding the issue indicate that Internet searches are permissible, but not required, and may provide insight into an examinee's emotional, behavioral, and cognitive functioning. (p. 3)

They noted that the recent American Academy of Psychiatry and Law guidelines for forensic assessment (Glancy et al., 2015) suggested such sources may be used, and Pirelli et al. offered their own recommendations. They argued that even the examinee's own words from postings should not be equated with the self-report data obtained in a forensic interview and that use of Internet data be considered on a case-by-case basis, weighing its probative and prejudicial value. They recommended that examinees and their lawyers should be informed up front that the Internet data may be used and, if found, that examinees be given a chance to discuss or refute such material.

CHAPTER SUMMARY

- Plan to observe the defendant in as many ways as feasible before, during, and after the exam.
- Provide appropriate notifications to the examinee and collateral sources. Prompt regarding the need for honesty and full effort, but do *not* warn about validity tests.
- Begin with open-ended questions.
- Notice and record any indications of impression management and psychopathology contemporaneously throughout the assessment.
- Pay attention to changes in apparent capabilities or cooperativeness during different topics in the interview.
- Identify and use collateral sources who observe the defendant in natural environments or a different motivational context, and, if necessary, obtain written permission to contact them or receive records.
- Remember the limitations of clinical and collateral sources and ask about possible biasing factors.
- If Internet or social media are anticipated to be used, include notification in one's informed consent and consider providing materials for the examinee to view and address during the exam.

NOTES

1. A fellow prisoner testified to this at Reséndiz's trial, portions of which the author attended.
2. J. V. Ray et al. (2013) conducted a meta-analysis and reported that those scoring high on psychopathy measures scored higher on measures of negative response bias. However, because subjects in these studies were anonymous. there was no external incentive to feign. Thus, they could not *malinger* given the absence of the first criterion for malingering: presence of an external incentive.
3. However, one reviewer (VC) of an earlier manuscript of this work reported she is paid for administering the M-FAST in Social Security Administration evaluations.

3

CST Instruments and General Clinical Measures

This chapter will report and discuss the most commonly used CST assessment instruments and traditional clinical measures for assessing negative response bias in competency evaluations. The MMPI-2, MMPI-2-RF, and PAI will receive considerable attention in this chapter, and dedicated response style measures are covered in the following chapters. The most widely used response style measures, as reported in six surveys, are shown in Table 3.1. The last two columns (Rubenzer, 2018) refer to a subset of the data presented in Chapter 10.

COMPETENCY ASSESSMENT INSTRUMENTS

CST forensic assessment instruments range from an informal competency-focused interview to highly structured standardized tests like the Evaluation of Competence to Stand Trial–Revised (ECST-R; Rogers, Tillbrook, & Sewell, 2004), MacArthur Competence Assessment Tool–Criminal Adjudication (MacCAT-CA; Hoge, Bonnie, Poythress, & Monahan, 1999), and Competence Assessment to Stand Trial for Defendants with Mental Retardation (CAST-MR; Everington & Luckasson, 1992). Straddling these extremes is the Fitness Interview Test–Revised (FIT-R; Roesch, Zapf, & Eaves, 2006), which has standardized questions, broad coverage of competency abilities, and a means of quantifying impairment in different areas, but no summary scores or norms.

Most competency measures are face valid (ask straightforward questions, such as "What is the role of your attorney?") and are defenseless should a defendant decide to feign. Rogers, Sewell, Grandson, and Vitacco (2002) found that both the MacCAT-CA and the Georgia Court Competence Test were vulnerable to

Table 3.1 Response Style Test Practices From 2003 to Present

	Lally (2003)	Archer et al. (2006)	Sharland & Gfeller (2007)	Neal & Grisso (2014)	Martin et al. (2015)	Rubenzer (2018)	
Participants	Forensic Psychologists	Forensic Psychologists	Neuropsychologists	Forensic Examiners	Neuropsychologists	CST Examiners	
						TM	WS
TOMM	A 53%	75.2%	75.3%	9.9%	77.8%	94.5%	2.16
M-FAST		42.2%		9.3%	2.2%	78.4%	1.92
SIRS-2[a]						74.5%	1.80
SIRS	R 58%	86.2%			3.5%	78.0%	1.72
MMPI-2	R 64%		75.1%	8.1%[b]	29.7%	68.8%	1.35
Validity Indicator Profile[c]	A 53%	54.1%	40.8%		4.7%	53.2%	1.28
Inventory of Legal Knowledge[d]						53.2%	1.26
Rey 15 Item Test	A 68%	46.8%	74.5%		16.1%	60.9%	1.17
ECST-R ATP[e]				(6.8[f])		51.1%	1.02
MMPI-2-RF						48.9%	0.98
Reliable Digit Span[g]						43.2%	0.86
SIMS[h]					10.1%	43.2%	0.82
Dot Counting Test[i]			39.6%		24.7%	41.9%	0.65
Word Memory Test[i]			40.7%		58.2%	25.6%	0.44
Medical Symptom Validity Test[j]					28.2%	15.9%	0.39
Coin in the Hand[k]						11.6%	0.21
NV-MSVT[l]					12.0%	9.3%	0.21
Memory Complaints Inventory[m]					6.9%	9.5%	0.14

NOTE: Figures cited are percentages of respondents reporting the use of a given measure at least some of the time (*total mentions* = *TM*), except for Lally (2003) and Rubenzer (2018), second column. For Lally, the figures denote the percentage of respondents who endorsed the test as "Recommended" (R) or "Acceptable" (A). WS = weighted sum: *Never* = 0. *Rarely* = 1. *Sometimes* = 2. *Often* = 3. *Almost always* = 4. *Always* = 5. All studies except Neal and Grisso sampled psychologists, primarily in the United States. Neal and Grisso sampled psychiatrists as well as psychologists, from abroad as well as from the United States.

[a]Rogers, Sewell, & Gillard (2010).

[b]Figure reported included all versions of the MMPI, including the adolescent version.

[c]Frederick (1997).

[d]Musick & Otto (2010); Otto, Musick, & Sherrod (2010).

[e]Evaluation of Competency to Stand Trial–Revised, Atypical Presentation Scales; Rogers, Tillbrook, & Sewell (2004).

[f]The figure reported here was actually for the ECST-R competency scales. The usage of the ATP scales may be substantially lower.

[g]Greiffenstein, Baker, & Gola (1994).

[h]Structured Inventory of Malingered Symptoms; Widows & Smith (2005).

[i]P. Green (2005).

[j]P. Green (2004a).

[k]Kapur (1994).

[l]P. Green (2008).

[m]P. Green (2004b).

Box 3.1

Significantly below chance: If a multiple-choice test has four possible answers, an examinee could score approximately 25% correct by guessing, knowing nothing at all about the subject of the test. Of course, if 100 such subjects guess blindly, some would score below 25% correct, and some above. But very few would score below, say, 15% or above 35%. A score that is statistically below chance is usually defined as occurring in less than 5% ($p < .05$) of test takers who respond randomly.

feigning. Indices were generated to assess improbably poor performance or performance inconsistent with increasing difficulty of items, but none of these were successful. The ECST-R uses some open-ended questions that lack obvious face validity. Thus, a defendant may not perceive their purpose and be distracted by the face content. Although this is a potentially desirable feature, the available evidence is that the ECST-R's approach was not successful (Rogers et al., 2002; Vitacco, Rogers, & Gabel, 2009; see also Norton & Ryba, 2010). Nonetheless, I have had defendants that clearly feigned on validity measures score normally on the ECST-R, providing highly desirable evidence of competence. The ECST-R also contains a small battery of response style scales referred to as the Atypical Presentation (ATP) scales. These focus on reports of psychiatric symptoms in connection with the court system and their impact on functioning as a defendant. No other validity measure does so. The ATP scales will be examined in more detail in Chapter 6.

The CAST-MR is a CST assessment instrument for intellectually disabled (ID) examinees that has no formal response style indicators to detect negative response bias. However, because its first two sections are in multiple-choice format, it can be utilized as a *forced-choice test*, with three choices for each item instead of the more commonly used two response options. Thus, an examinee should score approximately 33% correct simply by guessing. Defendants who score *significantly* below chance provide very strong evidence of feigning.[1] However, significantly below chance performance is uncommon even for feigners (Berry & Schipper, 2008; Greve, Binder, & Bianchini, 2009). Potentially more useful are the norms for ID defendants who were independently judged competent or incompetent. A defendant who obtains raw scores half those of ID defendants found incompetent to stand trial, and who has never been diagnosed with intellectual limitations, lives independently, and has a driver's license, is probably not presenting in a credible manner. There is no research on this use of the CAST-MR, however, so conservative interpretation is advised.

GENERAL CLINICAL MEASURES

Several influential authors have opined against routine testing of intelligence or administration of psychopathology or personality tests in CST evaluations (Melton et al., 2007; Mossman et al., 2007). Although IQ scores are relevant to

CST if limited intelligence is at issue (see Chapter 8), valid scores depend on good effort from the examinee. Further, IQ scores will provide less direct evidence of competency-related knowledge and capacity than scores from dedicated CST measures.

On the other hand, some psychopathology inventories, particularly the MMPI-2 (Butcher et al., 1991) and MMPI-2-RF (Ben-Porath & Tellegen, 2008), have excellent embedded response bias measures. The PAI (Morey, 2001) rivals the MMPIs in validity assessment, while the Millon Clinical Multiaxial Inventory–III (MCMI-III; Millon, Davis, & Millon, 1997) has limited empirical support for its validity scales (Berry & Schipper, 2007; Sellbom & Bagby, 2008). Regarding the Rorschach, Ganellen (2008) concluded, "No specific indicators on the Rorschach have received enough empirical support to be considered an accurate, reliable marker of malingering" (p. 101). Neither the MCMI nor the Rorschach appears to be used often in CST assessment. The rest of this chapter will focus on the MMPI-2, MMPI-2-RF, and PAI.

The Minnesota Multiphasic Personality Inventory–2 (MMPI-2)

The MMPI-2 (Butcher et al., 1991), published by Pearson, is a 567-item self-report true-false format inventory of psychiatric problems, attitudes, and behavior. An introductory kit for hand scoring costs $989.85, but one could get started with just a manual ($65.75) and the *Q Global* platform, which is web-based and has no usage fee. Mail-in scoring is available, as are both a web-based and a local software option for $17.15 to $21.55 per extended score report, depending on the platform and quantity.[2] A forensic interpretive report is available (Q Global) for $61.00 per report, with a discount ($56.00) for quantity. The MMPI-2 is billed as appropriate for examinees 18 and older.

Although the MMPI-2 is regarded as an effective measure of response style in many forensic settings (Lally, 2003), some attempts to distinguish feigning on the original MMPI among criminal defendants were not successful (e.g., Walters, White, & Green, 1988). This chapter will focus on findings regarding the MMPI-2 and MMPI-2-RF in criminal justice populations and for conditions that are frequently present in CST examinees.

The 1991 MMPI-2 manual included recommended interpretations for only a single "fake bad" validity scale, the Infrequency (*F*) scale. T scores above 70 were said to be of "questionable validity," while those over 90 were deemed "probably invalid." High scores were not viewed as necessarily indicative of feigning, as high scores could be obtained through confusion or poor cooperation.

Over time, a sizable MMPI-2 literature on feigning developed, which encompasses a variety of "fake bad" scales (Table 3.2). Rogers, Sewell, Martin, and Vitacco (2003) reviewed 65 feigning studies and 11 diagnostic studies using the MMPI-2, not limited to criminal defendants. The authors endorsed F and *Ds* (the Dissimulation scale) as effective validity scales, with F showing the largest effect

Box 3.2

T scores: A type of standard score. The average (mean) score for a sample is 50. A score that is one standard deviation (*SD*) above the average score is 60; two *SD*s above the average is 70. Similarly, a score one *SD* below the average score is 40; two *SD*s below the average is 30.

Table 3.2 MMPI-2 Indexes and Cutoff (Raw) Scores to Detect Feigning

Index	Description	Cutoff Score	Accuracy	Stringent Cutoff
F	(Infrequency Scale) Items that are rarely endorsed by "normal" people who are not psychiatric patients. May be elevated by careless responding or intentional faking of psychiatric disorder, especially psychosis.	>20	86%	>24
F(b)	(Infrequency back) Similar to F scale, but for items on the back side of the answer sheet. Helps identify protocols where the subject loses interest halfway through and fills out the rest of the test randomly.	>18	82%	>20
F(p)	(Infrequency psychopathology) Items that are rarely endorsed by psychiatric patients—a more specific version of F; includes fewer legitimate symptoms of psychiatric illness than F.	>7	84%	>7
F-K	The raw score of K subtracted from the raw score of F.	>12	84%	>15
O-S	The sum of "obvious" items ("I hear voices") minus the sum of subtle items ("I think Washington was greater than Lincoln").	>156	85%	>240
Ds	(Dissimulation Scale) Items that reflect erroneous stereotypes of neuroticism.	>19	76%	>35
Ds-r	(Dissimulation Scale–Revised) Items that reflect erroneous stereotypes of neuroticism.	>19	79%	NA
FBS	(Fake Bad Scale) Designed to identify faking in personal injury claimants; its items include reports of bodily complaints combined with a portrayal of oneself as an honest and virtuous person.	≥29[a]	NA	NA

NOTE: All cutoff scores and accuracy figures are from Rogers et al. (2003) except where noted and are raw (not T) scores. Accuracy rates apparently weighted false negatives and false positive errors equally, in contrast to the recent approach of minimizing false positives or holding this error rate to a given value, such as 5% or 10%. Stringent cutoff scores are from Greene's (2000) summary of Caldwell's data set, cited and presented in Rogers et al. These were set to define the upper 2% of a very large clinical sample, albeit one in which no assessment of response style was apparently made.

[a]Figure from Ben-Porath, Greve, Bianchini, & Kaufmann (2008).

Box 3.3

Cohen's *d*, Hedges' *g* (and *d*): Two measures of the size of the difference in scores between two samples. To calculate them, subtract one mean (average score) of sample from the other, then divide the difference by the pooled standard deviation (a measure of variability within each sample).* Generally, Cohen's *d* and Hedges' *g* (and *d*) are referred to as *effect sizes*. Effect sizes larger than 0.8 are generally considered "large," as they indicate a substantial difference in the average score between two samples compared with the variation within each sample (Cohen, 1988). However, Rogers (2008b) argued that for forensic practice, a higher standard of $d \geq 1.25$ be required to denote a "large" effect size.

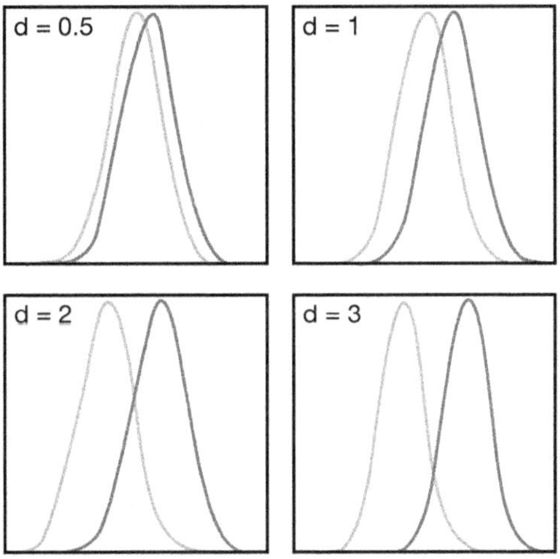

Figure 3.1 Illustration of Different Values of Cohen's *d*. This file is licensed under the Creative Commons Attribution–Share Alike 3.0 Unported license with an identified author of "Skbkekas." The image has been converted from color to grayscale.

size, but with widely ranging cutoff scores across studies. *Fb* (F back) had a lower average effect size than F, was deemed somewhat redundant with F, and had high false positive errors in some diagnostic groups. *Fp* (Arbisi & Ben-Porath, 1995), a scale developed to have little overlap with legitimate psychiatric symptoms, was effective across diagnostic groups (Cohen's $d = 2.02$), and the optimal cut score (raw >7) showed less variation than other validity scales. Similar virtues were described for Ds using a cutoff score of >35, and the authors also favored it for use of an *erroneous stereotype* detection strategy,[3] in contrast to the *rare symptoms* approach of F, Fb, and Fp.

However, several authors have concluded that Fp is insensitive to malingering of nonpsychotic conditions, including attention deficit hyperactivity disorder (ADHD; Harp, Jasinski, Shandera-Ochsner, Mason, & Berry, 2011) and PTSD

(Greiffenstein, Fox, & Lees-Haley, 2007; but see Goodwin, Sellbom, & Arbisi, 2013; Mason, Shandera-Ochsner, Williamson, Harp, Edmundson, Berry, & High, 2013; Rubenzer, 2009), and self-reported cognitive or memory problems (Gervais, Ben-Porath, Wygant, & Green, 2007; Gervais, Ben-Porath; Wygant et al., 2010; Jones & Ingram, 2011; Tsushima, Geling, & Fabrigas, 2011; Whitney, Davis, Shepard, & Herman, 2008; Whitney, 2013). However, Wygant et al. (2007) reported Fp predicted *performance validity test* (PVTs; tests that guage if the examinee has exerted good effort) performance in a criminal sample.

A number of studies have examined MMPI-2 validity scales among criminal defendants or prisoners (Barber-Rioja, Zottoli, Kucharski, & Duncan, 2009; Gassen, Pietz, Spray & Denney, 2007; Heinze, 2003; Iverson, Franzen, & Hammond, 1995; Kucharski, Johnsen, & Procell, 2004; Kucharski & Thomas, 2007; Lewis, Simcox, & Berry, 2002; McCusker, Moran, Serfass, & Peterson, 2003; McNulty et al., 2003; Rosenfeld et al, 2010; Steffan & Morgan, 2008; Steffan, Morgan, Lee, & Sellbom, 2010; Toomey, Kucharski, & Duncan, 2009). The validity scales examined vary between studies, but nearly all studies examined F and Fp. Optimal cutoff scores and diagnostic statistics have varied considerably among studies, even though most shared use of a common criterion (SIRS classification). Iverson et al. (1995), in a simulation study using federal inmates and psychiatric patients, recommended a cutoff score for F of T > 89, which achieved a sensitivity of 89% and specificity of 98%. At the other extreme, Lewis et al. (2002) reported a cutoff score of F > 107 produced a sensitivity of 67% with perfect (100%) specificity. However, none of the other studies in criminal samples achieved a specificity of 90% or greater at any cutoff score, which may reflect problems in the assignment to the honest samples. For Fp, optimal cutoff scores ranged from >70 (Gassen et al., 2007) to >100 (Heinze, 2003). Gassen et al. reported a sensitivity of 86% and specificity of 81% for >70, but McCusker et al. (2003) reported a specificity of only 48% at this same cut. Specificities equaling or exceeding 90% were reported only at a cutoff of 100 by some (Lewis et al., 2002; McCusker et al., 2003), and Heinze reported even this high cutoff achieved a specificity of only 85%.

Among the subset of studies cited here that examined CST referrals, several (Lewis et al., 2002; Heinze, 2003; Rosenfeld et al., 2010) apparently did not exclude inconsistent profiles as indicated by the MMPI-2 Variable Response Inconsistency (VRIN) or True Response Inconsistency (TRIN) scores. Kucharski et al. (2004) excluded cases with an elevated VRIN (≥13) but not TRIN. This leaves a small sample of studies (Barber-Rioja et al., 2009; McCusker et al., 2003; Gassen et al., 2007; Kucharski et al., 2007; Toomey et al., 2009) that can provide reliable data on the validity scales and their diagnostic statistics, and Toomey et al. did not report them. Finally, several studies (Barber-Rioja et al.; McCusker et al.; Kucharski et al.) classified all subjects that did not meet the SIRS criterion (three scales in the *probable* feigning range, or one in the *definite* range) as honest. Combined with the modest sensitivity (≤ 50%) of the SIRS, this has serious consequences for setting cutoff scores: Many apparent false positives for the MMPI-2 scales may actually be false negatives for the SIRS (Frederick, 2000a; Frederick & Bowden,

2009b). Attempts to maximize classification accuracy based on these statistics will predictably lead to inflated cutoff scores on the MMPI-2. Consider a simplified example in which half the sample is honest, the other half feigning. Assume also that:

1. The honest subjects are all classified accurately, as the test has very high specificity;
2. The test has a sensitivity of 50%, so that half the feigners are missed and are false negatives.

Now, let's consider the apparently honest group as classified by the test. This consists of the truly honest subjects, plus the false negatives: feigners whom the test failed to detect. In this example with a base rate of 50%, feigners who were not caught account for 25% of the total sample. Together, honest and successful feigners account for 75% of the total sample. Now the kicker: Fully 1/3 (25%/(25%+50%)) of the apparently honest subjects are actually feigners. This spoils the honest sample. Attempts to set a cutoff score on a different test to achieve a low false positive rate (e.g., 5%) are bound to grossly overestimate the appropriate score in an attempt to "pass" the wrongly classified honest responders. The problem is most severe for a high base rate condition, but it remains significant at lower base rates: At .25, 14.3% of subjects classified as honest are false negatives, at .15, 8.1% are, and at .10, 5.3% are wrongly classified as honest.

Of the CST sample studies cited here, only Gassen et al. (2007) identified an indeterminate group on the SIRS and did not lump that group with honest responders. They reported sensitivity and specificity for only a single cutoff score for F (>104; sensitivity = 93%; specificity = 92%) and Fp (>70; sensitivity = 86%; specificity = 81%). Incredibly, the reliable MMPI-2 validity scale data on CST examinees to determine cutoff scores appear to be limited to this single study. Finally, I note that the cutoff score provided for Fp is considerably lower than recommended by Rogers et al. (2003) and has a lower specificity (81%) than the ≥90% standard recommended by Greve and Bianchini (2004). Thus, a higher score for making a firm conclusion of feigning would be appropriate.

The various MMPI-2 validity indicators are moderately to highly intercorrelated (Ben-Porath & Tellegen, 2008; Nelson, Sweet, Berry, Bryant, & Granacher, 2007), which tends to work against their ability to provide incremental validity over each other. Of the studies that included only consistent MMPI-2 profiles, only Toomey et al. examined incremental validity, and reported Fp and Fb did not improve classification over F alone.

Meyers, Millis, and Volkert (2002) created an index by combining seven established MMPI-2 validity scales and indices. Subsequent studies (Greve, Bianchini, Love, Brennan, & Heinly, 2006; Tolin, Steenkamp, Marx, & Litz, 2010) have affirmed the index's validity but have not shown it superior to existing indices.

Megargee (2004) observed that the F and Fp scales contain items that might be endorsed by offenders because of background or environmental factors endemic to being incarcerated. In response, he developed the Offender Criminal Infrequency

Table 3.3 Diagnostic Statistics for Fc

	Gassen et al. (2007)		Kucharski & Duncan (2007)		Barber-Rioja et al. (2009)	
	Sensitivity	**Specificity**	**Sensitivity**	**Specificity**	**Sensitivity**	**Specificity**
>14	96.6%	84.6%	88%	89%	91%	82%
>15					88%	83%
>16					84%	87%
>17					81%	87%
>18					81%	89%
>19					75%	93%

NOTE: Kucharski et al. reported statistics for cuts lower than >14; Barber-Rioja et al. reported statistics for both lower and higher cutoff scores.

Scale (Fc) from MMPI-2 items. Gassen et al. (2007) reported Fc outperformed Fp, producing the highest classification accuracy rate of all validity scales at a cutoff score of >14. An AUC of .967 and Cohen's *d* of 2.86 were reported with the SIRS as the criterion. These values were not significantly higher than some traditional validity scales and indices (F, F-K, Fb, Ds, Ds-r), but they were higher than for Fp and FBS. Kucharski and Duncan (2007) reported Fc showed incremental validity over F, while F did not add to Fc, and Fc and F were highly intercorrelated (r = .87). Barber-Rioja et al. (2009) reported Fc outperformed Fp and Fb, and equaled or exceeded F. Sensitivity of Fc (59%) was lower than for F (69%) and Fb (81%), although specificity was better.[4] Fc showed incremental validity over all other scales in a hierarchical logistic regression analysis, while no scale demonstrated incremental validity over Fc. However, the authors noted that Fc is not published, that there were only two published studies (prior to their paper) supporting its use, and that forensic use may be premature. However, given three published, very supportive studies, this conclusion may be overly conservative. Still, as shown in Table 3.3, the highest specificity reported in Gassen et al. and Kucharski et al. (for >14) falls shy of the 90% standard, and a cutoff of >19 may be required to do so (Barber-Rioja et al.). However, this is based on a single study.

Bacchiochi and Bagby (2006) created and provided initial validation data on the *Malingering Discriminate Function Index* (M-DFI) on large samples of simulators and psychiatric patients. The M-DFI was designed to be more resilient to coaching than the standard validity scales. However, three subsequent known

---

Box 3.4

Known group design: A study in which the participants are determined to be honest or feigning through the best available classification procedure. In the literature addressing feigning of psychopathology, the SIRS was often employed as the criterion.

---

group studies (Tolin, Steenkamp, Marx, & Litz, 2010; Toomey et al., 2009; Steffan & Morgan, 2008) found the M-DFI did not outperform standard MMPI-2 validity indicators, and Toomey et al. found it to have a significantly lower AUC and lower sensitivity than the F scale.

While the MMPI's most familiar validity scales target exaggeration of psychotic symptoms, two newer validity scales have been shown to be sensitive to feigning of cognitive symptoms, as indexed by failure on PVTs. The Fake Bad Scale (FBS; Lees-Haley, English, & Glenn, 1991) was originally developed to identify pseudo-PTSD (claimed PTSD without a valid stressor/trauma) in a personal injury setting. Subsequent research has found it to correlate substantially with scores on PVTs, in contrast to traditional MMPI validity indices (Larrabee, 2003; Nelson et al., 2007; Ruocco et al., 2008, Sellers, Byrne, & Golus, 2006; Wygant et al., 2007; but see Rogers, Gillard, Berry, & Granacher, 2011; Whitney et al., 2008). It has been controversial (Ben-Porath, Greve, Bianchini, & Kaufmann, 2009, 2010; Butcher, Gass, Cumella, Kally, & Williams, 2008; Gass & Odland, 2014; Gass, Williams, Cumella, Butcher, & Kally, 2010; C. Williams, Butcher, Gass, Cumella, & Kally, 2009), but a recent meta-analysis (Nelson, Hoelzle, Sweet, Arbisi, & Demakis, 2010) reaffirmed its validity, particularly in forensic contexts with claimed traumatic brain injury. Lee, Graham, Sellbom, and Gervais (2012) found that previously expressed concerns about gender bias in the FBS are not clinically meaningful.

Two validity scales, the *Response Bias Scale* (RBS; Gervais et al., 2007) and *Henry Heilbronner Index* (HHI; Henry, Heilbronner, Mittenberg, & Enders, 2006) were developed using failure on PVTs as the criteria for item selection. Subsequent 39-item and 28-item versions of the RBS were created using multiple regression, and the latter is scoreable on the MMPI-2-RF. Several recent studies (Gervais et al., 2007; Gervais et al., 2010; Rogers et al., 2011; Tarescavage, Wygant, Gervais, & Ben-Porath, 2013; Tsushima et al., 2011; Whitney, 2013; Whitney et al., 2008; Wygant et al., 2011) have shown that RBS and HHI were more predictive of PVT performance than the F family scales, and they typically show incremental validity. However, effect sizes tend to be lower (Cohen's *d*s typically around 1.0) than those observed for the F scales when they are used to separate feigned psychopathology

---

Box 3.5

Positive predictive power (PPP): The percentage of examinees who score positive (fail) a validity test who are actually feigning; the accuracy rate for those who fail. This is the most meaningful statistic for an examinee who fails a validity test, but it requires knowledge of the base rate. PPP gives the probability that an examinee is feigning/not performing validly.

Negative predictive power (NPP): The probability that an examinee who scores negative (passes) a validity test is indeed performing genuinely. This is the most relevant statistic for an examinee who passes a validity test, but it requires knowledge of the base rate. NPP equals the probability that the defendant is performing genuinely.

---

from genuine presentations. Whitney (2013) reported that cutoff scores for RBS and HHI did not yield sufficiently high positive predictive power (PPP) and negative predictive power (NPP) rates. The most frequently recommended cutoff score for RBS on the MMPI-2 has been raw score $\geq$17. However, sensitivity at this score is typically low (13% to 59%; *M* = .34%), PPP modest (52%; Whitney, 2013), while specificity is variable (81% to 99%; *M* = 91%; Dionysus, Denney, & Halfaker, 2011; Gervais et al., 2007; Whitney et al., 2008; Whitney, 2013; Wygant et al., 2011; J. C. Young, Kearns, & Roper, 2011). Figures for HHI are generally comparable, with a frequently recommended cutoff score of $\geq$ 8, but Whitney (2013) reported an associated specificity of only 54%.

MMPI-2 SUMMARY

Pros:

- Many varied and validated response style scales that cover multiple domains.
- Can provide much additional, relevant information beyond response style.
- Does not require significant examiner time if scored by an assistant or computer.
- While the average reading level grade to comprehend items is rather low, some items contain vocabulary or syntax that will be difficult for those with intellectual disabilities or reading limitations.

Cons:

- May require 2 hours or more to complete, which must be supervised.
- Tedious and taxing on examinee.
- Very limited reliable data regarding cutoff scores and diagnostic statistics with CST examinees.
- Relatively expensive unless hand-scored.
- Some potentially valuable response style scales (RBS, Ds) must be hand-scored.

The Minnesota Multiphasic Personality Inventory–2–Restructured Form (MMPI-2-RF)

The MMPI-2-RF (Ben-Porath & Tellegen, 2008) is a substantial revision of the MMPI-2 in multiple ways. It shares many of the same administration and scoring platforms with its predecessor, although there is no forensic interpretive report, and pricing is similar.

Most of the RF's validity scales are derived and refined from the MMPI-2's scales, although there is a new validity scale, *Fs*, designed to assess feigning of somatic problems. Two of the venerable fake bad scales, F and Fp, underwent substantial revisions, removing items that did not meet the original conceptions of the scales. The revised validity scales have been subjected to examination and performed well in a number of clinical groups, including criminal defendants (Sellbom, Toomey, Wygant, Kucharski, & Bagby, 2010; Wall, Wygant, & Gallagher, 2015; Wygant et al., 2010), civil litigants (Gervais et al., 2010; Rogers et al., 2011; Tarescavage et al., 2013; Wygant et al., 2011; Wygant, Ben-Porath, Arbisi, Berry, Freeman, & Heilbronner, 2009; Youngjohn, Wershba, Stevenson, Sturgeon, & Thomas, 2011), neurological samples (Schroeder, Baade et al., 2012), military samples (Jones & Ingram, 2011), and psychiatric inpatients (Purdon, Purser, & Goddard, 2011; Sellbom & Bagby, 2010).

When directly compared, validity scales from the RF have exceeded the validity of their MMPI-2 counterparts (Gervais et al., 2010; Tyner, 2009). Chmielewski, Zhu, Burchett, Bury, and Bagby (2016) found not only that MMPI-2-RF validity scales improved classification among 742 disability claimants over their MMPI-2 counterparts, but that, as a group, the RF validity scales added incremental validity to *all* the MMPI-2 response scales, including those (e.g., Ds, Fb) that did not survive the transition to the RF. Among RF scales, F-r provided the best discrimination, while Fs also performed well. In contrast, Ingram and Ternes (2016) reported that in a meta-analysis of RF validity scale studies,[5] Fp-r had the highest effect size (Hedges' $g = 1.43$; 95% CI = 1.16–1.69) across studies, although the other validity scales also had strong effect sizes, and those for RBS and FBS-r showed less variability across moderators than F-r and Fp-r. Purdon et al. (2011) reported that acutely psychotic examinees tended to elevate the MMPI-2-RF's validity scales, including Fp-r and RBS, to about 70 on the average. FBS-r was less affected.

The MMPI-2-RF manual (Ben-Porath & Tellegen, 2008) indicates ranges of interpretation for each of the fake bad scales. These are presented, somewhat simplified, in Table 3.4. Because somatic malingering is not a major concern in CST evaluations, I will omit discussion of this scale.[6] Scores of 120 or greater on F-r, and 100 or greater on Fp-r, are deemed to render the profile and clinical scales invalid. Although the manual does not include this specific language for FBS-r (cutoff ≥100), the primary interpretive options for all three scales are either *inconsistent responding* or *over-reporting* for the cutoffs referenced in this paragraph. However, elevations on FBS-r and RBS are said to invalidate scales similar to their content: somatic and cognitive complaints for FBS-r and cognitive complaints for RBS.

The FBS was reduced from 43 to 30 items for inclusion in the MMPI-2-RF and renamed the *FBS-r* or alternatively, the *Symptom Validity Scale* (SVS). Schroeder, Baade et al. (2012) found FBS-r to have the highest sensitivity (48%; cutoff >89T) among MMPI-2-RF validity scales to Slick neurocognitive malingering classification when specificity for validity scales was held to 90% across neuropsychological

Table 3.4 MMPI-2-RF Validity Index Official Cutoff Scores

Index	Interpretive Rule	Interpretation(s)
Cannot Say (?)	≥15	Scores on some scales may be invalid
	1–14	Scores on shorter scales may be invalid
Variable Response Inconsistency-R (VRIN-R)	≥80	Invalid profile
	70–79	Interpret validity and substantive scales cautiously
True Response Inconsistency (TRIN-R)	≥80	Invalid profile
	70–79	Interpret validity and substantive scales cautiously
Infrequency (F-r)	≥120	Invalid profile
	79–119	Interpret substantive scales cautiously
Infrequency Psychopathology (Fp-r)	≥100	Invalid profile
	70–99	Interpret substantive scales cautiously
Infrequency Somatic (Fs)	≥100	Scores on somatic scales may be invalid
	80–99	Interpret somatic scales cautiously
Symptom Validity Scale (SVS/FBS-r)	≥100	Some scales may be invalid[a]
	80–99	Interpret cognitive and somatic scales cautiously[a]

NOTE: All scores listed are T scores. Elevations on all scales can occur due to carelessness or lack of comprehension, and this is an interpretive possibility unless these are ruled out by low VRIN-r and TRIN-r scores. RBS is not described in the MMPI-2-RF manual.

[a]Scales that contain items asking about cognitive and somatic (bodily) problems.

(including a psychiatric) patient groups. These authors also found no significant difference in mean scores between men and women on the FBS-r.

Other validity indices have been modified for scoring on the MMPI-2-RF. Henry, Heilbronner, Algina, and Yasemin (2013) described a revision of the HHI for the MMPI-2-RF and reported promising diagnostic statistics in a litigating sample. Meyers et al. (2014) reported on a revision of the original Meyers Index

---

Box 3.6

The Slick criteria: A set of criteria proposed by Slick, Sherman, and Iverson (1999) to objectively diagnose *malingered* cognitive impairment. They require the presence of an incentive to perform poorly, such as obtaining disability benefits, and either implausible test performance or inconsistencies between the examinee's presentation, self-report, or test scores with other facts or data.

(MI; Meyers, Millis, & Volkert, 2002), both of which combine scores from other MMPI "fake bad" validity scales: On the MMPI-2-RF version (MI-r), each validity score (F-r, Fp-r, Fs, FBS-r, RBS) equal or above 75 is given 1 point, and each score at or above 90 is given 2 points. An MI-r above 4 is predictive of PVT failure. Data are presented for examinees with mTBI, chronic pain, and PTSD.

Two new neuropsychological symptom measures were included in the MMPI-2-RF: the *Neurological Complaints* (NUC) scale, which measures self-reported neurological complaints such as dizziness, and the *Cognitive Complaints* (COG) scale, which measures self-reported problems such as concentration and memory difficulties. Youngjohn et al. (2011) found that NUC and COG, and the somatic scale *Malaise*, were better predictors of PVT failure than the MMPI-2-RF validity scales, including FBS-r, in their sample of head-injured litigants. Gervais, Ben-Porath, and Wygant (2009) reported COG strongly correlated with subjective emotional and cognitive complaints but not with actual cognitive performance. Bolinger, Reese, Suhr, and Larrabee (2014) also reported NUC and COG had no relationship to neuropsychological performance, but found they correlated highly with the MMPI-2-RF validity scales.

Only four studies to date (Grossi et al., 2016; Sellbom et al., 2010; T. D. Wall et al., 2015; Wygant et al., 2010) have specifically addressed MMPI-2-RF validity scales' performance with criminal defendants. Sellbom et al. reported that F-r and Fp-r were most effective for classifying 127 defendants (74% CST referrals) classified as feigning or honest by the SIRS. Analyses were run both with dichotomous classification from the SIRS and with eight indeterminate cases omitted. The results were quite similar, with AUCs from .89 to .93. Both F and Fp independently contributed to correct classification on the SIRS. Cutoff scores from the manual (F-r $\geq$ 120; Fp-r $\geq$ 100) were generally supported and achieved good sensitivity. However, the authors recommended a higher cutoff for Fp-r ($\geq$110) and cautioned that PPP remained below 80% at base rates of .15 and .30. F-r was considerably more sensitive (89%) than Fp-r (67%) at the recommended cuts, but less specific (91% vs. 97%). Although FBS-r was not as effective as the other scales, this was expected given the nature of the criterion (SIRS classification), and it still produced large effect sizes (*ds* = 1.59 to 1.74) and showed incremental validity over Fp-r.

Wygant et al. (2010; see also Wygant et al., 2007) found that all the MMPI-2-RF's validity scales had substantial effect sizes (*d*s = .97 to 1.65) in predicting a single PVT failure in civil and criminal forensic samples. Although RBS outperformed the other validity scales in the civil sample, it did not do so among pretrial criminal defendants, and RBS did not provide incremental validity over F-r and Fp-r in predicting PVT failure. In the criminal sample, all MMPI validity scales were highly intercorrelated, and they correlated highly with most of the MMPI-2-RF's clinical scales as well. An RBS cutoff score of T $\geq$ 100 produced a sensitivity of 59% and specificity of 89% in the criminal forensic sample, and $\geq$110 produced respective figures of 44% and 95%.

T. D. Wall et al. (2015) found the Fs scale best distinguished simulators from psychiatric patients, with considerably better sensitivity (75%) than

Fp-r and F-r at a cutoff score that achieved 90% specificity (T >100). However, they did not caution their simulators to avoid detection or provide an incentive for credible performance, and their incarcerated psychiatric patients were presumed to be responding honestly—a highly questionable assumption.

Grossi et al. (2016) focused on the ability of RBS to predict failure on the TOMM among 155 male pretrial defendants. They found a moderately strong relationship (AUC = .76; d = 1.46), although all the MMPI-2RF over-reporting scales were highly correlated and F-r performed as well as RBS. Grossi et al. found at the standard cutoff score (≥100), RBS had poor sensitivity (28.6%) but excellent specificity (97.8%). These are not desirable figures for a screening test, as a great many feigners will be overlooked. The authors also examined sensitivity and specificity at lower cutoff scores. A cutoff score of ≥88 maintained specificity over .90 (92.5%), with an associated sensitivity of 47.6%. Scores equal to or greater than 63 had very good sensitivity (85.7%) but weak specificity (37.3%). While RBS has not proved its unique value among pretrial defendants as a whole, it may have unique value among those who present as only having cognitive deficits apart from intellectual disabilities.[7]

The MMPI-2/RF as a Performance Validity Test (PVT)

In addition to the fake bad validity scales, the MMPI-2 and MMPI-2-RF have three validity scales to assess the degree of engagement and consistency the examinee demonstrated. CNS simply provides a numerical count of the items that were unanswered or answered both true and false, which, if excessive, can invalidate shorter scales and even the entire protocol. VRIN/VRIN-r assesses whether the examinee responded consistently to very similar, positively correlated items. TRIN/TRIN-r item pairs are negatively correlated, so that answering true (or false) to both suggests a yea-saying (acquiescent) or nay-saying response style. CNS, VRIN, and TRIN do not target over- or under-reporting, and are non-content-based (validity) scales. Ben-Porath and Tellegen (2008) wrote that high scores on VRIN-r are possible for a number of reasons, including poor attention or effort, lack of comprehension, or misplacement of scoring marks. They regarded TRIN-r (as opposed to VRIN-r) elevations as more likely due to poor cooperation than to benign carelessness or lack of comprehension.

Mason et al. (2013) reported that substituting 50% or 100% random item responses led to elevations on all the MMPI-2-RF's validity scales, especially F-r,

---

Box 3.7

Important Point

Moderate elevations (<80T) on VRIN-r or TRIN-r can cause false positives on Fp (and Fs).

Fp-r, and Fs. Burchett et al. (2016) examined the effect of replacing the answers from actual protocols with increasing proportions of random, acquiescent, and nay-saying responses from 0% to 100%. They found most of the validity scales were substantially impacted, although FBS-r and K-r were not. Modest elevations on VRIN-r and TRIN-r resulted in some examinees being wrongly being labeled "false fakers," in that they failed one or more fake bad validity test without exceeding the standard cutoff scores for VRIN-r or TRIN-r. Burchett et al. concluded:

> We recommend the following: (1) With modest VRIN-r elevations (70–79T)—notably, in the True (acquiescent) direction—clinicians should proceed with particular caution when interpreting Fp-r and Fs. (2) With modest TRIN-r elevations (70–79T), clinicians should proceed with particular caution when interpreting Fp-r and Fs. (p. 10)

Gu, Reddy, Green, Belfi, and Einzig (2016) reported that prior studies (E. A. Wise, 2009; Wygant et al., 2010; Sellbom et al., 2010) using criminal justice examinees found that between 10% and 21% of MMPI-2 protocols were invalid (either VRIN or TRIN $\geq$ 80) due to inconsistent responding. Gu et al. found that 12% of their CST restoration examinees exceeded the cutoff for VRIN-r, and 22% did so for TRIN-r. There was some overlap so that 31% of 156 protocols were deemed invalid due to inconsistent responding. Gu et al. reported both VRIN-r and TRIN-r were affected by low education and IQ (measured concurrently), and correlated with inconsistent responding on the SIRS Inconsistency scale. Scores on the TOMM did not add to the prediction after education and IQ were considered, likely because poor effort, if present, was already represented in the IQ scores. Psychiatric symptoms also predicted performance on TRIN-r, leading the authors to conclude as follows:

> Random and fixed responding (as gauged by TRIN-r) are not only affected by education and intellectual functioning, but also by intentional exaggeration and aspects of psychopathology. Measures of intellectual functioning and effort and response style should be considered for administration in conjunction with self-report personality measures to rule out rival hypotheses of invalid profiles. (Gu et al., 2016, p. 1)

Elevated TRIN-r scores should probably not be attributed to malingering or even poor cooperation without corroboration from PVTs or other data. For example, an ID examinee, who naively endorses most items, including those he or she doesn't understand, would likely score high. Now, this could be viewed as poor cooperation, because there may be an element of carelessness or a willful bias toward endorsing items which, after the first page or so, obviously tend to be keyed "true." But an attribution of poor cooperation may not be optimal.

Whether a competency examiner chooses to use a lengthy self-report measure will likely depend on systemic issues, such as the defendant's reading level and whether the examiner can arrange for the defendant to be properly supervised during testing. The MMPI-2's reading level and length will be a barrier for many defendants, and both the MMPI-2 and RF are relatively expensive unless one opts for hand scoring. However, the MMPI-2 and RF have a variety of excellent response style scales and, with the addition of the SVS, RBS, and Fs, are sensitive to most forms of exaggeration detectable from self-report. However, most data suggest smaller effect sizes and lower sensitivity for scales sensitive to cognitive underperformance than the F family for feigned psychopathology, so self-report measures cannot replace PVTs.

MMPI-2-RF SUMMARY

Pros:

- Similar strengths and limitations to MMPI-2, but better discriminant validity.
- 229 items shorter than the MMPI-2.
- Response style scales generally improved over those for the MMPI-2.

Cons:

- Still somewhat controversial, although this pertains more to the clinical scales than the validity indices.
- Does not include means to detect over-reporting of legitimate symptoms or distress from them.
- Expensive per use for computer scoring.

The Personality Assessment Inventory (PAI)

The PAI is a 344-item self-report inventory of psychiatric symptoms and of clinically relevant constructs. Published by Psychological Assessment Resources, Inc., it is based on recent theoretical constructions of psychopathology and sophisticated scale development procedures and requires a 4th-grade reading level. A specimen kit, which includes 25 answer sheets, costs $353.00. For hand scoring, forms are $62.00 for 25 and profile forms are $44 for 25 ($4.24/administration for both forms). Mail-in scoring is available for $227.00 for 10 answer sheets ($27.00 each), while the PAI software portfolio costs $726.00, which provides unlimited interpretive reports and on-screen administrations at $4.40 per use. Online administration through PARiConnect costs $5.00 per administration; score-only reports cost $6.00, and interpretive reports cost $17.00. The PAI has three established fake bad indicators: the *Negative Impression Management* (NIM) scale, the *Malingering Index* (MAL), and the *Rogers Discriminate Function* (RDF; Rogers, Sewell, Morey, & Ustad, 1996).

Sellbom and Bagby (2008) reviewed 15 published studies that examined the validity of the PAI response style indicators. They reported that although the RDF had the largest effect size in simulation studies, its effect size was essentially zero in the three known group studies. The NIM had the highest correlation with external fake bad indices, such as the SIRS. Nonetheless, the authors reported limited sensitivity, particularly for sophisticated feigners or those feigning anxiety. They recommended that NIM T scores below 77 suggest malingering is unlikely, while those ≥77 indicate feigning should be further evaluated. NIM scores of ≥110 and MAL ≥5 were reported to "very likely" indicate feigning.

Hawes and Boccaccini (2009) conducted a meta-analysis of 36 studies examining feigning on the PAI. They found that NIM, across studies, separated feigners from genuine clinical patients with a Cohen's d of 1.09. At an optimal cutoff score of ≥81, it produced an average sensitivity of 73% and a specificity of 83%. MAL showed a nearly equivalent effect size ($d = .92$), with a sensitivity of 58% and specificity of 86% at an optimal cutoff of ≥3. The *Rogers Discriminate Function* (RDF) did not perform well in studies with offenders. Hawes and Boccaccini reported that coaching did not appear to diminish the effectiveness of NIM and MAL, and that they were effective at detecting feigned anxiety and depression, although the effect sizes were smaller (ds = .90 to 1.25) than for more serious psychopathology (ds = 1.89 to 2.32). However, they also cautioned that observed effect sizes tended to decrease with better ecological validity of the studies, and although they included recommended cutoff scores on NIM and MAL, with associated diagnostics statistics, these were collapsed across studies: Some studies used a nonclinical control group, which predictably leads to larger effect sizes and specificities. Cutoff scores cited by Hawes and Boccaccini were selected to maximize overall classification, which may not be appropriate if false positive errors are deemed more serious than false negatives. Classification rates for other cutoff scores from Hawes and Boccaccini are shown in Table 3.5.

A number of studies have examined performance of PAI indices in criminal samples (Boccaccini, Murray & Duncan, 2006; Edens et al., 2007; Gaines, Giles, & Morgan, 2013; Hill, 2009; Kucharski et al., 2007; Mogge, Lepage, Bell, & Ragatz, 2010; Rogers et al., 1996; Rogers et al., 1998). Boccaccini et al. (2006) reported

Table 3.5 Sensitivity and Specificity of PAI Validity Indices

Scale/Cutoff Score	Sensitivity	Specificity
NIM		
≥77	.75	.77
≥81	.73	.83
≥92	.59	.80
≥100	.33	.98
MAL		
≥2	.76	.65
≥3	.58	.86
≥4	.35	1.00
≥5	.28	.99

NIM increased prediction of SIRS classification over the MMPI-2 F scale among federal pretrial defendants. Kucharski et al. found only the NIM predictive of SIRS classification and reported that 54.1% of those excluded from the primary analysis because of elevated *Inconsistency* or *Infrequency* scale elevations failed the SIRS. This suggests, as Gu et al. (2016) argued for the MMPI-2-RF, that inconsistent or content-invalid responding may be a manifestation of feigning. Edens et al. reported all the PAI validity indicators discriminated simulators and suspected malingerers from genuine forensic patients, with NIM performing best and even besting the SIRS. Unfortunately, many of the studies in criminal samples did not examine diagnostic statistics but focused on demonstrating significant correlations or incremental validity.

Two new scales or indices make use of items or scores across the major clinical scales. Mogge et al. (2010) created and provided initial validation for the *Negative Distortion Scale* (NDS), which utilizes items with extreme item response frequencies from the PAI's eight psychopathology scales. The NDS discriminated suspected malingerers from genuine forensic inpatients (groups defined by dichotomized SIRS classification), and it added incremental validity to existing PAI validity indices. Thomas, Hopwood, Orlando, Weathers, and McDevitt-Murphy (2012) found the NDS to have the highest effect size among PAI fake bad indicators for separating simulators from students not in treatment but qualifying for a PTSD diagnosis, and to be relatively robust to coaching. Rogers, Gillard, Wooley, and Kelsey (2013) replicated these findings in a simulation study and reported a large effect size (d = 1.81) and relatively low correlations with other PAI validity scales. They concluded NDS showed promise for both ruling in and ruling out response bias. Table 3.6 summarizes the available cutoff score data.

Table 3.6 Cutoff Scores, Sensitivity, and Specificity for NDS

	Sensitivity			Specificity		
Cutoff Scores	Mogge et al. (2010)	K. M. Thomas et al. (2012)	Rogers et al. (2013)	Mogge et al. (2010)	K. M. Thomas et al. (2012)	Rogers et al. (2013)
11	.88	.78	.98	.57		.56
12	.88			.57	.77	
13	.82		.89	.71		.71
14	.73			.74		
15	.71	.70	.89	.77	.90	.77
16	.61			.89		
17	.61			.91		
18	.50			.91		
19		.64	.79		.97	.90
25			.55			.94

Note: Values from K. M. Thomas et al. were mislabeled in the original article (C. Hopwood, personal communication, August 26, 2015). I also obtained the NDS mean and *SD* to convert T scores to raw score values from this exchange (M = 4.23; SD = 4.17).

Beginning in this table, I will express sensitivity and specificity in tables in a decimal format (e.g., .50) rather than as percentages, but the meaning is the same (.50 = 50%).

Gaines, Giles, and Morgan (2013) created the *Multiscale Feigning Index* (MFI), which averages scores on the seven clinical scales that inmates are likely to elevate if feigning (e.g., *Schizophrenia, Paranoia, Anxiety*), as opposed to those they might want to avoid elevating (*Alcohol* or *Drug Abuse, Antisocial* and *Borderline* personality scales). The MFI outperformed all the PAI's standard validity indicators when predicting SIRS classifications, and it produced a sensitivity of 69% and specificity of 94%.

The PAI response fake bad indices have produced quite mixed results in distinguishing honest and simulating or malingering mTBI samples, with some authors finding them ineffective or poorly predictive of PVT performance (Armistead-Jehle, 2010; Haggerty, Frazier, Busch, & Naugle, 2007; Whiteside, Dunbar-Mayer, & Waters, 2009; Whiteside, Galbreath, Brown, & Turnbull, 2012), and others (Lange, Pancholi, Bhagwat, Anderson-Barnes, & French, 2012; Keiski, Shore, Hamilton, & Malec, 2014) reporting fairly strong effect sizes (*d*s = 1.0 to 1.4). Lange et al. reported that several clinical scales (*Somatoform, Anxiety, Depression, Schizophrenia*) had larger effect sizes than NIM. Simulators who were instructed to feign psychiatric problems in addition to cognitive and somatic complaints were better detected than those who were instructed to feign only cognitive and somatic problems.

A few recent studies have examined PAI validity index performance in specific diagnostic groups. Rogers, Gillard, Wooley, and Ross (2012) reported that traumatized inpatients who passed the M-FAST showed considerable elevations on the NIM: Those diagnosed with PTSD obtained a mean score of 71.96; those with both PTSD and dissociative identity disorder averaged 85.85. Rogers et al. nonetheless reported large effect sizes between these patients and matched patients asked to feign disability. MAL and RDF were found particularly helpful, as severe pathology of the patients did not elevate these indices. Rios and Morey (2013) reported the PAI-Adolescent validity scales distinguished feigned ADHD from those so diagnosed, with RDF being most successful.

Summarizing, the PAI's well-established response style measures (NIM, MAL) tend to produce lower effect sizes than the MMPI-2 and MMPI-2-RF validity scales. NIM does not have the specificity of Fp/Fp-r, although MAL performs well in this regard. NDS is very promising and has sufficient support for use in forensic assessments using the data presented in Table 3.6.

PAI SUMMARY

Pros:

- Considerably shorter than MMPI-2.
- Requires minimal clinician time.

- Likert scale format may be more palatable for brighter or obsessive examinees.
- Excellent source of clinical information if the profile is valid.
- Less expensive per use than MMPI-2/RF if computer administration and scoring are used.

Cons:

- Validity scales appear less potent than for MMPI-2/RF.
- NIM scale has a significant portion of items that reference dissociative symptoms, potentially leading to false positives in this group.
- Likert scale format may be more confusing or difficult for examinees with cognitive limitations or limited reading competence.

CHAPTER SUMMARY

Most CST instruments lack any defense against feigning or poor effort. If the defendant can read adequately and is not ID, and the evaluation circumstances allow, the MMPI-2 and MMPI-2-RF are strong choices to assess feigned psychopathology, and they provide some capacity to assess feigned cognitive problems. Both contain an arsenal of very good to excellent response style indicators. A relative weakness, however, is they do not cover overendorsement of legitimate psychiatric symptoms. The MMPI-2-RF, in addition to being 229 items shorter than its predecessor, appears to exceed it in response style assessment. The PAI is also a solid contender, although its validity scales appear less effective than the MMPI's. An advantage of these tests is that, if valid, they may provide valuable information about symptoms and functional impairments that would not be obtained on instruments like the M-FAST or SIRS. Table 3.7 shows selected indices that have shown 90% (.90) specificity in multiple relevant studies and associated cutoff scores, sensitivities, and citations. The reader should remember the methodological shortcomings cited in the text, which will tend to inflate cutoff scores and underestimate sensitivity and specificity. Nonetheless, I do not recommend readers adopt other less stringent cutoff scores until better data are available.

Table 3.7 Selected Test Indices With Recommended Cutoff Scores and Diagnostic Statistics

Test/Index	Criteria/Cutoff Score	Includes SMI, ID?[a]	Sensitivity	Specificity	Citations
MMPI-2 F[b]	>106	SMI	.67–.78	.76–1.00	Lewis et al., 2002; McCusker et al., 2003; Kucharski & Duncan, 2007
MMPI-2 Fp[b]	>100	SMI	.35–.52	.85–1.00	Lewis et al., 2002; McCusker et al., 2003; Heinze, 2003
MMPI-2 RBS	>17 raw		.13–.50	.88–.99	Gervais et al., 2007; Whitney et al., 2008; Dionysus et al., 2011; J. C. Young et al., 2011
MMPI-2-RF F-r	≥120	SMI	.27[c], .64–.89	.88–.92	Sellbom & Bagby, 2010; Sellbom et al., 2010
MMPI-2-RF Fp-r	≥100	SMI	.43[c], .72–.74	.90–.97	Sellbom & Bagby, 2010; Sellbom et al., 2010
PAI NIM	≥110	SMI	.33	.98	Hawes & Boccaccini, 2009
PAI MAL	≥4	SMI	.35	.99, 1.00	Hawes & Boccaccini, 2009
PAI NDS	≥19	SMI	.64, .79	.90, .97	Mogge et al., 2010; K. M. Thomas et al., 2012; Rogers et al., 2013

NOTE: Figures do not apply to defendants with severe cognitive impairment or SMI unless otherwise noted. Many studies have the methodological shortcomings cited in the text, which will tend to inflate cutoff scores and underestimate sensitivity and specificity.

[a]SMI = serious mental illness; ID = intellectually disabled.

[b]Cutoff scores reported based only on studies of criminal samples.

[c]Coached subjects.

NOTES

1. * The *pooled* standard deviation is similar to averaging the standard deviation of the two samples. There appear to be several formulas for calculating it, some of them complicated. Fortunately, several free websites allow an uninitiated user to easily calculate effect size indices like Cohen's *d*.

   It is important to distinguish chance-level responding and responses that are significantly below chance (Frederick & Speed, 2007). Some people who guess blindly to a three-response test will score above or below 33%. The distribution of these scores is described by the binomial theorem. The VassarStats website allows a user to easily find the probability of observing a score given the number of response choices and items. Technically, one is interested in the probability of observing a particular score *or lower* if one is interested in below chance performance.
2. Mail-in service also requires purchase of official answer sheets, which cost $23.70 for 25.
3. An erroneous stereotype detection strategy uses popular misconceptions of a mental disorder to generate items. For example, the Ds scale was created by having subjects try to answer the (original) MMPI as they thought someone who was neurotic would.
4. Figures were apparently based on hierarchical regression analysis.
5. However, Ingram and Ternes (2016) did not include studies that reported their finding in raw scores.
6. However, the Fs does contain three items that are potentially relevant to feigned incompetency, in that they ask about having blank spells, sleepwalking, and not knowing what is going on around them.
7. RBS has not been evaluated with ID examinees.

4

Instruments for Assessing Feigned or Exaggerated Psychopathology

Defendants may falsely claim to hear voices, to be depressed, or to experience any number of psychiatric symptoms. A number of specialized instruments have been designed to assess feigning in this domain.

STRUCTURED INTERVIEW OF REPORTED SYMPTOMS (SIRS)

The SIRS (Rogers et al., 1992) is a 172-item structured interview. It was published by Psychological Assessment Resources but is no longer being sold. It remains relevant because of controversies involving the SIRS-2 revision, because much from the original was retained in the SIRS-2, and some examiners may choose to use the SIRS classification scheme rather than that of the revision. The SIRS-2 booklets can be used to administer and score the original version.

The SIRS has often been referred to as the gold standard of malingering assessment, and many studies of other response style measures have used SIRS classification as the criterion. The SIRS was *recommended* for use in assessing malingering in Lally's (2003) survey of forensic diplomats and was the most frequently used malingering instrument in Archer et al.'s (2006) survey of forensic psychologists and a more recent survey of CST examiners (Chapter 10, this volume).

Gothard et al. (1995) found the SIRS to provide nearly perfect classification of feigners in a criminal setting. Other authors, however, have reported very disappointing results (Pollock, 1997; Edens, Poythress, & Watkins-Clay, 2007). The SIRS's ability to discriminate feigned depression, anxiety, and PTSD from genuine patients was demonstrated in simulators (Rogers, Kropp, Bagby, & Dickens, 1992) and in compensation cases (Rogers, Payne, Berry, & Granacher, 2009).

The SIRS does not adequately address several forms of feigning that may be encountered among competency referrals, such as feigned intellectual disability, memory impairment, or ignorance of the court system. Even among those presenting with primarily psychiatric symptoms, the SIRS manual (Rogers et al., 1992) reported sensitivity of only 48.5%. This means the SIRS would fail to identify more than 50% of those feigning.

A recent meta-analysis (D. Green & Rosenfeld, 2011) found the SIRS to have better sensitivity than reported in the manual, with an average sensitivity of 75% across studies, but a much higher average false positive rate than reported in the manual: 11% versus 0.5% to 5.0%. However, all but one of the studies conducted after the four initial validation studies reported in the manual used different criteria for classification than specified in the manual, such as discriminant function analysis. The higher false positive rates are likely due to more impaired clinical samples, such as dissociative identity disorder (DID; Brand, McNary, Loewenstein, Kolos, & Barr, 2006; Rogers, Payne, Correa, Gillard, & Ross, 2009) and intellectually disabled (ID) persons (Farkas, 2008; Hurley & Deal, 2006), than used in the initial validation studies. About one third of ID examinees failed the SIRS in Farkas (2008) and Hurley and Deal (2006). D. Green and Rosenfeld noted that the *Improbable Failure* (IF) scale, which consists of very easy cognitive items that might be useful in assessing performance validity, had not received much research.

Among the few studies that used the SIRS's standard scoring rules, Green and Rosenfeld reported a mean weighted sensitivity of 48.6%, with a mean weighted specificity of 94.6%—very close to the figures reported in the manual. They also found the SIRS's Total Score at a cutoff of $\geq$76 showed the highest effect size of any scale (Cohen's d = 1.90) when contrasted with clinical controls, but it also had a substantial false positive rate in samples of ID, dissociative, and incarcerated mentally ill examinees. Finally, effect sizes showed large variability from one study to another, particularly in criminal forensic samples: Whereas Gothard et al. (1995) found perfect classification and a very large effect size (d = 3.26), Edens et al. (2007) reported the SIRS was not effective in distinguishing malingerers from genuinely mentally ill offenders (d = 0.11), although Rogers and Bender (2003) criticized the methodology of this study. Two subsequent studies (D. Green, Rosenfeld, Belfi, Rohlehr, & Pierson, 2012; Rosenfeld, Green, Pivovarova, Dole, & Zapf, 2010) found the SIRS/SIRS-2 to perform as well as or better than any other validity test examined.

SIRS SUMMARY

Pros:

- Validated in both known group and simulation studies.
- Shown to generalize (apply validly) across race and gender.

- Measures multiple strategies of symptom exaggeration, including those not tapped by other instruments (over-reporting of genuine symptoms).
- Has been regarded as the gold standard for assessment of feigned psychopathology.
- Inexpensive per use (about $6).

Cons:

- Appears to successfully detect only about half of those feigning psychopathology.
- Relatively long and time-consuming to administer and score; many unscored items.
- Appears prone to false positives with ID and possibly DID examinees.
- Has been superseded by the SIRS-2 and is no longer sold by the publisher; might be portrayed as obsolete.
- Not well researched for assessing cognitive feigned impairment.

Structured Inventory of Reported Symptoms–2 (SIRS-2)

The SIRS-2 (Rogers et al., 2010) is a significant revision of the original test. Items are unchanged, but new indices have been created and the *Total Score* index dropped. There are now two indeterminate classifications: *Indeterminate-Evaluate* and *Indeterminate-General*. The former indicates a need for further evaluation of feigning, but the latter does not. The SIRS-2 is published by Psychological Assessment Resources, and a specimen kit, in either English or Spanish, costs $339.00. Assessment booklets are $264.00 for 25, for a per administration cost of $10.56. The publisher reports the SIRS-2 is appropriate for ages 18 to 100, and the test takes 30 to 40 minutes to administer and 20 minutes to score.

The SIRS-2 revision appears to have been stimulated by findings of high false positives among hospitalized, traumatized patients with dissociative symptoms (Brand et al., 2006; Rogers et al., 2009) on the original SIRS. Brand, Tursich, Tzall, and Loewenstein (2014) reported the SIRS-2 was more specific, but less sensitive, than the original SIRS in distinguishing dissociative patients from coached simulators. Weiss, Rosenfeld, and Farkas (2011) reported that the SIRS-2 scoring rules resulted in far fewer false positives (7%) among ID individuals than the original SIRS criteria (23.3%).

The SIRS-2 has received critical attention that the original largely avoided. Because the SIRS-2 has added criteria to qualify for feigning, sensitivity should be lower than before. Nonetheless, the SIRS-2 manual reports sensitivity as 80%, much better than for the original. Questions have been raised about the reported statistics and lack of peer review of the new decision rules (DeClue, 2011; D. Green & Rosenfeld, 2011; Rubenzer, 2010). DeClue noted that if the cases classified as indeterminate (not clearly honest or feigned) on the SIRS-2 are included in the analysis, the SIRS-2's sensitivity is only 49%. He noted that some subject characteristics were not reported and that his requests to review the original data were refused by the publisher (DeClue, 2011). This led DeClue to state the SIRS-2 is "very vulnerable" to be ruled inadmissible due to lack of peer review, cross-validation, and inability to fully examine the data upon which the SIRS-2 decision rules rely. However, I was not able to find any instances in which this occurred. In the one case in which SIRS-based testimony was challenged (*Dorgan v. O'Connor*, 2011), the trial judge allowed the testimony and the judgement was upheld on appeal.[1] In addition, queries to two forensic psychology listservs asking members for knowledge of any cases in which the SIRS-2 was excluded produced no positive responses.

D. Green, Rosenfeld, and Belfi (2013) compared the diagnostic accuracy of the SIRS and SIRS-2 decision rules in both community simulators and defendants admitted for competency restoration. For inpatients, presentation status was based on the agreement of psychiatrist and psychologist evaluators who had access to extensive collateral information as well as test data. The two SIRS scoring schemes produced congruence on classification of 58.8% of patients as genuine, 11.3% as feigning, and 9.4% as indeterminate. An additional 20.5% were indeterminate on one SIRS but not the other. To examine diagnostic statistics, indeterminate cases were classified as genuine. In contrast, the figures cited in the SIRS manuals excluded the 23% of cases that had an indeterminate classification. Sensitivity was considerably higher for simulators (SIRS = 75.0%; SIRS-2 = 66.7%) than for defendants suspected of malingering (SIRS = 47.4%; SIRS-2 = 36.8%). Conversely, the specificity was good, with the SIRS-2 showing a small advantage (specificity = 94.3% vs. 92.0%) over the original SIRS. D. Green et al. reported that the newly added MT index was not effective and that the old SIRS Total Score performed better. The authors reported that if *Indeterminate-Evaluate* cases on the SIRS-2 were classified as feigning, sensitivity increased, but only to 52.6%, with a predictable drop in specificity. Thus, nearly half of those suspected of feigning went completely undetected. However, these cases may have feigned cognitive impairment or ignorance of the court system rather than psychopathology. Still, Brand et al. (2014) also reported that many simulators (44.2%) also escaped detection, not even being flagged as *Indeterminate-Evaluate*. This was despite the fact that they were simulating DID, a condition characterized by very high levels of symptom endorsement across multiple domains of psychopathology, and subjects were not cautioned to avoid detection.

Tarescavage and Glassmire (2016) compared the sensitivity of the SIRS and SIRS-2 among 95 CST restoration patients suspected of malingering by staff and corroborated by stringent cutoff scores on the MMPI-2-RF or M-FAST. They found the SIRS had a sensitivity of 87.1%, whereas the SIRS-2's respective figure was 53.8%. Concordance between the SIRS and SIRS-2 classifications of feigning, indeterminate, and genuine was only 53.9%, with the primary discrepancy being that a great many of those deemed feigning by the SIRS were classified as indeterminate on the SIRS-2. Although specificity was considerably higher for the SIRS-2 (86.7% vs. 72.7%), the authors implied this was due to methodological limitations of their study (use of nonconsecutive referrals). The authors concluded, "Given the substantial sensitivity losses found in the current study and by (D.) Green et al. (2013), independent research does not support that the SIRS-2 is as useful for identifying feigned psychopathology as the SIRS" (p. 13). They also noted that feigning remains a distinct possibility for the substantial number of indeterminate classifications on the SIRS-2.

D. Green et al. (2012) reported the relative contributions of the SIRS-2 and PVTs in assessing invalid presentation among CST examinees. Several such tests, including the TOMM, Rey 15 Item Test, Dot Counting Test, but not the Validity Indicator Profile (VIP; Frederick, 1997) Verbal scale, matched the SIRS-2 in diagnostic accuracy. However, the SIRS-2 identified only 5.1% of test-takers as feigning, whereas psychiatrists, at the time of the initial evaluation, suspected 21.1%, and quite a few examinees who passed the SIRS-2 failed two or more PVTs.

Grossi et al. (2016) examined the SIRS-2's IF scale, which consists of very easy cognitive problems, among a large group of pretrial defendants. They found an AUC = .72 in predicting TOMM classification, but at the manual's recommended cutoff score of ≥6, sensitivity was only 41.3% and specificity 78.7%. The authors examined other cutoff scores to see if more favorable statistics could be obtained. A cutoff of ≥1 was necessary to obtain a sensitivity of 80%, suitable for a screening test, but this produced a very low specificity of 28.9%. Grossi et al. concluded, as did Rogers and colleagues (Rogers, Payne, Berry, & Granacher, 2009), that IF should not be used as a screening test or with examines with IQs of 80 or below. Given the limited specificity at a cutoff of ≥6, it does not appear to be useful as a diagnostic test either.

In sum, the SIRS-2's new decision rules have reduced false positive findings, particularly in ID and possibly DID examinees.[2] However, this comes at a considerable cost, which is loss of sensitivity. Even so, the SIRS-2's sensitivity is comparable to the MMPI-2-RF's F-r and Fp-r scales. The SIRS-2 is not suited to detecting cognitive feigning and may not provide strong evidence of feigning (a *definite* feigning classification) in a substantial portion of those who feign psychopathology. The original SIRS has been studied in both simulator and known group studies and has demonstrated validity across race and gender. It has been validated on non-test criteria, including ward observations and collateral data. In contrast, most other symptom validity test (SVT) studies have used the SIRS itself as the criterion. However, the criticisms of DeClue (2011) and Rubenzer (2010) should be carefully considered before relying on the SIRS-2 as one's primary psychopathology validity indicator. Finally, although the SIRS/SIRS-2 is often described as a *diagnostic* (as opposed to *screening*) test, the manuals clearly state that scores should be interpreted within the context of additional information. Thus, like other validity tests, the SIRS and SIRS-2 are corroborative, not definitive, evidence of feigning.

SIRS-2 SUMMARY

Pros:

- Similar virtues to original SIRS.
- Shown to be less prone to possible false positives in some populations (ID, DID).

- If failed, produces strong evidence of feigned psychopathology.
- Less expensive than MMPI-2/RF unless they are hand-scored.
- The only psychopathology feigning measure that can be recommended for ID defendants.

Cons:

- Less sensitive than original SIRS; may misclassify a substantial number of feigners as genuine.
- Does not adequately assess feigned cognitive problems or feigned ignorance of the court system.
- Controversial given publisher's refusal to release raw data, critical reviews; could possibly face *Daubert* challenge and be excluded.

MILLER FORENSIC ASSESSMENT OF SYMPTOMS TEST (M-FAST)

The M-FAST (H. A. Miller, 2001) is a 25-item structured interview that is marketed as a screening test for feigned or exaggerated psychiatric symptoms. Published by Psychological Assessment Resources, the test takes only 5 to 6 minutes to administer and perhaps a minute to score and is appropriate for ages 18 to 71. A specimen set sells for $198.00 and includes 25 protocols. Replacement booklets cost $142.00 for 25, for a per administration cost of $5.68.

Although the M-FAST has scales that parallel those of the SIRS, the Total Score has received the most attention and is the only scale that consistently demonstrates strong internal reliability (.89 or better). The M-FAST Total Score correlates strongly with other measures of feigned or exaggerated psychopathology such as the MMPI-2 validity scales, particularly Fp ($r = .78$; H. A. Miller, 2001) and the SIRS *Rare Symptoms* ($r = .67$), *Reported/Observed* scale ($r = .66$; H. A. Miller, 2001), and SIRS *Total Score* ($r = .85$; Guy & Miller, 2004). Gaines (2009) reported that the M-FAST accounted for 78.5% of the variance in the SIRS.

The M-FAST has been examined in both simulation and known group designs, has been validated across gender and race, and has a nearly unblemished record of positive findings except among ID persons (Graue et al., 2007).[3] It has a well-defined factor structure and a single malingering factor (H. A. Miller, 2001), and all but one M-FAST item had strong loadings on it in a replication (Vitacco et al., 2008). The M-FAST may be more sensitive at detecting feigned schizophrenia and bipolar disorder (sensitivities = .86 to .88) than feigned major depression or PTSD (.62 to .63; Guy, Kwartner, & Miller, 2006), although better findings have also been reported in some samples (Guriel-Tennant & Fremouw, 2006; Messer & Fremouw, 2007) and among disability claimants (Alwes, Clark, Berry, & Granacher, 2008). Patients with psychotic disorders do not generally obtain elevated scores, but mean scores for patients with depression tend to be mildly elevated (Guy et al., 2006). Most studies have supported use of the recommended cutoff score, although among acute psychiatric patients, Veazey, Wagner, Hays, and Miller (2005) found a cutoff score of ≥8 to produce the best classification rates using the PAI Malingering Index ≥3 as a criterion instead of the SIRS. The M-FAST does not seek to assess feigning of somatic or cognitive problems, and Sollman, Ranseen, and Berry (2010) reported it had poor sensitivity (10%) for feigned ADHD but excellent specificity (100%) using the standard cutoff score (≥6). Guriel-Tennant and Fremouw (2006) found that coaching reduced the M-FAST's sensitivity among subjects simulating PTSD from 84% to 52%. Vitacco, Rogers, Gabel, and Munizza (2007) found the M-FAST identified *every* pretrial defendant who failed the SIRS, and the Total Score had a very large effect size ($d = 2.69$). Studies examining the M-FAST are summarized in Table 4.1.

Glassmire, Tarescavage, and Gottfried (2016) argued that previous M-FAST studies with psychiatric patients or criminal justice examinees relied on volunteer subjects, so that those who were too impaired or dangerous to give informed consent or to be evaluated were excluded. The authors suggested that this selection process resulted in samples that are higher functioning than the population they are meant to represent, and that diagnostic statistics based on them may be overly optimistic. In their own archival study, they examined the records of forensic examinees who had been administered both the M-FAST and the SIRS. Most of these (81%) were referred for assessment of possible feigning. The authors also scored the SIRS-2 from the SIRS protocol. They found that of examinees who scored 6 or above on the M-FAST, 66% failed the SIRS, and 42% failed the SIRS-2. They reported that examinees with an M-FAST score of 16 or above all failed the SIRS, while a cutoff score of 19 was needed to guarantee failure of the SIRS-2. The authors found no incremental validity for the M-FAST subscales over the Total Score other than the one-item Suggestibility scale. If endorsed, the Suggestibility item indicated a 90.5% likelihood of failing the SIRS if the M-FAST Total Scale was also ≥6.

Although some researchers (e.g., Jackson et al., 2005; H. A. Miller, 2001; Vitacco et al., 2007; Rogers et al., 2010) have stated that the M-FAST be used only as a screener,[4] others (Boone, 2013; Frederick, 2011; Gaines, 2009; Glassmire, Tarascavage et al., 2016; Tarescavage & Glassmire, 2016) have suggested the M-FAST can play a broader role. Frederick noted that with the full diagnostic statistics reported in the manual, the examiner might reasonably interpret a very high score (e.g., 12 or above) as substantial evidence of feigning. At the same time, Frederick cautioned that use of the most widely recommended cutoff score (≥6) would result in substantial false positive rates at low base rates (e.g., 5%). However, this is true of any screening test that has less than perfect specificity. Frederick and Bowden (2009b), who noted that higher cutoff scores could be used to address this problem, provided a means for calculating the PPP and NPP at all possible base rates and for all scores.[5] Several studies (Alwes et al., 2008; Jackson et al., 2005; Vitacco et al., 2007) have reported the M-FAST's standard cutoff score of ≥6 to have 90% or better specificity for the SIRS's standard criteria or even a more stringent standard (Gaines, 2009). While Glassmire, Tarascavage et al.

Table 4.1 M-FAST Forensic Studies Summarized

Study	Type	Sample	Feign *n*	Criteria	Type Control	Control *n*	Control Criteria	Indeterminate Group?	Sensitivity	Specificity	*r*	*d*	AUC
H. A. Miller (2004), H. A. Miller (2005)[a]	KG	Hospitalized ♂ defendants found ICST	14	SIRS 2 & ≥76	N/A	36	All not +	N	.93	.83	.81	2.73	.95
Guy & Miller (2004)	KG	Maximum security prisoners	21	SIRS 2 & ≥76	N/A	29	All not +	N	.83 .72 (≥9)	.86 1.00 (≥9)	.83	2.06	.92
Jackson et al. (2005)[c]	Sim	TX jail inmates (52% ♀)	43	N/A	CST R	41	N/A	N	.76	.90		1.47	
Jackson et al. (2005)[b]	KG	Vernon male CST R	8	SIRS ≥3/1	CST R	41	All not +[c]	N				2.80	
Veazey et al. (2005)	KG	Inpatient psychiatric patients	5[d]	PAI MI[e] ≥3		39[c]	All not +	N	.80 (≥6) .60 (≥9)	.85 (≥6) .92 (≥9)			
Guy et al. (2006)[f]	Sim	Student simulators	190		psychiatric patients	146	[g]		.62 (MDD) –.88 (Schiz)	.79 (MMD, Bip) –.85 (PTSD)			
Vitacco et al. (2007)	KG	♂ CST examinees	21	SIRS 3/1	100	79	All not +	None in study	1.00	.90		2.69	
Guriel et al. (2006)	Sim	Student simulators PTSD	56 (C) 57 (Unc)					N/A	.52 (C) .84 (Unc)				
Messer & Fremouw (2007)	Sim	80% ♀ psychology students	41			24	Students + on DAPS	N/A	.78 (C)	.792			
Alwes et al. (2008)	KG	Disability claimants	23	SIRS 3/1 *OR* ≥76	172		Genuine on SIRS	113	.826	.906		3.0	

Alwes et al. (2008)	KG	Disability claimants	75	Fail 2+ PVTs	178	Passed all 3 PVTs	55[h]	.432	.876	1.0
Gaines (2009)	KG	Maximum security inpatient psychiatric jail inmates psych	38	SIRS ≥4 *OR* >76	39	SIRS <3 and <76	23	.92	.92	
Glassmire, Tarascavage et al. (2016)		Forensic inpatients[i]	66	SIRS 3/1 or ≥76	34[j]	All not +[j]			.804 (≥12)	

NOTE: KG = known group; Sim = simulation design; CST = competency to stand trial examinees; CST R = competency restoration patients; "2 & ≥76" = 2 SIRS scales in *Probable* feigning range and Total Score ≥ 76; "≥3" = 3 or more SIRS scales in the *Probable* range; "3/1" = 3 or more scales in the *Probable* range or one scale in the *Definite* feigning range; "All not +" = all subjects who were not positive on inclusion criteria; ICST = incompetent to stand trial; MDD = major depressive disorder; Bip = bipolar disorder; Schiz = schizophrenia; PAI MI = Personality Assessment Inventory Malingering Index; DAPS = Detailed Assessment of PTSD Symptoms; "C" = coached; "Unc" = uncoached.

[a]This same data and analysis appear to be presented in H. A. Miller (2005), although the figures for sensitivity and specificity are transposed.

[b]Did not include item 5 in analyses.

[c]This is presumed, as the criterion used was not described in the publication.

[d]Calculated from figures in Veazy et al., Table 1.

[e]The PAI MI actually had a lower correlation with the M-FAST Total Score than NIM and even PIM.

[f]Used data from H. A. Miller 2004; Guy & Miller 2004; Veazy et al., 2005.

[g]Malingering was ruled out using criteria from H. A. Miller 2004; Guy & Miller 2004; and Veazy et al. for subjects from each of these studies.

[h]Failed one PVTs.

[i]Only subjects who scored positive on the M-FAST (≥6) were included in the study.

[j]Various criteria were examined in this study.

(2016) suggested a cutoff score of 16, so that there were no false positives relative to the SIRS, Glassmire (personal communication, December 18, 2016) acknowledged that apparent false positives for the M-FAST may have actually been false negatives for the SIRS. H. A. Miller (2001) reported that no psychiatric patient who passed the SIRS ($n = 56$)[6] scored 11 or more on the M-FAST. Guy and Miller (2004) reported that none of their 29 maximum security inmates who passed the SIRS scored above 8 on the M-FAST. Further, Gaines (2009) performed an archival study on inpatient psychiatric forensic patients and found that none of their 39 subjects classified as genuine on the SIRS[7] scored above 11 on the M-FAST.

Given the limited sensitivity of the SIRS and especially the SIRS-2, it is overly conservative to set the M-FAST cutoff scores to achieve no false positives relative to the SIRS. Recall that D. Green and Rosenfeld (2011) found a mean sensitivity of 48.6% for the SIRS's standard criteria, so that many disagreements between the SIRS and M-FAST probably reflect the SIRS's 51.4% false negative rate. Setting an M-FAST cutoff score so high that no subject passes the SIRS virtually guarantees a high percentage of false negative errors. A convention in response style assessment is to set a cutoff score to achieve a false positive rate of no more than 5% to 10% (Greve & Bianchini, 2004), but given the SIRS's limited sensitivity, this is overly conservative for setting M-FAST cutoffs.

Turning to the issue of sensitivity, if the M-FAST is used as the sole screen for feigned psychopathology, using a cutoff score of ≥6, significant numbers of feigners will escape initial detection. Among simulators, the M-FAST, using a cutoff score of 6, has a false negative rate relative up to 38% (for major depressive disorder), and the sensitivity for both feigned major depression and PTSD did not reach .90 or better until the cutoff score is lowered to 3 (Guy et al., 2006). Glassmire, Tarascavage et al. (2016) found 36% of psychiatric patients who passed the M-FAST failed the SIRS. Thus, if the M-FAST is to be used as a screener, examiners should consider lower cutoff scores and their own local base rates.

Given that the SIRS has limited sensitivity and imperfect specificity, the existing validity studies provide an indirect and rough guide to the M-FAST's actual sensitivity and specificity. In fact, it is by no means clear that the SIRS is more accurate than the M-FAST, as they have never been directly compared. The M-FAST is approximately one seventh as long as long as the SIRS (25 vs. 172 items) and takes minimal clinician time both to administer and to score. Unlike the SIRS, item analysis was used to substantially reduce the original item pool to the most effective items. Its use of continuous scores, and published diagnostic statistics for all possible scores, potentially allows for use as both a screener and a diagnostic test (Frederick, 2011). However, to date it has not been validated against strong, non-test criteria.

M-FAST SUMMARY

Pros:

- Well-validated, cost- and time-effective measure of feigned major psychopathology.

- Validated in both known group and simulation studies, across race and literacy, with comparable results.
- Can be used as a screening test or, with caution, as part of a diagnostic assessment.
- Diagnostic statistics are provided for all raw scores.

Cons:

- Not suitable for ID defendants or those too limited or confused to provide reliable answers.
- Manual and some authors have portrayed it only as a screening test, leading to possible challenge if used as a diagnostic test.
- Does not assess memory or cognitive complaints; may be less effective with less severe psychiatric disorders (depression, ADHD).
- Does not assess over-reporting of genuine symptoms (frequency, distress level).

STRUCTURED INVENTORY OF MALINGERED SYMPTOMOLOGY (SIMS)

The SIMS (Widows & Smith, 2005) is a 75-item self-report questionnaire that attempts to gauge feigning of five different conditions: psychosis, depression, neurological symptoms, amnesia/memory, and low intelligence. Questions are in a true-false format at the 5th-grade reading level. The SIMS is sold by Psychological Assessment Resources, Inc., is billed as appropriate for ages 18 to 99, and requires 15 minutes to administer. A specimen set including 25 administration booklets costs $168.00, while 25 paper answer forms cost $86.00 ($3.28 per administration). There is also software for on-screen administration ($582.00) that offers a small discount on the per administration/scoring cost ($3.24).

The SIMS has been examined in simulation and known group studies, and in several criminal forensic samples, but early studies were flawed by lack of suitable clinical comparison groups (Smith, 2008). Those studies that had a clinical comparison group (Alwes et al., 2008; Clegg, Fremouw, & Mogge, 2009; Edens, Otto, & Dwyer, 1999; Edens et al., C. Harrison, 2008; Lewis et al., 2002; Poythress, Edens, & Watkins, 2001; Vitacco et al., 2007; Wisdom, Callahan, & Shaw, 2010) reported specificities from 37% to 65% using cutoff scores of 14 or 16.

Some SIMS studies have examined the performance of the various subscales (Edens, Otto, & Dwyer, 1999; Giger, Merten, Merckelbach, & Oswald, 2010; Graue et al., 2007), although the Total score has received the most attention and often performs best, often with very large effect sizes (Cohen's d = 1.0 to 3.5; Smith, 2008). The *Low Intelligence* subscale was unable to discriminate ID persons from those feigning the condition (Graue et al., 2007) and should not be used for this purpose. Edens et al. (1999) found the SIMS scales very sensitive to simulated psychopathology and cognitive problems, but also found that the *Affective Disorder* and *Low Intelligence* scales had high false positive rates among subjects with a history of psychiatric treatment or moderate elevations on the SCL-90.

Giger et al. (2007) reported the SIMS *Amnestic Disorders* and *Neurological Impairment* scales performed very well in identifying those simulating amnesia for a mock crime, although their effectiveness was reduced by coaching, and no control group of genuinely amnestic defendants was included. Jelicic and colleagues (Jelicic, Hessels, & Merckelbach, 2006; Jelicic, Peters, Leckie, & Merckelbach, 2007) found coaching about psychiatric symptoms did not much diminish the SIMS's accuracy. However, coaching about test detection strategies, combined with coaching of psychopathology symptoms, did (Jelicic, Ceunen, Peters, & Merckelbach, 2011).

Wisdom et al. (2010) classified personal injury claimants with a clear external incentive according to the Slick criteria (Slick et al., 1999). Besides utilizing a more rigorous criterion, these authors also examined diagnostic statistics for multiple cutoff scores. The SIMs manual and prior studies reviewed by Wisdom et al. have suggested Total scores on the SIMS of greater than 14 or 16 as preliminary evidence of feigning. Because the SIMS is presented as a screening test, it is most important to have high sensitivity and high negative predictive power to correctly exclude those who are not feigning. Most studies have found the SIMS performs quite well in these areas, typically identifying 85% to 100% of psychiatric feigners but misclassifying many presumed genuine patients. However, some of the SIMS studies that produced high false positives had a weak criterion (the psychiatrist's judgment of feigning status), with no articulation of what this judgment was based on, or the SIRS, which may have substantial false negative errors. Wisdom et al. also examined the capacity of the SIMS to serve as a diagnostic (as well as a screening) test. Examining multiple cutoff scores, they reported a SIMS Total score of 24 correctly excluded all genuine patients, while identifying 55% of feigners. This compares well with many validity tests.

However, C. Harrison (2008) found the SIMS performed modestly in separating psychiatric patients from simulators (Cohen's $d = 1.2$), and that a cutoff score of 23 resulted in a specificity of only 43%. Specificity did not reach 90% until a cutoff score of 40 was applied, leading Harrison to question the value of the SIMS even as a screening instrument.

Alwes et al. (2008) reported that while the SIMS Total score was quite sensitive to psychiatric feigning in personal injury and disability examinees, it was less sensitive to cognitive feigning and that at higher base rates (e.g., 30%), NPP fell to 85%. Thus, passing the SIMS did not rule out cognitive malingering as assessed by PVT performance. Benge et al. (2012) found the SIMS of limited use in distinguishing pseudo-seizures from genuine epileptic patients.

Rogers, Robinson, and Gillard (2014) created scales from the SIMS paralleling the Rare Symptoms and Symptom Combination factors found for the SIRS, and the resulting scales performed as well as the SIMS Total score. Subjects were adult psychiatric inpatients at the Timberlawn trauma unit, many with a diagnosis of PTSD or DID. Patients were asked to either respond honestly or exaggerate. The authors recommend a much higher cutoff score for the Total score (>44) than the >14 recommended by Smith (2008). In the Rogers et al. sample, impressive sensitivity (60%) and specificity (98%) were reported for the higher cutoff score. However, these figures must be interpreted in light of the patient sample (inpatient, trauma; many failed the SIRS in Rogers et al., 2009), so that the cutoff recommended is probably very conservative for other populations.

A recent review (van Impelen, Merckelbach, Jelicic, & Merten, 2014) of 26 studies since 2005 (*N* = 2,292) concluded the SIMS is sensitive to feigning of both psychiatric and cognitive problems (Cohen's *d*s = 2.5, 2.4, respectively), "fairly robust" to prior knowledge and coaching of psychopathology (citing six studies), but vulnerable to coaching about SVTs, which greatly reduces its ability to discriminate (Cohen's *d* = 1.0). It is also prone to false positives in schizophrenics and those with intellectual disabilities. They reported the SIMS Total score correlates substantially with symptom measures (.50 to .72), such as the SCL-90, which suggests a lack of discriminate validity. However, this could also be interpreted as showing the SCL-90 is suffused with indiscriminate willingness to endorse psychiatric problems. Van Impelen et al. also cited Merckelbach and Smith (2003), who found substantially lower alpha coefficients for the subscales (.24 to .59) than reported by Smith and Burger (1997). These scores are well below the criterion of .80 recommended as a minimum for forensic measures by Heilbrun (2001), and van Impelen et al. discouraged use of the subscales. Van Impelen et al. also noted that the SIMS contains bizarre items that may render it transparent as a validity measure, yet they also criticized it for having items that are valid psychopathology symptoms, particularly depression, yet scored as indications of exaggeration. They cited Kobelt, Göbber, Bassler, and Petermann (2012), who reported disproportionate false positives among depressed patients (57% vs. 4% to 24% in other groups). Finally, the authors suggest a cutoff score of >16 for screening purposes, >19 for patients at risk for elevations (schizophrenics, depressed patients) and in forensic settings, and >24 for use with such groups when used as part of a response style battery (and, presumably, as evidence of feigning). Unfortunately, they did not provide diagnostic statistics for these cutoff scores.

In sum, the SIMS Total score has shown excellent sensitivity as a screening measure for psychopathology *and* cognitive malingering, but it is prone to false positives in schizophrenics, depressed, ID, and probably dissociative examinees. Only a single study has addressed feigning of depression, despite there being a subscale of this nature. The primary strength of the SIMS is ruling out feigning, as its high sensitivity and negative predictive power allow it to detect nearly all feigners, even those feigning cognitive problems other than ID, *unless they are forewarned (or particularly wary) about validity testing.* At lower cutoff scores (>14, >16), the SIMS is not strong evidence of negative response bias. It does not have an inconsistency scale, which means that feigning cannot be readily distinguished from poor comprehension or disengagement. Like the M-FAST, further research should examine the SIMS's potential as a diagnostic test and report diagnostic statistics at different cutoff scores. At present, reported cutoff scores for use as a diagnostic test vary widely (>19 to >44), and users who wish to use the SIMS as evidence of feigning should keep abreast of the data on this issue.

SIMS SUMMARY

Pros:

- Brief self-report inventory that is inexpensive and requires little time of the examiner or examinee.
- Has shown strong validity/effect sizes in most studies.
- Equally good at detecting feigned psychopathology and cognitive presentations.
- Very high sensitivity at lower cutoff scores (>14, >16), which is desirable for screening purposes; excellent ability to rule out feigning.
- Subscales can help identify what particular symptoms are being over-reported.

Cons:

- No internal validity checks (consistency scales).
- Little demonstrated value to subscales.
- Cutoff scores have varied, especially for use as a diagnostic test.

Table 4.2 SVT cutoff scores and Diagnostic Statistics

Test	Criteria/Cutoff Score	Includes SMI, ID?[a]	Sensitivity	Specificity	Citations
SIRS	Per manual	SMI	.486	.946	D. Green & Rosenfeld, 2011
SIRS-2	Per manual	SMI, ID	.37 (KG), .325–.75 (Sim)	.93–1.00	D. Green et al., 2013; Brand et al., 2014; Weiss et al., 2011; Tarescavage & Glassmire, 2016; DeClue, 2011
M-FAST	≥12	SMI	.22–.47[b]	.824–1.00	H. A. Miller, 2001;[c] Gaines, 2009;[d] Glassmire, Tarascavage et al., 2016;[c] Guy & Miller, 2004[c]

[a]Does not include seriously mentally ill or intellectually disabled subjects unless indicated.

[b]Calculated relative to the SIRS.

[c]Defined SIRS failure as two scales or more in the *probable* range and Total Score > 76.

[d]Defined SIRS failure as four scores or more in the *probable* range.

CHAPTER SUMMARY

While in the past the SIRS had been frequently described as the gold standard of feigned psychopathology, the accumulation of data and release of the SIRS-2 make for a different playing field. The SIRS-2 has received criticism the original SIRS largely avoided and has been shown in several studies to be rather insensitive to feigned psychopathology—but no more than other indices such as the MMPI-2-RF's Fp-r that have high specificity. The M-FAST is a very cost-effective tool that can play a larger role than that of a mere screening test. Two of three studies found no subject who scored ≥12 passed the SIRS. The SIMS may also have a role to play here, but cutoff scores for diagnostic purposes have varied widely, and its lack of a consistency scale limits its potential to serve as a diagnostic test. Table 4.2 summarizes the available data.

NOTES

1. This was a civil, not criminal, case.
2. I say the SIRS-2 *possibly* reduced false positive findings in dissociative examinees because I don't believe it has been demonstrated that such examinees always respond validly. This issue is discussed in Chapter 8.
3. Although Hill (2009) reported much lower sensitivities that others, subjects in this study were told their results would be kept confidential and would not affect their treatment. Therefore, if subjects believed the examiners, it was not possible for them to malinger. This study also produced atypically low sensitivity findings for the SIMS.
4. Rogers et al. (2010) went so far as to state:

   > Feigning screens should not be used as a "shortcut" to the determination of feigning. Such misuse is prohibited by American Psychology Association (2002) Ethical Standard 9.02 (a). The typical excuse of expediency cannot be used to explain or justify this deliberate misuse of feigning screens. (p. 44)

   APA 9.02 (a) states: "Psychologists base the opinions contained in their recommendations, reports, and diagnostic or evaluative statements, including forensic testimony, on information and techniques sufficient to substantiate their findings." It is perhaps worth noting that use of screening tests for assessment of feigning could deeply cut into the SIRS-2's market share.
5. A spreadsheet to do this, and to display the Test Validation Summary, is available for download at http://www.richardfrederick.com/files.
6. Calculated from the total sample size (n = 86) and reported base rate of .35. Those passing the SIRS were those who did not have more than one scale in or above the *probable* range or whose Total Score <76.
7. Fewer than three scales in or above the *probable* feigning range and Total Score <76.

5

Tests of Feigned or Exaggerated Cognitive Impairment

There has been tremendous growth in the research on performance validity tests (PVTs), tests designed to assess an examinee's motivation and effort on cognitive or motor tasks, over the past 20 years. This chapter will review only those PVTs that are most widely used by forensic psychologists or are viewed as especially promising by the author. The interested reader is referred to the neuropsychological literature, where new articles appear constantly, and several fine books that address response style (Boone, 2007a; Carone & Bush, 2013; Larrabee, 2007) are available.

Whereas early PVTs were often very brief, like the Rey 15 Item Test (FIT), a number of freestanding tests, such as the TOMM, Word Memory Test (WMT), and Validity Indicator Profile (VIP), were developed, some of which might require almost an hour of administration time. Although several of these are now well-validated and widely accepted, Boone (2009) recommended ongoing validity assessment for the duration of test administration. She proposed the utilization and development of *embedded* PVTs for all cognitive measures included in the test battery. A prime example is *Reliable Digit Span* (RDS; Greiffenstein, Baker, & Gola, 1994) that is scoreable from the standard WAIS-R/III/IV Digit Span subtest. Embedded PVTs have drawn considerable research and clinical interest because they (a) enhance the sensitivity of the entire malingering battery without requiring extra administration time; (b) can provide direct information about the validity of performance on specific tests; (c) may be less susceptible to coaching than freestanding PVTs; and (d) can be used to evaluate performance validity in the absence of specialized techniques (Greve, Bianchini, & Brewer, 2013). However, embedded PVTs tend to be less sensitive than freestanding PVTs (Armistead-Jehle & Buican, 2013), so that a sizable number (e.g., three or more) of them should be used. This chapter reviews the best-researched embedded PVT, the RDS, freestanding PVTs, and one brief and somewhat controversial validity test, the Rey 15 Item Test (Rey, 1941, 1958).

THE REY 15 ITEM TEST (FIT)

The FIT (Rey, 1941, 1958) consists of 15 ordered items, in five rows, which a test-taker is asked to reproduce after a short delay. It is one of the earliest, simplest, quickest, and widely used validity tests. There is no publisher or manual, and no cost per use.

The FIT has been criticized as being insensitive to malingering, prone to false positives with cognitively impaired populations, and lacking face validity as a memory test (Farkas et al., 2006; Guillette, Hart, Giuliani, & Leninger, 1994; Schretlen, Brandt, Krafft, & van Gorp, 1991; Vallabhajosula & van Gorp, 2001). However, Merten, Green, Henry, Blaskewitz, and Brockhaus (2005) found the FIT less identifiable as a malingering test than several competitors. Iverson (2006) suggested the use of the FIT might be unethical in situations where it was chosen because of its low sensitivity (e.g., by a psychologist retained by a personal injury lawyer). Vallabhajosula and Van Gorp (2001) concluded the FIT did not meet *Daubert* criteria, stating it is "unacceptably insensitive" to malingering.

Vickery, Berry, Inman, Harris, and Orey (2001) reported a meta-analysis of the FIT and the other most widely researched validity tests. The FIT was found to be significantly less discriminating than two digit-based forced-choice tests and the 21-Item Test (Iverson, Franzen, & McCracken, 1991, 1994), with a Cohen's $d = .77$. Average sensitivity was 43.3%, with a specificity of 92.5% using a cutoff of <9. The sensitivity was about half the value of the best test in the comparison,

---

Box 5.1

THE *DAUBERT* CRITERIA

In the landmark case of *Daubert v. Merrell Dow Pharmaceuticals* (1993), the United States Supreme Court provided guidelines to judges tasked with assessing the reliability of scientific evidence. These included:

1. Whether the theory or technique employed by the expert is generally accepted in the scientific community;
2. Whether it has been subjected to peer review and publication;
3. Whether it can be and has been tested;
4. Whether the known or potential rate of error is acceptable; and
5. Whether the research was conducted independent of the particular litigation or dependent on an intention to provide the proposed testimony.

Table 5.1 Diagnostic Statistics of the FIT at Two Cutoff Scores From Reznek (2005)

Cutoff Score	Entire Sample		Excluding ID	
	Sensitivity	Specificity	Sensitivity	Specificity
<8	.09	.92	—	.95
<9	.36	.85	—	.90

the Digit Memory Test (Hiscock & Hiscock, 1989), and the specificity was lower as well.

Reznek (2005) combined individual-level data from preexisting studies that reported such data. He reported the FIT had good specificity for most conditions, except intellectual disability, and recommended a conservative cutoff score of < 8. However, this produced such low sensitivity (9%) that the test is rendered nearly useless. Sensitivity was considerably better using the traditional cutoff of <9 (36%; Table 5.1), although the false positive rate doubles from 5% to 10% when intellectually disabled (ID) subjects are excluded.

Frederick (2000) and Frederick and Bowden (2009a) used Mixed Group Validation (MGV; Dawes & Meehl, 1966; Frederick, 2000) to estimate the FIT's diagnostic statistics in a large sample of criminal defendants. MGV takes account of the limitations of the criterion and has a number of potential advantages over *known group* designs, such as the ability to validate a new test with an imperfect criterion. In the more recent analysis, Frederick and Bowden estimated the FIT (cutoff <9) had a sensitivity of 46.7% in 723 criminal defendants, with a very low false positive rate of 4%.

Subsequent to Reznek's review, Farkas et al. (2006) reported the FIT showed a sensitivity of 36% to those identified as feigning on the TOMM in a sample of civil litigants, but a specificity of 100%. The FIT cutoff score used was not identified. D. Green (2010) found a score of <9 on the FIT to have a sensitivity of 39% for simulators and 44% for defendants identified as feigning incompetence, respectively, with specificities of 82.4% for both a community and an honest pretrial, hospitalized sample. The FIT equaled the TOMM among simulators (subjects instructed to feign), but was superior to it, *and equaled the SIRS*, in distinguishing suspected feigners from genuine forensic patients. However, Denney (2007) reported that less than half as many defendants failed the FIT (25.6%) as the TOMM (61.5%) or WMT (60.5%).

Goldberg, Back-Madruga, and Boone (2007) reviewed the FIT and noted that it is not affected by even severe depression, but psychosis does lower performance. Although several studies reported that even severely brain-damaged subjects are able to pass the FIT, ID persons and those with severe global cognitive impairment and low education often do not, and D. Green et al. (2012) found the FIT score affected by apathy.

Goldberg et al. reported several attempts to increase the perceived difficulty of the FIT while decreasing its actual difficulty, but they noted these versions had not been cross-validated. Boone, Salazar, Lu, Warner-Chacon, and Razani (2002) made one such effort, adding a recognition trial in which examinees are asked to identify stimuli seen in the recall portion from distractors. The score is derived by summing the recall and recognition scores and produced somewhat better accuracy than the original scoring method. Stimmel, Green, Belfi, and Kalver (2012) examined Boone et al.'s procedure with criminal defendants. They found a significant increase in sensitivity (44% to 64%) but an increase in false positive errors from 17.6% to 25.3%. Glassmire, Toofanian Ross, Kinney, and Nitch (2016) found the recall and recognition FIT had the highest Cohen's *d* (3.66) of all PVTs examined in distinguishing hospitalized schizophrenics from pretrial forensic patients who failed PVTs. The standard FIT was the second most discriminating ($d = 2.82$), outperforming the TOMM's Trial 2 ($d = 1.96$).

Two sets of authors (D. Green 2010; Marshall & Happe, 2007) reported that idiosyncratic FIT errors, including elaborations, reversals of letters (e.g., *d* for *b*), and errors in sequences, are rare even in psychiatric and developmentally delayed samples and thus might serve as highly diagnostic signs of intentional failure when present.

If the FIT is to be used, it should probably be administered prior to other cognitive tests, before examinees have a frame of reference for its lack of difficulty. Also, several authors advocated modifications of the traditional instructions (which imply it is a difficult task) to avoid giving a deceptive statement that may not be credible. Although it is often viewed as a screening test, the FIT is poorly suited for this role because of its low sensitivity, and many actual feigners will go undetected. Conversely, with high specificity outside of ID, demented, and seriously impaired samples, it can provide solid evidence of poor motivation or effort if those conditions can be eliminated from consideration. Finally, Frederick (2011) noted the FIT's minimal investment of time, cost, and portability (stimuli could be reproduced on the spot) as significant advantages.

FIT SUMMARY

Pros:

- Quick, cheap, convenient cognitive validity test; unmatched in these considerations.
- If ID and severe cognitive impairment can be excluded, good specificity.
- If examinee is known not to be cognitively impaired, the FIT is the fastest test to obtain fairly strong evidence of feigning/poor effort.

Cons:

- Not a published test, no manual.
- Not sensitive, not an appropriate screening test.

- Not suitable for ID, severely impaired, or very poorly educated examinees.
- Given a critical review on the issue of admissibility (Vallabhajosula & van Gorp, 2001), could face a *Daubert* challenge.

THE DOT COUNTING TEST

The Dot Counting Test (DCT; Rey, 1941, 1958; Boone, Lu, & Herzberg, 2002) consists of groups of dots, some in organized groups, others not. The examinee is asked to count them as quickly as possible. The DCT was one of Rey's malingering tests described by Lezak (1983/1995). The DCT is now published by Western Psychological Services and is advertised to take 5 to 15 minutes to administer and to be appropriate for examinees aged 17 and up. A specimen set costs $153.50, while score forms cost $37.50 for 50 (per administration cost of $.75).

Vickery et al.'s (2001) meta-analysis found the DCT showed a lower average effect size than a number of other such tests. This analysis was based on a wide variety of DCT scoring criteria, so it may underestimate the DCT's optimal performance. Numerous scoring rules have been proposed for the DCT, including total counting time, the difference between grouped and ungrouped counting time means, total errors made, performance curve analysis, and combinations of counting times and errors. Binks, Gouvier, and Waters (1997) examined a number of possible scoring schemes among naive and coached simulators, with a control group of neuropsychiatric patients. Although they found support for the difference between the ungrouped and grouped mean response time ($M_U - M_G$) and *performance curve* anomalies, the total number of counting errors proved most robust.

Boone et al. (2002) examined 100 suspected malingerers from personal injury and criminal forensic samples. The authors, who found that both counting time and number of errors were effective response style indicators, created a *combination score* (also known as *E score*) that sums the mean time to count the grouped and ungrouped dots and number of errors (E score = $M_G + M_U$ + Errors). This index produced perfect sensitivity and 90% specificity or better for all diagnoses except moderate dementia, but the sample did not include ID examinees.

Back et al. (1996) found the DCT was affected by cognitive impairment and age, but only 13% of their schizophrenic subjects failed using criteria of $M_G > 4.8$ seconds and $M_U - M_G < 2$ seconds. The severity of psychosis was not related to DCT performance. Goldberg et al. (2007) reviewed prior studies and concluded depression had no effect on DCT scores, while schizophrenia increased false positive rates and required adjustments to $M_U - M_G$ and E score criteria. Rudman, Oyebode, and Bentham (2011) noted that the E score disadvantages subjects with cognitive slowing.

Two additional studies examined DCT performance in cognitively impaired samples. Hurley and Deal (2006) reported ID subjects made an average of 3.1 (*SD* = 1.9) counting errors, and that a total counting time of ≥180 seconds was the only index to have an acceptable false positive rate (2.6%). Rudman et al. (2011)

reported that $M_G < M_U$ had 100% specificity among demented patients, the only PVT that did. However, neither Hurley and Deal nor Rudman et al. examined sensitivity. Other authors (Boone et al., 2002; Frederick, Sarfaty, Johnston, & Powel, 1994) have reported $M_G < M_U$ to have low sensitivity. Victor, Kulick, and Boone (2013) reported that emerging data suggest that the DCT's sensitivity is below 50% for individuals feigning mild traumatic brain injury (mTBI).

Pertaining to CST examinations, D. Green et al. (2012) reported the DCT E score discriminated suspected CST malingerers from defendants judged genuine as well as the SIRS, with a sensitivity of 41.7% and specificity of 85.7%. Scores on the DCT were not correlated with rated *Apathy* on the Brief Psychiatric Rating Scale, whereas FIT scores were.

In sum, the DCT does not appear to be affected by depression or apathy, but standard cutoff scores should not be used with psychotic subjects. It appears to have modest sensitivity and is prone to false positives in ID defendants on indices other than total counting time.

DCT SUMMARY

Pros:

- Not affected by depression, apathy.
- $M_G - M_U$ generally has good specificity.
- Has been studied in forensic/CST samples.
- Capacity to assess feigned cognitive impairment in ID persons using total counting time.
- Probably not easily recognized as a validity test.

Cons:

- Modest sensitivity.
- Little ongoing research.
- Scores affected by psychosis, cognitive deficits.

RELIABLE DIGIT SPAN (RDS)

Greiffenstein et al. (1994) derived RDS from the Digit Span subtest of the Wechsler Adult Intelligence Scale–Revised (Wechsler, 1981). RDS is the sum of the longest string of forward digits repeated correctly in both trials, added to the parallel measure for digits backward. Thus, if an examinee repeated 4 digits forward correctly and 3 digits backward, *on both trials*, RDS = 7.

Duncan and Ausborn (2002) examined RDS in a sample of 187 adult male pretrial defendants, using staff diagnoses based on both considerable validity testing and 30 to 45 days of inpatient observation. They found that an RDS ≤7 had a sensitivity of 67.9%, but low specificity (71.6%). Lowering the cutoff score to ≤6 resulted in respective figures of 56.6% and 90.3%. Not surprisingly, RDS was substantially correlated with contemporaneously assessed IQ scores, even within honest and malingering groups. No other studies of RDS using a pretrial/CST sample were located.

Goldberg et al. (2007) concluded that depression, obsessive-compulsive disorder, and somatoform conditions do not affect RDS and other digit span indices, although psychosis does, raising false positive rates to near 20%. Jasinski, Berry, Shandera, and Clark (2011) meta-analyzed 24 studies of digit span measures, including RDS and the WAIS age-corrected scale score (ACSS), as measures of negative response bias. They reported an average Cohen's $d = 1.34$ for RDS and 1.08 for ACSS, which did not differ significantly. However, few psychiatric patients and no intellectually disabled subjects were included. Schroeder and Marshall (2011) reported that 96% of both psychotic and nonpsychotic psychiatric patients scored 7 or above on RBS. Schroeder, Twumasi-Ankrah, Baade, and Marshall (2012) examined more than 20 published studies on RDS, examining sensitivity and specificity for different groups at cutoff scores of ≤7 and ≤6. They concluded that the widely used cutoff score of ≤7 produced inadequate specificity in a variety of clinical groups. On the other hand, ≤6 produced good specificity in most clinical groups but not in those with intellectual disability, dementia, cardiovascular accident, or borderline IQ. Sensitivity was estimated at 30% and 35% when calculated by weighted averages and Bayesian methods, respectively, with specificities of 96% and 97%. While Schroeder et al. included psychiatric patients in the group for which the diagnostic figures apply, only one study (Schroeder & Marshall, 2011) included psychotic patients.

Silk-Eglit, Stenclik, Miele, Lynch, and McCaffrey (2015) recently found that RDS was the most discriminating of the embedded PVTs they examined in mTBI claimants, with a relatively good sensitivity of 64% and a specificity of 92%. Glassmire, Toofanian Ross et al. (2016) examined both the original RDS and RDS-R, the latter of which adds the sequencing subtask of the WAIS-IV Digit Span subtest, among schizophrenic patients that passed four PVTs (TOMM, VIP, DCT, and FIT). They found RDS and RDS-R performance was strongly dependent on IQ.

The RDS is one of the quickest PVTs but is susceptible to false positives in examinees with cognitive impairment or schizophrenia unless low cutoff scores are used. However, its low sensitivity means that several other such tests will need to be employed.

RDS SUMMARY

Pros:

- Cheap, no test forms or manuals to buy beyond WAIS materials.
- Quick (less than 5 minutes).

- Good specificity if ≤6 is used as cutoff absent schizophrenia or moderate to severe cognitive impairment.
- Most discriminating of embedded PVTs among cognitively intact examinees.

Cons:

- Low sensitivity, not well suited to be a screening test.
- Lack of a manual and publisher could be held against it in an admissibility hearing.
- Digits backward and sequencing require considerable mental effort—possibly more than required in the rest of the CST exam.

TEST OF MEMORY MALINGERING

The TOMM (Tombaugh, 1996) consists of 50 pictures of common objects. The examinee is shown each picture and is then tested for his or her recognition of the pictures, and the process is repeated. A third trial, referred to as the Retention Trial, is optional. The TOMM is sold by Pearson, is billed as taking 15 to 20 minutes to administer, and is advertised as appropriate for ages 16 to 84. A specimen set costs $234.00 and includes 25 answer forms, while 25 additional answer sheets cost $50.00.

The TOMM was the most frequently used validity test in Sharland and Gfeller's (2007) survey, as well as the most highly rated for accuracy. It was the second most frequently used malingering measure in Archer et al.'s (2006) survey of forensic psychologists, whereas it was deemed as merely "acceptable" in Lally's (2003) survey. I found (see Chapter 10, this volume) the TOMM was the most frequently used PVT among CST examiners but that it nonetheless was used about half as often as the SIRS and SIRS-2 combined. Among the TOMM's advantages are its wide acceptance, substantial research base, and consistent cutoff scores for most populations. Importantly, performance on the TOMM is relatively unaffected by anxiety and depression (Ashendorf, Constantinou, & McCaffrey, 2004; Rees, Tombaugh, & Boulay, 2001; Yanez, Fremouw, Tennant, Strunk, & Coker, 2006) and pain (Etherton, Bianchini, Greve, & Ciotac, 2005). Duncan (2005) reported TOMM scores were unaffected by psychosis, although psychosis with distractibility did lower performance. Four of 29 psychotic examinees with distraction scored below 45 on Trial 2 and the Retention Trial, for an apparent false positive rate of 13.8%. Of course, this assumes these examinees did put forth their best effort.

The TOMM has been studied in multiple criminal forensic samples and contexts (Delain, Stafford, & Ben-Porath, 2003; D. Green, 2010; D. Green et al., 2012; Heinze & Purisch, 2001; Heinze, 2003; Weinborn et al., 2003). Pivovarova, Rosenfeld, Dole, and Green (2009) examined the ability of the TOMM to discriminate between 29 community simulators and 88 day hospital patients, most diagnosed with SMI. Simulators were told to feign mental illness so to be found incompetent to stand trial. The TOMM had an Area Under Curve (AUC) of .80, identified 62.1% of simulators, and had very good specificity (94.2%) with genuine psychiatric patients, both classified with a cutoff score of <45 on Trial 2. D. Green (2010) found the TOMM effective at distinguishing simulators from genuine patients but not effective at distinguishing suspected malingerers from examinees who showed no indication of feigning.

Several groups of authors have calculated diagnostic statistics for the TOMM based on prior research. Sollman and Berry (2011) reported a meta-analysis of 21 TOMM studies that met their inclusion criteria. They reported an average sensitivity of 65.4%, an average specificity of 93.8%, and average Hedge's *d* of 1.59 for Trial 2, the only TOMM index examined. Frederick and Bowden (2009b) used Mixed Group Validation (MGV; Dawes & Meehl, 1966; Frederick, 2000) to summarize 24 studies of the TOMM and estimate diagnostic statistics. Sensitivity was estimated at 85.5%, and the false positive rate was estimated at 4.9% (specificity = 95.1%). However, MGV tends to yield better diagnostic statistics than other designs, as illustrated by the contrast between Sollman and Berry's and Frederick and Bowden's results. Mossman et al. (2015) used a Bayesian approach to MGV in an attempt to overcome the limitations of the standard MGV approach. They reported that across 89 articles, excluding studies involving dementia or ID subjects, TOMM Trial 2 had a median sensitivity of 58% among identified feigners (as opposed to 86% for simulators) with a very low median false positive rate of 0.12%.

Potential users should be aware that different cutoff scores may be appropriate for some diagnoses. Dementia may cause failure on the TOMM (Teichner & Wagner, 2004). For ID examinees, some authors (Graue et al., 2007; Hurley & Deal, 2006; Shandera et al., 2010) have suggested lowering the standard cutoff score (<45) for Trial 2 and the Retention Trial to <30, while others reported that the standard cutoff scores produce few false positives (Love, Glassmire, Zanolini, & Wolf, 2014; Simon, 2007), at least in ID persons living independently. It should be noted that the subjects in Simon (2007) had already been adjudicated competent and so may have been preselected on capacity. Smith et al. (2014) reported that even in neurologically impaired samples with an IQ of 75 or lower, a Trial 2 cutoff of ≤48 had perfect specificity. Others (Greve, Bianchini, & Doane, 2006; Jones, 2013; Mossman, Wygant, Gervais, & Hart, 2017; Stenclik, Miele, Silk-Eglit, Lynch, & McCaffrey, 2013) have suggested less stringent cutoff scores (e.g., <48 or <49) for less impaired populations, such as for examinees with mTBI several months after injury. Mossman et al. (2017) reported 99% specificity in a large sample of disability and personal injury examinees for a cutoff score of <47, while the traditional cutoff score of Trial 2 <45 identified only one third of feigners.

Specificity among seriously mentally ill (SMI) patients was considerably lower than in neuropsychological control groups, ranging from 80% to 100% (Duncan, 2005; Gierok et al., 2005; D. Green, 2010; D. Green et al., 2012; Hubbard, 2007; Hunt, Root, & Bascetta, 2014; Marcopulos et al., 2014; Pivovarova et al., 2009;

Weinborn et al., 2003). Hubbard reported that TOMM failure among honest psychiatric patients was more frequent among patients with positive symptoms of schizophrenia (25.8%) than among those with negative symptoms (12.5%). Marcopulos et al. (2014) reported a number of psychiatric patients failed the TOMM despite an apparent lack of secondary gain, which they defined as facing legal charges. They noted that failure was associated with being older, with being female, and with diagnoses indicating schizophrenia-spectrum illness and cognitive impairment.

Multiple studies have found the TOMM to be less sensitive to feigned cognitive impairment than other modern stand-alone PVTs (Armistead-Jehle & Gervais, 2011; Gervais, Rohling, Green, & Ford, 2004; P. Green, 2011; Mossman, Wygant, & Gervais, 2012; Mossman et al., 2017; Tan, Slick, Strauss, & Hultsch, 2002; Whitney, 2013). However, Greiffenstein, Greve, Bianchini, and Baker (2008) argued that the TOMM is disadvantaged relative to the WMT, which uses three scales as its primary effort indicators, while the TOMM utilizes only Trial 2. When all three TOMM scales were utilized for classification, they reported equal sensitivity to the WMT. Greve, Ord, Curtis, Bianchini, and Brennan (2008) argued that the TOMM discriminates between genuine and feigned presentations as well as the WMT, but it simply was more conservative in its cutoff scores. Fazio, Sanders, and Denney (2015) recently reported that the TOMM (using Trial 2 *or* Retention Trial <45) had a sensitivity of 68.2% to *probable* feigned cognitive impairment relative to the Slick criteria among CST and restoration patients referred for neuropsychological assessment, and a specificity of 86.8%.

Among criminal defendants, Ardolf, Denney, and Houston (2007) reported that the TOMM showed a failure rate equal to the WMT and higher than most other validity tests, and Hubbard (2008) reported the TOMM had equal sensitivity (93%) and a greater effect size than the WMT. This may be because defendants, as opposed to civil litigants, tend to portray more severe psychopathology and cognitive impairment (Boone, Lu, Back et al., 2002; Merckelbach, Smeets, & Jelicic, 2009; Wygant et al., 2007). Other authors (D. Green, 2010; Heinze & Purisch, 2001; Pivovarova et al., 2009) have reported lower sensitivities (55.6% to 66%) among simulators portraying incompetence than suspected malingerers (40.9%; D. Green, 2010; D. Green et al., 2012).

Several approaches have attempted to increase the TOMM's sensitivity. Greve and Bianchini (2006) reported that a cutoff score <45 on the Retention Trial in addition to Trial 2 increased the proportion failing the TOMM from 17.3% to 21.3% in their traumatic brain injury (TBI) sample (see also Wisdom, Brown, Chen, & Collins, 2012) and recommended that the Retention Trial be used routinely. Others have researched Trial 1, either to use as a brief screening measure or as a means to increase the TOMM's sensitivity (Bauer, O'Bryant, Lynch, McCaffrey, & Fisher, 2007; Denning, 2012; Hilsabeck, Gordon, Hietpas-Wilson, & Zartman, 2011; Kulas, Axelrod, & Rinaldi, 2014; O'Bryant, Engel, Kleiner, Vasterling, & Black, 2007; O'Bryant et al., 2008; Schroeder, Buddin, et al., 2012; Wisdom et al., 2012). It has been hypothesized that test-takers initially do not know how easy or difficult a test is but gradually calibrate their performance over the course of the administration to be credible. Thus, the first trial, and perhaps the first 10 items, may be the most sensitive portion of the test. Wisdom et al. (2012) reported that a score of ≥45 on Trial 1 agreed 99.3% of the time with passing scores on Trial 2 and Retention Trial. Denning (2012) summarized 18 studies examining diverse clinical and forensic samples and found that a Trial 1 cutoff score of <41 produced an average sensitivity of 77% and average specificity of 92% judged against performance on TOMM Trial 2 or the Slick criteria. Reporting new data, Denning found that both approaches (Trial 1, first 10 items of Trial 1 [TOMMe10]) produced accuracy rates as good as or better than traditional indicators (see also Kulas et al., 2014) and concluded that Trial 1 has now been sufficiently cross-validated to be used in practice. Fazio, Denning, and Denney (2016) examined the TOMM T1 among 119 inpatient criminal defendants referred for neuropsychological evaluation and concluded as follows:

> The use of TOMM1 ≤40 is statistically equivalent to the standard decision rules of the full TOMM; this combined with the expansive body of literature with other populations which evaluated use of TOMM1 at similar cut-offs leads to the conclusion that TOMM1 can be used in lieu of the full TOMM in a criminal forensic population. (p. 11)

However, studies that used an SMI control sample (Duncan, 2005; Gierok et al., 2005; Marcopulos et al., 2014) reported variable specificities for Trial 1. Duncan reported excellent specificity (95.3%) at <41 on Trial 1 for SMI patients without concentration difficulties, but 76% specificity for those with such problems. Gierok et al. reported respective figures of 75% for <41 and 100% for <36. Marcopulos et al. found a specificity of 84.2% for a cutoff of <41 in civilly committed patients who had no external incentive and passed the TOMM, and a specificity of 95.4% for <36. Thus, Fazio et al.'s recommendations for Trial 1 should be applied cautiously with defendants presenting with SMI rather than neurocognitive deficits. Conversely, Mossman et al. (2017) concluded that scores of 46 or higher on Trial 1 suggest good effort, whereas no score on Trial 2, even 50, provided strong evidence of such.

Another recent approach is to incorporate measures of consistency between answers on the TOMM's three trials. This approach, referred to by some as the Albany Consistency Index (ACI), has shown improved sensitivity over the TOMM's standard decision rules (Davis, Wall, & Whitney, 2012; Gunner, Miele, Lynch, & McCaffrey, 2012; Schroeder et al., 2013; but see Buddin et al., 2014; Kulas et al., 2014) and greater resistance to coaching (Davis et al., 2012). Schroeder et al. found the ACI had the highest AUC (.926) of multiple TOMM indices, including Trial 1. Relative to the WMT, Gunner et al. (2012) found the ACI increased sensitivity to 71%, compared with 31% for the standard TOMM criteria.

Buddin et al. (2014) noted that the ACI treats improvement on items from early to late trials as evidence of unreliability, whereas this could represent legitimate learning between trials (examinees are given feedback on whether or not their responses are correct). They proposed the *Invalid Forgetting Frequency Index*

(IFFI), which removes points due to learning from the inconsistency score, and provided evidence the IFFI equaled or outperformed the ACI and TOMM's usual scores on some, but not all, diagnostic statistics. The ACI and IFFI have not been examined in SMI samples.

The TOMM would seem to be susceptible to coaching given its relative simplicity and reliance on a single detection strategy. Further, Bauer and McCaffrey (2006) reported that the TOMM had the most coaching material on the Internet among PVTs, including some websites that included test stimuli and cutoff scores. However, two groups of authors (Powell, Gfeller, Hendricks, & Sharland, 2004; Jelicic, Ceunen, Maarten Peters, & Merckelbach, 2011) found the TOMM surprisingly resistant to coaching.

The TOMM has much to recommend its use in CST evaluations, including a strong research base, broad acceptance, and fairly good specificity in SMI samples. It also has cross-validated cutoff scores for ID examinees, and new scoring schemes appear to increase its sensitivity. However, the TOMM has a significant limitation that cannot be overcome by recent refinements to its decision rules: It has no internal check to distinguish between low effort and low ability. Although the ACI and use of Trial 1 appear to increase sensitivity and accuracy, these have not been studied in psychiatric samples. Finally, the TOMM's standard cutoff scores are overly conservative for some diagnostic groups (e.g., mTBI, chronic pain), resulting in low sensitivity.

TOMM SUMMARY

Pros:

- Very well validated and very well accepted in both forensic psychology and neuropsychology.
- Does not require a computer for administration.
- Fairly robust to psychiatric and mild to moderate cognitive impairment, pain.
- With addition of Trial 1 and Albany Consistency Index, nearly as sensitive as WMT.
- Requires very little effort to perform adequately—primarily sensitive to motivation.

Cons:

- Susceptible to failure by demented or severely cognitively impaired examinees; no internal validity check to distinguish between poor effort and poor ability.
- Cutoff scores for ID examinees have been quite variable across studies.

- Requires so little effort to pass that it is likely to be insensitive to suboptimal, superficial effort.
- The TOMM's popularity, single detection strategy and amount of coaching material on the web make it potentially more vulnerable than most PVTs to coaching.

VALIDITY INDICATOR PROFILE (VIP)

The VIP (Frederick, 1997) has Verbal and Nonverbal sections, both similar to intelligence test items. The VIP was the outgrowth of studies by Frederick and colleagues (Frederick & Foster, 1991; Frederick, Sarfaty, Johnson, & Powel, 1994) on a two-response choice version of the Test of Nonverbal Intelligence, with items randomized in respect to difficulty. For analysis, a running average score of 10 items of similar difficulty is created, producing a curve that illustrates the test-taker's performance (percent correct) as items increase in difficulty. A Verbal (vocabulary) subtest was subsequently added. The VIP is published by Pearson and is billed as appropriate for ages 18 to 69. The Verbal subtest can be completed in 20 minutes, the Nonverbal in 30. A specimen set costs $192.00 for the Q-global platform ($205.00 for Q Local) and includes three answer sheets and interpretive reports. Additional interpretive reports cost $25.50 or $26.95 for Q-global and Q Local platforms, respectively. Profile reports (without interpretive content) cost $19.75 or $21.00, and additional answer sheets cost $23.00 for 25.

Early VIP publications, such as that by Frederick and Crosby (2000), presented mathematical indices on which VIP decisions rules were based. These were replaced by more accessible strategies by Frederick (2003).

VIP performance is summarized in a two-by-two table (Figure 5.1) with variables of *Intent* and *Effort* as the axes. *Intent* denotes if the test-taker exhibited motivation to perform well, as indicated by scoring better on the easier items than on items beyond the test-taker's ability, indicating motivation or intention to perform well (vs. poorly).

Effort refers to the consistency of performance. Only those who show intent to perform well and do so consistently are classified as *Compliant* and valid. Conversely, only subjects who show an intention to perform poorly, and do so consistently, are classified as showing a *Suppressed* (formally called *malingering*) response style. Those who show good intent but erratic performance (*Inconsistent* style), or intent to fail and *perform inconsistently* (*Irrelevant* style), are also classified as invalid but do not provide clear evidence of malingering or even feigning. Instead of relying on normative groups to define implausible levels of performance, the VIP uses the individual's own performance, referred to the *personal floor effect* (Frederick, 2003), on items of varied difficulty. A number of response style indices are also produced by the interpretive software, including one (the Adjusted score) that is claimed to allow fairly precise estimation of the examinee's IQ. Decision rules are clearly described in the manual.

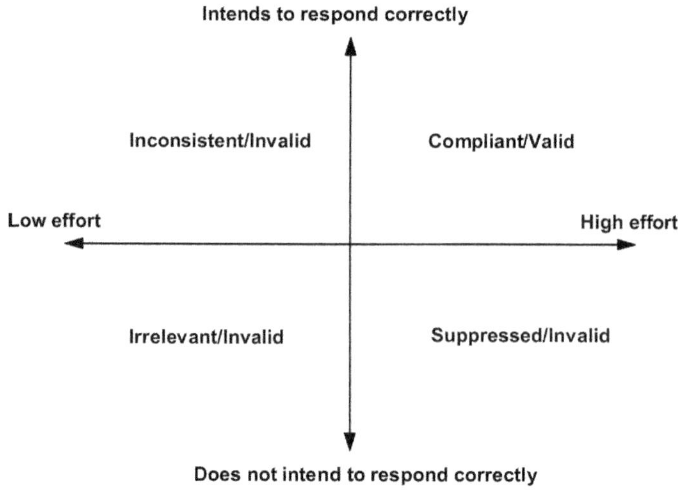

Figure 5.1 VIP Typology of Response Styles
Reproduced with permission from Frederick & Bowden (2009a).

Frederick and Crosby (2000) reported on findings from a simulation and a cross-validation study consisting of 61 TBI examinees, 52 coached simulators, and 49 head injury claimants with lack of documented injury who were deemed at risk for malingering. No clear diagnostic statistics are reported for the first study, whereas sensitivities of 67.3% and 73.5% were reported for the Verbal and Nonverbal subtests, respectively, in the cross-validation sample, with specificities of 83.1% and 85.7%. However, examination of the data indicates the VIP was much less effective in distinguishing suspected malingerers than simulators from honest TBI patients. In fact, a higher percentage of brain-injured patients were classified as *Invalid* (37%) on the Verbal subtest than were suspected malingerers (27%). Forty-five percent of suspected malingerers failed the Nonverbal subtest, as did 27% of TBI patients. Good agreement (kappa = .70) between the Verbal and Nonverbal subtests was reported.

Ross and Adams (1999) noted limitations in the manual's presentation of diagnostic statistics (inclusion of randomly generated profiles) and the VIP's normative base, limited sensitivity to malingering, and the need for further validation, but they also noted the VIP's unique assets and sophisticated conceptual basis. Frederick (2003) provided a summary of VIP research to that point. He noted the difficulty in forming pure criterion groups and cited diagnostic statistics, although these appear to be based on the earlier studies and included normal controls, likely inflating the specificities. Several reviews (Gamache, 1998; Gebart-Eaglemont, 2001; Ivens, 2001; Ross & Adams, 1999) were cited, as well as criticism by Lees-Haley, Dunn, and Betz (1999), who asserted the VIP's classification system unnecessarily muddles the detection and diagnosis of malingering. Frederick (2003) acknowledged that malingerers might produce any of the VIP profiles, including a *Compliant* pattern, which is usually indicative of good motivation and effort. Rogers and Bender (2003) noted that only a tiny proportion of simulators and malingerers are correctly classified as malingering (*Suppressed*) on the Verbal (7.7%, 2.0%, respectively) and Nonverbal VIP subtests (5.8%, 2.0%). Finally, Sollman and Berry (2011) identified 16 studies examining the VIP but did not include the VIP in their meta-analysis because of the difficulty of calculating mean VIP scores.

Rogers and Bender (2003) cited data from the VIP manual and noted that persons with borderline intellectual functioning were as likely as simulators to produce invalid profiles on the VIP. Although acknowledging that ID subjects often produce *Inconsistent* or *Irrelevant* VIP profiles, Frederick (2003, 2011) asserted the VIP can be used with persons with *suspected* intellectual disability, absent a documented history of severe cognitive impairment. The manual reports 50% of 20 ID subjects with an IQ of 65 or greater produced a *Compliant* profile on the Verbal subtest, whereas only 35% did so on the Nonverbal subtest. Among those with an IQ of 64 or lower, very few produced *Complaint* profiles. D. Green et al. (2012) found several VIP Verbal subtest indices (*Total Score, Adjusted Score*) were substantially correlated (*rs* = .64 to .65) with IQ estimates among defendants judged to be genuine (average IQ = 86.1; *SD* = 15.0; range = 57 to 125), although the correlation with the Adjusted score was much lower than the figure cited in the VIP manual. VIP *Compliant* classifications fell steadily as IQ decreased, reaching 45.5% for those with borderline IQ and 38.5% in the lowest group. VIP indices were not affected by the scores on the Expanded Brief Psychiatric Rating Scale (A. Thomas, Donnell, & Young, 2004) *Apathy* factor, which might have been expected given the VIP's emphasis on performance consistency, and the fact that *Apathy* did affect performance on the less demanding FIT.

Hunt et al. (2014) reported that community residential psychiatric patients diagnosed with schizophrenia or schizoaffective disorder produced mostly invalid VIP profiles. The VIP Nonverbal subtest was especially problematic, with a specificity of 17%. The Verbal subtest fared better, as 40% of examinees obtained a *Compliant* profile. However, limitations in the reporting or methodology limit the value of this study.[1] The authors noted that the VIP is lengthy and largely self-administered, and compared with the TOMM, may suffer from the lack of interaction with an examiner to maintain focus and motivation. The Nonverbal test, perhaps more than any other PVT, requires the examinee to concentrate and think intently; because of the tests' organization, some of the items may be well beyond the examinee's ability, yet are presented early in the test. Given that the two VIP subtests have been examined in different studies, potential users should evaluate them separately.

The Verbal VIP

Several studies (D. Green, 2010; Pivovarova et al., 2009; Rosenfeld et al., 2010) examined the ability of the VIP Verbal subtest variables to discriminate between community simulators and day hospital patients, most diagnosed with SMI, in a partially shared data set. Simulators were told to feign "*mental or emotional problems* [emphasis added] that might make you appear *incompetent to stand trial*." Although they were told they could fake any way they wanted, the instructions seem to emphasize feigning mental illness, not intellectual limitations. Pivovarova et al. used the VIP Verbal subtest to classify subjects into either *Valid* (*Compliant*) or *Invalid* (*Inconsistent, Irrelevant, Suppressed*) response styles. This classification had a sensitivity of 73.1% but a much lower specificity (71.6%) than the TOMM. The VIP *Point of Entry* index, which is based on responses to the easiest 10 items, had the best discrimination (AUC = .78) and produced a sensitivity of 61.5% and specificity of 93.8%. No other VIP indices added to a discriminant function. Rosenfeld et al. (2010) reported the VIP Verbal subtest increased classification accuracy over an abbreviated version of the SIRS and the MMPI-2 F, Fp, and Obvious-Subtle scales in some stepwise discriminant analyses and in all regression tree analyses. However, the authors acknowledged that these results reflect optimization of a limited data set and might not generalize. D. Green (2010) reported the VIP Verbal variables *Slope, Point of Entry*, and *Total Score* produced sizable Cohen's *ds* (.68 to 1.05) for separating simulators from community psychiatric patients.

D. Green (2010; D. Green et al., 2012) next examined a group of suspected malingerers among hospitalized CST examinees previously deemed incompetent. She found *none* of the VIP Verbal subtest variables produced significant AUC with the criterion—the treating psychiatrist's assessment of genuineness, based on "access to a wealth of information beyond psychological testing." The VIP's performance was similar to the TOMM's but inferior to the FIT's.

The Nonverbal VIP (NV-VIP)

Frederick, Crosby, and Wynkoop (2000) examined the NV-VIP among 737 pretrial defendants, the majority undergoing competency evaluation or restoration treatment. However, the analysis was hampered by the poor sensitivity of other validity measures employed and the inability to clearly attribute poor VIP performance to motivation, psychopathology, or cognitive limitations. Frederick and Bowden (2009a) reanalyzed data from Frederick et al. (2000) using MGV and reported that the *intent to perform poorly* classification (*Suppressed* and *Irrelevant* classifications) on the Nonverbal subtest had a sensitivity of 86% and specificity of 100% among 527 pretrial examinees. Using the MMPI-2 *Variable Response Inconsistency* (VRIN) scale as an index of inconsistent responding, a VIP classification of *poor effort* (*Inconsistent* or *Irrelevant* styles) had a sensitivity of 62.5% and false positive rate of 5.6%. These data were presented as supporting the VIP's two-variable classification scheme, although an analysis that simply contrasted all *Invalid* classifications with *Compliant* profiles produced comparable diagnostic statistics.

The assumptions of MGV were subsequently challenged by one of the study's co-authors in Jewsbury and Bowden (2013), who noted that MGV can be used confidently only when the conditional independence of the two tests in the analysis (predictor and criterion) can be justified prior to the study, either empirically or theoretically. The study by Frederick and Bowden (2009a) was cited as an example of a violation of this assumption, probably quite severe, where overestimation of sensitivity and underestimation of the false positive rate was likely.

The only other study to examine the Nonverbal VIP in a forensic (disability) sample (Farkas et al., 2006) found good sensitivity but much lower specificity (50% with the TOMM as the criterion) than in Frederick's studies, although this could reflect the TOMM's limited sensitivity or disengagement of psychiatric patients from a demanding task with no personal interaction.

Combined Studies

Three studies examined both VIP Verbal and Nonverbal subtests in disability, somatoform, or academic accommodation samples, respectively. Farkas et al. (2006) examined VIP classifications on both Verbal and Nonverbal subscales to the MMPI's F, Fp, and F-K scales and the TOMM in a group of 66 disability and personal injury claimants. Both the Verbal and Nonverbal scales showed surprisingly good agreement with MMPI-2 validity scales' classifications, but less agreement with TOMM results, contrary to expectations. Both VIP subtests detected 75% of those who failed the TOMM, whereas, as discussed earlier, the NV-VIP identified twice as many persons as invalid as did the TOMM. Among female patients with chronic fatigue, Cockshell and Mathias (2012) reported that the NV-VIP produced few (5.6%) invalid profiles (all *Inconsistent* style), which were not significantly different than among normal controls. The Verbal subtest had no false positives. Sopko (2012) reported the VIP Verbal subtest had a sensitivity of 39% for feigned ADHD or reading disorder, with a specificity of 1.00. The Nonverbal subtest was much more sensitive (64%) and only slightly less specific (95%).

VIP SUMMARY

The VIP's use of the test-taker's own performance as a baseline is an elegant approach that potentially allows differentiation of a test-taker's motivation and effort, which is crucial information for a diagnosis of malingering. However, it is not clear that the VIP can deliver. Frederick (2003) acknowledged that some simulators obtained profiles suggesting motivation to perform well. Thus, profiles that are interpreted as showing intent to perform well on the VIP might simply reflect a more sophisticated strategy of feigning. For example, a test-taker might try to calibrate his of her performance to the difficulty of the item, intentionally failing only on those items that pose some difficulty, or intentionally getting 40% of those wrong that are within his or her ability. In addition, the label of "effort" for the second dimension may be less than optimal. A test-taker who knows the answer but intentionally gives the incorrect one has engaged in at least one more process than a test-taker who straightforwardly gives the correct answer. A less inferential term would be *performance consistency*, which Frederick and Bowden (2009a) used as an alternative to *effort* and which is supported by correlations observed with MMPI consistency scales.

For the Verbal VIP, simulator studies have been supportive and used a severely impaired psychiatric control group. However, the only known group study with CST examinees (D. Green 2010; D. Green et al., 2012) reported the VIP Verbal scale was not significantly related to treating psychiatrists' assessments of malingering. Given that the criterion rating was not assessed for inter-rater reliability, and the well-validated TOMM also failed to demonstrate validity, these results are not definitive. The Nonverbal VIP's most supportive data are provided by its author (Frederick & Bowden, 2009b) and entailed a very large sample ($n = 527$) of competency examinees, but are from a single setting using a method of analysis (MGV) that one of the authors subsequently criticized.

The Nonverbal subtest may require more motivation and mental effort than some clinical groups (ADHD, schizophrenics, personality disorders) are apt to give (Hunt et al., 2014), and more than required for the tasks required in a CST, but not a neuropsychological, exam. Thus, some examinees may present with poor effort on the VIP despite having given adequate effort during the rest of the exam. Some defendants will present with memory problems rather than intellectual disability, which are not directly tapped by the VIP. Finally, the VIP's apparent inability to distinguish genuine from feigned intellectual disability limits its usefulness when this issue is in question. To summarize the VIP's assets and shortcomings:

Pros:

- The only published PVT to target feigned intellectual impairment.
- Use of examinee's own baseline performance is more precise than norms and presumably controls for some sources of error variance.
- Does not require significant examiner time to administer.
- Verbal and Nonverbal subtests; can provide rough estimates of intelligence in both domains.
- May be significantly more sensitive than TOMM to poor effort.
- May be able to distinguish intent to perform poorly from poor effort.

Cons:

- Unable to assess feigning or poor effort in ID and borderline IQ subjects unless they score below chance or worse on easier items than on harder items.
- Lack of feedback and interaction with examiner may lead to poor engagement and results that don't generalize to a different setting (the rest of the evaluation).

- More expensive per use than other PVTs.
- The NV-VIP may require more effort and is more taxing than any other aspect of a CST exam and thus elicit poor effort that is specific to the task.

PAUL GREEN'S PVTS

The WMT (P. Green, 2005), Medical Symptom Validity Test (MSVT; P. Green, 2004), and Nonverbal Medical Symptom Validity Test (NV-MSVT; P. Green, 2008) are all creations of neuropsychologist Paul Green, and although each is a separate test with distinctive parameters, they share numerous features. All three (a) are administered by computer and involve recognition, paired associates, and free recall memory tasks; (b) have been studied in multiple practices across the globe; (c) rely on patient diagnosis and profile analysis as well as standard cutoff scores, and have formal decision rules for classifying cases as showing genuine cognitive impairment or poor effort; (d) take account of the person's living and functional status; (e) aspire to greater sensitivity and specificity than the TOMM; (f) were primarily developed in a forensic (disability evaluation) context; (g) have been and are the subject of considerable evaluation in the published literature (the NV-MSVT less than the others); (h) have limited data in SMI samples (as opposed to neurological samples) and criminal justice samples; (i) rely heavily on differential prevalence studies, showing higher failure rates than other tests in populations at high risk for feigning and low failure rates in very impaired samples (intellectual disability and dementia); (j) can be used with children as young as 7 years of age (P. Green & Flaro, 2016); and (k) have their own administration, scoring, and interpretive programs. In addition to the effort subtests, all contain additional scales that provide meaningful data about memory if the examinee demonstrates good effort. An additional program, the Automated Interpretive Program (AIP; P. Green, 2010), offers larger normative groups than some of the individual programs, flow charts for the decision rules using the test-taker's scores, and a visual comparison between WMT and MSVT scores. However, the AIP has a one-time purchase price of $380. The survey reported in Chapter 10 found that the WMT, MSVT, and NV-MSVT were infrequently used by CST examiners, but they are well known and widely used within the neuropsychology community (Martin, Schroeder, & Odland, 2015).

The Word Memory Test (WMT). The WMT is a verbal learning task that uses 20 pairs of words as stimuli, then multiple response tasks to test memory and effort. One subtest is administered immediately after presentation of the stimuli, the others after a 30-minute delay. The first three subtests, the recognition trials and the consistency between them, are often referred to as the *easy* subtests and *primary effort indicators*, although all the subtests now contribute to response style assessment. The WMT is published by Green's Publishing at WordMemoryTest.com. A 1-year license for unlimited administrations and scorings, which includes the manual, costs $340.00, and subsequent license renewals cost $165 per year.

The WMT takes only a few minutes of examiner time to administer, but with the 30-minute distraction period between the initial and subsequent subtests, it requires a total time of about 45 minutes to complete. It can be administered in any of 19 languages, with several more languages available only on the oral version paper forms.

According to the WMT manual (P. Green, 2005), the WMT was administered to more than 1,250 consecutive adults referred for neuropsychological evaluation of compensation and disability claims. In addition, three psychologists in different geographical locations provided another, independent sample of 1,244 forensic cases and large samples of clinically referred children. Among the early findings was that claimants with mild brain injuries or questionable histories often scored worse than those with severe head injuries on the primary effort indictors—the recognition memory subtests and the consistency scale. Most cases were involved in some sort of compensation claim. Validation of the WMT included normal adults and sophisticated simulators, such as psychologists and neurologists, and often showed near-perfect detection (P. Green, 2005). Specificity has been demonstrated by showing that young children, persons with serious brain conditions, and children with fetal alcohol syndrome are able to pass the easy subtests (P. Green, 2005; P. Green & Flaro, 2003; Rienstra, Spaan, & Schmand, 2010). Even patients with bilateral damage to the hippocampus, the brain structure most closely associated with memory storage, scored in the valid performance range on the recognition trials, while showing the expected impairment on the WMT's "hard" memory subtests (Goodrich-Hunsaker & Hopkins, 2009; Carone, Green, & Drane, 2014; but see Rienstra et al., 2013).

The WMT has been the flagship instrument of a new generation of effort tests that strive for higher sensitivity than such tests exhibited in the past, while also showing high specificity and internal checks for distinguishing poor effort from very impaired ability. Hartman (2002) reported the WMT has a number of advantages over competing PVTs, in that it (a) is sensitive to effort and insensitive to cognitive dysfunction; (b) has face validity as a legitimate cognitive test; (c) taps abilities likely to be exaggerated; (d) has a strong normative base; (e) has validation studies that include normals, patient populations, simulators, and verified malingerers; (f) is difficult to coach; (g) is easy to administer; and (h) is supported by continuing research. Although the WMT was originally developed as an orally administered test, it has been computer-administered since 1996. Two studies have found the oral and written versions to be equivalent (Allen & Green, 2002; Hoskins, Binder, Chaytor, Williamson, & Drane, 2010). This would seem to make the oral WMT suitable for nonliterate subjects, but P. Green and Flaro (2003, 2015, 2016) recommended that the WMT not be used with persons who lack a 3rd-grade reading level.

The WMT has been central to one of the seminal findings in neuropsychology: that *effort* accounts for 50% of the variance in neuropsychological test batteries and overshadows the modest effects of brain injury (P. Green, 2007; P. Green, Rohling, Lees-Haley, & Allen, 2001; Fox, 2011; Meyers, Volbrecht, Axelrod, & Reinsch-Boothby, 2011; Moss, Jones, Fokias, & Quinn, 2003; Stevens, Friedel,

Mehren, & Merten, 2008). At the same time, its high failure rates in litigating samples have made it controversial.

There has been contention that the WMT's sensitivity was achieved at the cost of higher false positive errors (Batt, Shores, & Chekaluk, 2008; Greve et al., 2008; Martins & Martins, 2010), and that the WMT and TOMM exhibit similar ability to discriminate if all the TOMM's scales, including Trial 1, are employed (Greiffenstein et al., 2008). Greve et al. created groups based on known incentives and a number of cognitive and psychopathology validity tests. They concluded that the WMT had a significant false positive rate in a group of TBI patients, which included patients with moderate or severe brain injuries, and suggested modified (lower) cutoff scores to maintain specificity at 2% or 10%. Although the authors concluded the WMT was no more discriminating than the TOMM, a large portion of the sample (49.6%) was indeterminate on malingering status. P. Green, Flaro, and Courtney (2009) noted that the embedded PVTs Greve et al. used to classify patients are much less sensitive than the WMT, and that mTBI patients would not be expected to fail the WMT based on the minimal cognitive sequelae of such injuries. Further, P. Green (2015b) charged that Greve et al. refused to release their data for independent analysis.

The WMT has a reputation as the most sensitive PVT, and several studies have shown that it produces considerably higher failure rates in compensation samples than the TOMM (Armistead-Jehle & Gervais, 2011; P. Green, Berendt, Mandel, & Allen, 2000; Demakis, Gervais, & Rohling, 2008; Greve et al., 2008; Tan, Slick, Strauss, & Hultsch, 2002), sometimes almost five times greater. Such findings are ambiguous, however, because the real question is the ability to discriminate valid examinees from those who feign or exaggerate. Mossman, Wygant, and Gervais (2012) estimated the WMT's sensitivity at 65% and the AUC at .923 in a sample of 1,301 disability and personal injury claimants, most presenting with pain, anxiety, PTSD, or depression. Both figures are considerably higher than for the TOMM, but only Trial 2 of the TOMM was examined. Sollman and Berry's (2011) meta-analysis reported that WMT, MSVT, TOMM, and the Letter Memory Test (Inman et al., 1998) had statistically equivalent sensitivities. The authors reported an average sensitivity for the WMT of 75% and an average specificity of 69%—the latter figure being alarmingly low and significantly lower than for other validity tests. However, Sollman and Berry did not employ profile analysis, which should greatly increase specificity. However, sensitivity would also suffer if one restricts *hits* to those failing the test with an implausible profile. An implausible profile is one in which the subject scores relatively better on the harder tests than the easier ones, and is formally defined in the interpretive program.

As with the TOMM, persons with severe cognitive impairment, dementia (Merten, Bossink, & Schmand, 2007), or predementia (Martins & Martins, 2010) are at risk for failure on the WMT's primary effort indicators. To address this problem, two decision rules were added to the software program that compares the subject's performance on the various subtests. First, if the examinee fails the easy subtest criteria, a simple decision rule classifies profiles as suggesting *poor effort* or *a genuine memory impairment* profile (GMIP). Then the examiner notes whether the examinee's diagnosis is one that can explain failure on such easy tasks. Generally, only dementia or severe neurocognitive injury is deemed able to explain such failure.

Although profile interpretation has been incorporated into the software for some years, the WMT manual (published in 2005) does not address this, as noted by Frederick (2011, 2015b). P. Green, Montijo, and Brockhaus (2011) reported that among 78 dementia patients, all but one who failed the primary effort indicators produced a GMIP on the WMT (see also Martins & Martins, 2010). Eichstaedt et al. (2014) reported that some subjects with temporal lobe epilepsy failed the WMT's easy subtests, and in those with bilateral damage the failure rate reached 50%. However, profile analysis classified all but two subjects as having a GMIP, and the two who produced a *poor effort* profile were deemed to be accurately classified as such. Fazio et al. (2015) reported that use of profile analysis reduced WMT false positives among CST neuropsychological referrals from 31.6% to 5.3% relative to Slick criteria *probable* response bias classification but reduced sensitivity from 95.1% to 56.1%, less than observed for the TOMM. However, the authors applied additional criteria to define a GMIP and did not consider whether the examinee's diagnosis was consistent with severe cognitive impairment, as required by the WMT's current interpretive criteria (P. Green, 2015c).

The WMT has been widely researched in neuropsychological samples and well-reviewed (Hartman, 2002; Wynkoop & Denney, 2005), but it has been less widely used and researched in psychiatric or criminal forensic samples. Donders and Kirkwood (2013) noted that the WMT and profile analysis have not been validated in psychiatric samples. Gorissen, Sanz, and Schmand (2005) reported that 72% of chronic schizophrenics failed the WMT's primary effort indices, and 25% of psychiatric patients did so. However, no information was presented about possible external incentives for the psychiatric patients, and the authors did not perform profile analysis.[2] Gorissen et al. suggested that the high failure rate was attributable to negative symptoms of schizophrenia, measures of which correlated with effort indices. Schroeder and Marshall (2011) similarly concluded that WMT failures among psychiatric patients were due to motivational or attention deficits endemic to schizophrenia. Stevens et al. (2014) reported that 27% of schizophrenics failed the WMT's primary validity indicators (they did not use profile analysis), but they also concluded that failure appeared to be due to lack of engagement in the testing process, not to cognitive deficits.

Brockhaus (personal communication, February 21, 2013) provided MMPI, WMT, and Reliable Digit Span data on 116 German psychiatric patients. A preliminary analysis by this author shows that the great majority of different diagnostic groups, including schizophrenics, passed the WMT's primary effort indictors. Because the actual validity status of these patients was not independently assessed, one can estimate the *maximum* false positive rate in this sample by looking at the percentage who failed with a *poor effort* profile. The potential false positive rate varied from 2.7% (depressive disorders, $n = 73$) to 6.7% in schizophrenics ($n = 29$). However, both of the schizophrenic patients who produced poor effort profiles produced very high scores on the MMPI-2 Meyers Validity Index (Meyers, 2002), and thus had independent evidence of exaggeration or feigning.

Unlike some PVTs, such as the TOMM, the WMT appears to require fairly close attention and some mental effort to pass. Frederick and Bowden (2009a) distinguished between motivation and effort and presented evidence to suggest that both the WMT and the VIP required both *intention* to perform well and consistent *effort* to do so. Other tests, like the TOMM and FIT, were judged to be so easy that they required only the intention to perform well, with very little or no need to exert mental effort.

Studies suggest the WMT may be sensitive to emotional factors or sedating medication. Williamson, Holsman, Chaytor, Miller, and Drane (2012) reported that WMT failure among psychogenic non-epileptic seizure patients was associated with a history of childhood abuse, not financial incentives. Sedating medication (Loring et al., 2011) or distraction in vulnerable groups (Batt et al., 2008) may also cause failure on the WMT. Rohling (2013) countered that the Loring et al. findings showed that the majority (55%) of those who failed the WMT on lorazepam had a *poor effort* profile, similar to the proportion of such profiles in simulator groups, and the results were due to poor motivation and effort rather than to cognitive impairment.

The WMT has been studied in intellectually limited samples of both adults and children. Brockhaus and Merten (2004) reported that 31 of 32 testable ID patients passed the WMT's primary effort scales. Follow-up revealed that the one patient who failed, in fact, had feigned (R. Brockhaus, personal communication, February 4, 2013). Dean, Victor, Boone, and Arnold (2008) charged that Brockhaus and Merten's results were skewed by selection of subjects who were "testable" and did not have a co-occurring psychiatric disorder. Shandera et al. (2010) reported 75% of mildly developmentally disabled subjects scored below the WMT Consistency scale cutoff, which is sufficient to fail the primary effort criterion. The actual false positive rate was not reported, and the authors did not use profile analysis to identify genuine impairment profiles. Shandera's data were obtained and analyzed. Of the 18 ID subjects who failed the primary effort indicators, 12 (66.7%) produced a *genuine impairment* profile. P. Green and Flaro (2015) pointed out that the authors did not consider the disability status of the subjects, pointed to unexpectedly low WMT scores and profile features in both samples, and concluded Shandera et al.'s ID and healthy subjects were not motivated to perform well.

P. Green and Flaro (2015) reported that although more low-IQ adults (14.2%) undergoing parenting assessments failed the WMT than those with an IQ above 70 (4.9%), the difference was not significant. Of the two low-IQ subjects who failed the WMT, one was reportedly engaged in drug trafficking and did not want parental custody, and the other was described as very passive-aggressive and overtly uncooperative. Low-IQ adults did score significantly lower on most WMT subscales, including on two of the three primary effort indicators, but the latter scores were different by only 2 points and deemed not clinically significant. The authors stated, "The data strongly suggest that MR with an FSIQ in the range of 46 to 70 is not sufficient to explain failure on these performance validity tests by adults" (p. 293). However, given a very modest sample (n = 14), with a relatively high mean IQ (64.4), it seems premature to apply these findings to examinees in the 46 to 60 IQ range, or even below the mean of the sample.

Children have also been a significant part of the WMT's validation program. P. Green and Flaro (2003) reported most clinically referred children passed the WMT, and those who did not pass initially did pass when retested and offered a small incentive to perform their best. P. Green, Flaro, Brockhaus, and Montijo (2012) published data on a large sample of children described as having developmental disorders, but only about 10% of the sample was ID, and no separate analysis for this group is presented. P. Green and Flaro (2016) compared ID children (n = 19) with 554 child referrals who were not diagnosed with intellectual disabilities. Scores did not differ significantly on most WMT scales between ID (mean IQ = 63.3) and other clinically referred children (mean IQ = 85.5) except on the *Free Recall* subtest. No ID child with a 3rd-grade reading level on the WRAT-4 failed the WMT. Lorochette and Harrison (2012) reported that 6 of 63 normal-IQ, learning disabled adolescents failed the WMT easy subtests, although 5 of 6 produced a genuine impairment profile. They also reported that 3 of the subjects who failed the easy subtests had a reading level of 3.0 on the WIAT-II.

Fazio et al. (2015) recently examined the WMT's and TOMM's diagnostic statistics among forensic neuropsychological referral inpatients, many of whom were being assessed for CST or CST restoration. The WMT's primary effort indicators detected 95.1% of those who failed other effort tests, compared with 68.2% for the TOMM using both Trial 2 and Retention Trial. If those failing the WMT's effort indicators were also required to show a poor effort profile, the WMT had a lower sensitivity to feigned impairment than the TOMM (56.1% vs. 68.2%) but a higher likelihood ratio (10.7 vs. 5.2), an indication of better discrimination. Although the WMT without profile analysis reportedly had a false positive rate of 31.6%, P. Green (2015a) noted that several of the other effort tests that served as the criteria for classification have low sensitivity. The relatively high false positive rate reported for the TOMM (13.2%) supports this interpretation, as the most severe condition in the referral group was moderate TBI, which should not cause failure on either the TOMM or the WMT. The authors also examined the WMT's specificity using profile analysis but did not use the standard decision rules: They apparently did not require that failures on the primary effort indicators be explainable by the examinees' diagnoses. Only conditions suggesting severe cognitive impairment, such as dementia or severe head injury, are considered to qualify—even mild intellectual disability does not (P. Green & Flaro, 2015, 2016). Even so, the WMT with profile analysis produced a higher specificity (94.7%) than the TOMM (86.8%).

The Automated Interpretation Program for the WMT (and Green's other tests) includes WMT data on 33 developmentally delayed individuals with a mean IQ of 57.8 and a mean age of 13. P. Green (2012) encouraged the conjoint use of the WMT, MSVT, and NV-MSVT. He reported that when profile analysis is used on all three tests, no false positives are observed for the ID sample (n = 9), and Armistead-Jehle and Denney (2015) reported 98% of dementia simulators were detected.

In sum, the WMT has a strong research base with neurological samples and in forensic disability settings. The data pertaining to psychiatric populations with psychosis are limited, and high failure rates are reported, but they probably reflect disengagement and poor effort rather than true false positives. With ID subjects, the findings are mixed at present: P. Green and Flaro's (2003, 2015, 2016) and Larochette and Harrison's (2012) data are very supportive, in subjects with a grade 3.1 reading level or better, whereas Shandera et al.'s (2010) are not but suffer from incomplete analysis. It should be noted that the adults in the study by P. Green and Flaro (2015) were likely more highly motivated to perform well than many ID defendants, as they were seeking the return of their children. With neurological samples of greater than ID level intelligence, the WMT is a strong choice due to its sensitivity and, with profile analysis, its ability to distinguish poor ability and poor effort in about three quarters of simulators who fail the primary effort indicators. With psychiatric samples, data are limited, and, as for other PVTs, failures may reflect poor cooperation or engagement as well as feigning.

WMT SUMMARY

Pros:

- Highly sensitive to poor effort or poor motivation.
- Validated in multiple practice settings across the world using actual examinees.
- Excellent specificity in dementia and severe cognitive impairment when profile analysis is used.
- Requires little examiner time for administration or scoring.
- Relatively engaging, interactive for examinee.
- Good face validity as a memory test; contains three useful memory tests.

Cons:

- Limited data in SMI and criminal justice examinees.
- Current recommended administration requires use of computer.
- Examiner should leave room, yet monitor examinee, which can be difficult in criminal justice settings.
- Administration time, with distraction period, spans 45 minutes.
- Expensive initial buy-in, yearly renewal.

THE MEDICAL SYMPTOM VALIDITY TEST (MSVT)

The MSVT (P. Green, 2004) is a shorter, quicker, and easier version of the WMT. The list of words to be remembered is half as long, the words are simpler, and the stimulus word pairs are more clearly associated than in the WMT. The *Multiple Choice* subtest is dropped and the period between *Immediate-* and *Delayed-Recognition* subtests is reduced from 30 minutes to 10 minutes, yielding a total administration time of about 15 minutes. This makes the MSVT attractive for time-limited evaluations. Also available from Green's Publishing, a specimen kit for the MSVT comes with 30 on-screen administrations (which includes scoring and interpretive guidance) for $340. Additional administrations cost $6.00, or $3.50 with a WMT license. The MSVT can be administered in English, French, Spanish, Dutch, German, or Portuguese.

Carone (2009) reviewed the MSVT, noting the strengths and limitations discussed elsewhere in this section. Although Merten, Green, Henry, Blaskewitz, and Brockhaus (2005) found the MSVT transparent as an effort test (more so than the FIT), both they and Weinborn, Woods, Nulsen, and Leighton (2012) found the MSVT resistant to coaching.

The MSVT is infrequently used by CST examiners (see Chapter 10, this volume), probably because it is new and has not been marketed to forensic psychologists. It has much greater exposure in neuropsychology, where it has been employed as the criterion in numerous recent studies (Armistead-Jehle, 2010; Armistead-Jehle, Gervais, & Green, 2012; Chafetz, 2012; Chafetz, Prentkowski, & Rao, 2011; Kirkwood, Connery, Kirk, & Baker, 2014; Schutte, Millis, Axelrod, & Van Dyke, 2011; Whitney, Shepard, & Davis, 2013). Like the WMT, there are decision rules to classify profiles as being more like genuinely impaired groups or simulators. However, the MSVT interpretive program (version 1.3.1) lists three such criteria, while the Automated Interpretive Program (P. Green, 2010) uses only one (the difference in means between easy and hard subtests).

Several studies supporting the MSVT's validity, cutoff scores, and interpretive strategies in demented samples have been published (Howe, Anderson, Kaufman, Sachs, & Loring, 2007; Howe & Loring, 2009; Singhal, Green, Ashaye, Shankar, & Gill, 2009; P. Green, Montijo, & Brockhaus, 2011), most of which support a very low false positive rate even in this very impaired population. Although Rudman et al. (2011) concluded that the MSVT and several other SVTs were not suitable for demented patients, they apparently did not utilize profile analysis and did not respond to email queries on this issue. To date, nearly all subjects diagnosed with dementia produced a dementia profile if they failed the primary effort indicators, although Suesse, Wong, Stamper, Carpenter, and Scott (2015) reported 13.3% of their dementia sample did not.

The MSVT has been demonstrated to be easy enough to be passed by examinees with IQs below 75 if they are motivated to perform well (Chafetz, Prentkowski, & Rao, 2011)[3] and can read at least at the 3.1-grade level (P. Green & Flaro, 2015, 2016). As impressive, among low-IQ parents undergoing assessment for the return of their children, scores on *Immediate Recognition* and *Delayed Recognition* subtests were near the maximum possible (both 99.8% correct), with very small *SDs* (both = 1.0). Carone (2008) showed that children with moderate to severe brain injury or dysfunction passed the MSVT, whereas adults with mTBI, a group known for high rates of invalid responding and lack of legitimate cognitive impairment, often did not, implicitly demonstrating both specificity and sensitivity in different samples. Blaskewitz, Merten, and Kathmann (2008) found all but 1 of 73 children, aged 6 to 11, passed the MSVT. P. Green and Flaro (2016) reported ID children did not perform significantly worse than other clinically referred children on four of five MSVT scales, and the MSVT had no false positives in such children with a 3rd-grade reading level. Larson et al. (2015) reported 95% of children with fetal alcohol syndrome passed the MSVT. The MSVT interpretive program includes a group of 18 ID children with a mean IQ of 64, and the AIP includes 33 ID subjects with a mean IQ of 57.8. Because the MSVT is easier than the WMT, it is especially suitable for ID defendants.

Only one study has examined the MSVT in psychiatric patients with serious mental illness: C. Harrison (2008) reported the sum of MSVT scores across subtests had an AUC of .95 in separating simulators from patients, many of whom were in a state hospital. No normative data are provided for most adult psychiatric groups in the MSVT manual or interpretive programs.

Not all reports about the MSVT have been favorable. Axelrod and Schutte (2010) found that the MSVT's GMIP did not predict performance on a neuropsychological battery among Veterans Administration patients. Axelrod and Schutte (2011) recommended lower cutoff scores to bring the MSVT into better agreement with classifications of poor effort from the TOMM and California Verbal Learning Test Recognition subtest, implying that the MSVT made excessive false positive errors. However, they did not use profile analysis and acknowledged that greater sensitivity of the MSVT provides an alternative explanation for their results. Chafetz and Biondolillo (2013) reported that malingering disability claimants typically produced the GMIP on the MSVT, while claimants with IQs in the 60 to 75 range did not *because they didn't fail the easy subtests.* Bashem et al. (2014) reported that the MSVT was slightly less discriminating and sensitive than the TOMM in separating honest TBI patients from simulators, but slightly more specific, when profile analysis was employed.[4] The MSVT appears less sensitive than the WMT, and more transparent, with failure rates averaging 24.5% among disability claimants versus 32% for the WMT (P. Green, 2008). Feigners produce a *poor effort* profile less frequently on the MSVT (Armistead-Jehle & Denney, 2015; Chafetz & Biondolillo, 2013; Weinborn et al., 2012) than on the WMT or NV-MSVT, in only about half of cases, and thus a "dementia profile" is far from diagnostic of this condition. The MSVT appears less likely to identify invalid responding than the WMT, and when it does, the evidence may be less compelling. Sollman and Berry (2011) reported the MSVT showed a smaller average effect size than other modern SVTs, including the TOMM, the Letter Memory Test (Inman et al., 1998), and the WMT, although the average sensitivity (70%) and specificity (91%) were quite good. However, one of the three studies of the MSVT in the meta-analysis (Covert, 2008) did not report compensation status or response validity of clinical (mTBI) subjects. Thus, it does not meet one inclusion criterion (e.g., "objective evidence for honesty of a patient control group is required") specified by Sollman and Berry.

The MSVT may be preferred over the WMT with low-functioning defendants and ones who are unlikely to identify it as a validity test. In brighter, more educated, or wary defendants, the WMT, despite its greater administration time, should be preferred over the MSVT.

MSVT SUMMARY

Pros:

- Brief, well-validated PVT.
- Supportive data with ID examinees from multiple studies; best choice for this group if reading level is adequate.
- Requires little effort; not taxing or challenging for examinees.
- Some capacity to distinguish poor motivation from low ability in severely impaired groups.
- Requires only a few minutes of examiner time.

Cons:

- Less sensitive than WMT, less likely to produce a poor effort/implausible profile.
- May be recognized as a validity test by wary or brighter examinees.
- Limited data for criminal justice and seriously mentally ill examinees.
- Administration requires a computer.

The Non-Verbal Medical Symptom Validity Test (NV-MSVT). Despite its similarity in name to the MSVT, the Nonverbal MSVT (P. Green, 2008) is a completely different test, and one with advantages over its verbal counterpart. Designed to be a more sensitive nonverbal validity test than the TOMM, the NV-MSVT incorporates three internal checks to distinguish poor effort from very low ability. Availability and pricing are identical to those for the MSVT, and administration time is slightly longer.

P. Green (2011) found that among disability claimants, the TOMM and the NV-MSVT showed agreement in nearly 90% of cases. However, nearly 11% of cases failed the NV-MSVT while passing the TOMM, and only one claimant showed the opposite pattern. None of the 21 cases with moderate or severe head injury failed either the NV-MSVT or the TOMM, whereas 26% of those with a mTBI failed the NV-MSVT, and 10% failed the TOMM. Green presented evidence, including profile analysis on the NV-MSVT, failure on other concurrently administered validity tests (WMT and MSVT), and the head injury severity data cited earlier, to argue that the discrepant cases were false negatives for the TOMM. Armistead-Jehle and Gervais (2011) replicated this pattern of findings.

In civil disability samples, the NV-MSVT appears less sensitive than the WMT or the MSVT (P. Green, 2008), in that subjects are less likely to fail the primary validity indices. Yet, Weinborn et al. (2012) reported the NV-MSVT was quite sensitive to simulators and only modestly affected by detailed coaching. Armistead-Jehle and Denney (2015) found that 94% of 50 clinical psychology doctoral student simulators failed the NV-MSVT *and* produced a *poor effort* profile—much higher than the respective figures obtained for the WMT (73.5%) and the MSVT (54%).

Normative data are available on a variety of neuropsychological groups, but only a few psychiatric ones other than for children or adolescents. For example, the data for individuals with schizophrenia are based on only 7 patients with an average age of 14. There are substantial groups of adults with depression, grouped by whether they passed validity tests like the WMT. There is also a small group of 9 ID subjects with an average IQ of 56 in the NV-MSVT interpretive program, which is expanded to 20 in the Advanced Interpretation Program. P. Green and Flaro (2016) reported that among 26 ID children (mean IQ = 61.2), 3 (11.5%) failed the primary effort criteria, and all produced a poor effort profile. However, the authors reported 2 of the 3 children demonstrated severe oppositional-defiant traits or behavior at the time of the evaluation and, thus, were arguably not false positives. Two studies (Sollman, Ranseen, & Berry, 2010; Jasinski et al., 2011) have found excellent specificity with students with ADHD but modest sensitivity to feigned ADHD.

The NV-MSVT has been found to have high specificity in neurological patients, including the most challenging patients for a cognitive validity test—demented patients. Henry, Merten, Wolf, and Harth (2010) reported no false positives among 21 dementia patients and only 1 in a larger sample of neurological patients. Singhal et al. (2009) reported only 1 of 10 dementia patients failed the easy subtest indices, but this patient produced a GMIP.

Wager and Howe (2010) reviewed the NV-MSVT and concluded it met Hartman's (2002) criteria for PVTs. A few limitations should be considered, however. The NV-MSVT has not been studied in criminal forensic samples, and normative data on common psychiatric diagnoses are very limited. Profile analysis, based on both theoretical and empirical ordering of subtest severity, provides a crucial test of the distinction between poor effort and poor ability and has been cross-validated in severely impaired neurological samples, but further examination is needed for ID and psychiatric samples. This author's experience using the NV-MSVT in CST evaluations was that many test-takers needed closer supervision than described in the manual. It is not uncommon for defendants to require extensive prompting during the learning and immediate recognition trial to name the items they see, as required by the instructions. This behavior appeared to be associated with subsequent failure on the NV-MSVT and other indications of feigning.

NV-MSVT SUMMARY

Pros:

- Brief, nonverbal PVT that is well validated in neuropsychological samples.
- More sensitive than TOMM.
- Excellent internal checks to distinguish poor effort or motivation from low ability, including intellectual disability.
- Resistant to even detailed coaching.

- Takes little examiner time.
- Engaging, low effort, not taxing on examinee.
- If valid, provides a clinically useful assessment of nonverbal memory.

Cons:

- Limited data in psychiatric samples, none in criminal forensic samples.
- Not well known or widely used among CST examiners (as of November 2012),[5] although it is among neuropsychologists.
- Administration requires a computer.

CHAPTER SUMMARY

This chapter has presented an enormous amount of information on the various tests, some of which is summarized in Table 5.2. The various PVTs discussed here are well validated in neurological samples, less so in psychiatric ones. Significant false positive rates have been reported for the WMT, the VIP, and even the TOMM in SMI groups. However, in these studies, failures were usually defined in terms of malingering/feigning. As will be argued throughout this book a better focus is on the validity of the test results. Viewed in this light, the substantial portions of SMI patients who failed the WMT or VIP were not necessarily erroneous and, in fact, may have accurately reflected poor effort that otherwise might have gone unnoticed. Although there appears to be wide agreement on this interpretation, limited data bearing on the matter have been reported. Finally, a word on TOMM and Rey FIT failures in psychiatric samples is warranted. Frederick and Bowden (2009a) classified both as measures primarily of *intent*, not *effort*, because they are so easy that most examinees do not have to "try" to pass. Yet, significant numbers of psychiatric patients without apparent external motivations have failed these tests in some studies. If external motivations were indeed absent (which is hard to know for certain), this suggests that some such examinees are failing for motives other than malingering.

Although many PVTs are now described as *effort tests*, there has been no research to accurately measure how much mental effort different tests require. As indicated earlier, some PTVs, like the TOMM, probably require very little subjective mental effort in most examinees. At the other end of the spectrum, the Nonverbal VIP requires substantial mental effort, with the Verbal VIP and the WMT probably falling next on the continuum. Ideally, a PVT (or CST forensic assessment instrument) would require about as much mental energy as performing in the CST exam or in the actual role as a defendant as the case progresses. If the test requires more effort, the PVT may be prone to false positive errors: Some examinees will not put forth the needed effort to pass the test but can muster enough to function in the role of defendant. If the PVT requires less effort than the CST assessment tasks, it does not provide a valid assessment of the person's

Table 5.2 PVT Indices With 90% Specificity in Multiple Studies

Test/Index	Criteria/Cutoff Score	Includes SMI, ID?[a]	Sensitivity	Specificity	Citations
FIT	<9	SMI	.36	.90[b]	Reznek, 2005; Vickery et al., 2001
RDS	≤6		.30–.35	.96–.97	Schroeder, Twumasi-Ankrah et al., 2012
TOMM Trial 1	<41		.77	.92	Denning, 2012
TOMMe10	≥2 Errors		.50, .71	.90, .93	Denning, 2012, 2013, 2014; Kulas et al., 2014
TOMM Trial 2	<45	SMI	.654	.938	Sollman & Berry, 2011
TOMM Trial 2	<30	ID	.24, .56	.96	Graue et al., 2007; Shandera et al., 2010
TOMM Retention Trial	<45		.48–.50	.971–1.00	Schroeder et al., 2013; Buddin et al., 2014; Kulas et al., 2014
TOMM Retention Trial	<30	ID	.20, .60	.96, 1.00	Graue et al., 2007; Shandera et al., 2010
TOMM ACI	≥10		.71–.77	.853–1.00	Gunner et al., 2012; Schroeder et al., 2013; Buddin et al., 2014; Kulas et al., 2014
WMT	Fail A criteria	ID, SMI	.751	.694	Sollman & Berry, 2011
WMT	With profile analysis	Dem, ID, SMI[c]	—	.86–1.00[c,d]	Larochette & Harrison, 2012; Martins & Martins, 2010; Eichstaedt et al., 2014; Hampson et al., 2014; P. Green & Flaro, 2015, 2016
MSVT	Without profile analysis	ID, Dem	.90–1.00 Sim	.273–1.00	Merten et al., 2005; Chafetz et al., 2007; Singhal et al., 2009; Blaskewitz et al., 2008; Rudman et al., 2011

(*Continued*)

Table 5.2 CONTINUED

Test/Index	Criteria/Cutoff Score	Includes SMI, ID?[a]	Sensitivity	Specificity	Citations
MSVT	With profile analysis	ID, Dem[c]	.40–.766[c,e,f]	.94–1.00	Singhal et al., 2009; Bashem et al., 2014; Chafetz & Biondilillo, 2013; Weinborn et al., 2012; Larson et al., 2015; P. Green & Flaro, 2015, 2016; Suesse et al., 2015
NV-MSVT	With profile analysis	ID, Dem	.88, .96 Sim .47–.92 KG	.885, 1.00	Singhal et al., 2009; Henry et al., 2010; Armistead-Jehle & Gervais, 2011; P. Green & Flaro, 2016; Armistead-Jehle & Denney, 2015

NOTE: Figures do not apply to defendants with severe cognitive impairment or SMI unless otherwise noted. Sim = simulator group; KG = known group.

[a]SMI = serious mental illness; ID = intellectually disabled; Dem = dementia.

[b]Specificity figure does not apply to ID examinees or those with dementia.

[c]Figure is for subjects with a 3.1 or greater reading level on WRAT-4.

[d]This range of figure excludes Eichstaedt et al.'s (2014) group of bilateral temporal lobe epilepsy patients because of its small size ($n = 3$). Further, the subjects who failed in the studies with lower specificities were reported to show other indications of poor effort/validity.

[e]Sensitivity figures include both for failing A criteria and for doing so with an implausible profile.

[f]The highest value cited is from a simulator study. Typical values from actual examinees tended to be much lower, around .45.

ability to engage in other, more demanding tasks. Lastly, the amount of effort required to complete a given PVT likely depends on the examinee's knowledge and intellectual ability: Grouped dot counting is a nearly effortless task for persons of average intelligence and basic arithmetic skills; it would not be effortless for someone who lacks those qualities.

NOTES

1. No information is provided about the disability status of subjects or whether they were told the results would be confidential. Regarding the instructional set, little is said other than to state subjects were paid $5 for their participation, and that they would be paid whether or not they finished the testing protocol. One cannot help but wonder if this contributed to the poor performances reported. Indeed, 9% of subjects produced a *Suppressed* profile on the Nonverbal subtest.
2. I contacted the lead author about possibly obtaining their data for this analysis, but I was informed that they had not administered the multiple-choice, paired-associates, and free-recall subtests (M. Gorissen, personal communication, January 30, 2013).
3. Chefetz compared Social Security examinees who were applying for disability versus those applying for rehabilitation services or to regain parental rights. The only subjects who failed the SVT also were applying for disability payments.
4. Thus it appears that for "hit," a simulator would have to both fail the primary effort indicator and produce an implausible profile. Sensitivity would presumably be much higher if one did not require an implausible profile. However, for patients with moderate or severe head injuries, such a finding would be ambiguous.
5. Data in Rubenzer (2018) were collected in November 2012.

6

Measures of Feigned or Exaggerated Incompetence

Previous chapters have addressed response style indices that are widely employed in clinical psychology, forensic psychology, and neuropsychology. This chapter reviews instruments specifically designed to assess feigned incompetence to stand trial. Two instruments reviewed here focus on feigned ignorance of the legal system and its workings. In contrast, the first test discussed contains items like those found on the SIRS, but contextualized to the situation of a defendant in the criminal justice system.

THE EVALUATION OF COMPETENCE TO STAND TRIAL–REVISED (ECST-R) ATYPICAL PRESENTATION SCALES

The Atypical Presentation (ATP) scales (Rogers, Tilbrook, & Sewell, 2004) are a brief battery of response bias scales at the end of the ECST-R protocol. The ECST-R is sold by Psychological Resources, and a specimen kit, which includes the manual, administration binder and materials, and 25 answer sheets and score profiles, costs $312.00. A packet of 25 answer forms costs $97.00, for a per use cost of $3.88. The ATP questions ask the examinee about psychotic and nonpsychotic symptoms experienced in the courtroom and, separately, the impairment they cause in focusing on the case. The ATP scales contain 28 items, take about 6 minutes to administer, and are primarily designed to act as a screen for feigned incompetence. They are appropriate for examinees aged 18 and older.

In what the manual refers to as the primary validity study, Rogers, Jackson, Sewell, and Harrison (2004) compared simulators to competency restoration patients at a state hospital. A small group of suspected malingerers (n = 8), based on failing SIRS, were also considered. The ATP scales designed to detect feigning all showed very large effect sizes (ds = 1.37 to 2.35) that were consistent across simulators and identified malingerers. Sensitivities at recommended cutoff scores were 72% to 90%, and specificities were 60% to 91%. The specificities are quite good for a screening test, but the sensitivities are lower than ideal. The authors also examined an index (the sum of ATP Psychotic symptoms, Nonpsychotic symptoms, and Impairment scales) for use as a "collaborative evidence" of feigned incompetency. A cutoff score on this index of >14 had a sensitivity of 95%, a specificity of 73%, and an NNP of 98% at the base rate of 21%. The ATP scales performed comparably to the M-FAST and the SIMS, two well-validated screening tests.

Vitacco, Rogers, Gabel, and Munizza (2007) examined the ATP scales among 100 forensic patients, 29 of whom were identified as feigning on the SIRS. The ATP scales again showed large effect sizes, with excellent sensitivity and very good specificity. The best-performing scale, *Psychotic Presentation*, had a sensitivity of 95% and a specificity of 73%. It produced an NNP of 98% with a cutoff score >1 at a base rate of 21%, with discrimination again comparable to the M-FAST and SIMS. Unfortunately, the authors did not report cross-validation for the index reported by Rogers et al. (2004).

Two studies reported positive results in student simulator designs. Norton and Ryba (2010) found the ATP scales effectively distinguished student simulators from students responding honestly but had substantial false positive rates. Further, the ATP scales showed smaller effect sizes (ds = .80 to 1.40) than the ECST-R's competency scales, all of which had very large effect sizes (ds = 1.48 to 1.95). However, this finding could be an artifact of using a normal control group rather than mentally ill defendants. Springman and Vandenberg (2009) found the ATP scales quite resistant to coaching, which included instructions to avoid endorsing bizarre items, in student simulators. A cutoff score >5 on the composite index explored by Rogers et al. (2004) misclassified 47% of honest responders as malingerers but detected 97% of both uncoached and coached simulators. Large effect sizes were reported for both uncoached (Cohen's d = 1.97) and coached (Cohen's d = 2.12) simulators and a student control group. Of course, this is much less impressive than if the control group had been SMI patients.

The ATP scales tap several possible styles of feigning incompetence, but they emphasize reports of psychiatric symptoms manifested in the courtroom. There is no protection against defendants who present as cognitively impaired, as ignorant of the court system, as amnesic for the crime, or who confine reports of psychiatric impairment to outside the courtroom. Nonetheless, the ATP scales are brief and have good evidence of validity; if used as part of the ECST-R, they pose no additional cost and require modest additional time. Hopefully, further research will examine whether the ATP scales can play a diagnostic role in response style assessment.

ATP SUMMARY

Pros:

- Brief, requires no additional material or cost beyond the ECST-R.
- Performed very well as a screening test in several studies.
- Unique focus on mental illness in the context of adjudication.
- Has been researched in multiple CST-related samples.

Cons:

- Only two studies using SMI control subjects.
- Does not assess some frequent presentation styles of defendants feigning incompetence.
- Very limited data to support its use as evidence of feigning.

INVENTORY OF LEGAL KNOWLEDGE (ILK)

The ILK (Musick & Otto, 2010; Otto, Musick, & Sherrod, 2010) is a 61-item true-false structured interview, published by Psychological Assessment Resources, that utilizes both below-chance performance and normative comparisons to assess performance level. Despite its name, the ILK does not purport to measure legal knowledge, only the feigned lack of it. A specimen kit including 25 answer sheets costs $158.00, and additional answer sheets cost $63.00 for a packet of 25 ($2.52 per administration). The ILK is billed as appropriate for ages 12 to 99 and as taking 15 minutes to administer.

A few years after the ILK was released, CST examiners (see Chapter 10) reported using it nearly as often as the TOMM and more often than the FIT. ILK scores correlate substantially with cognitive validity tests like the FIT and the TOMM (Otto, Musick, & Sherrod, 2011). Normative data are available for defendants in competency restoration programs and for general forensic patients. However, data for only a small sample ($n = 17$) of defendants judged to be genuinely incompetent are presented. This is the most crucial comparison group for the ILK, since the task of the examiner will be to distinguish those examinees who are feigning from those with genuine CST-related impairment. Although the publisher recommends a cutoff score of 47 or less for suspected feigning, the mean score of genuinely incompetent defendants was reported to be 40.6 ($SD = 8.53$). Thus, nearly all incompetent defendants would be misclassified. Rubenzer (2011a) advised against using the recommended cutoff score for this reason (see also Gottfried, Hudson, Vitacco, & Carbonell, 2017; Rogers, Robinson, & Henry, 2017; Watson & Kivisto, 2017) and suggested that only significantly below-chance performance be used as evidence of feigning until more supportive data are presented. However, using below-chance performance means that the ILK's sensitivity to malingering will likely be below 20%—arguably too low to be useful.

No norms are available for ID defendants, and Gottfried and Carbonell (2014) recently provided evidence that the ILK performance is correlated ($r = .47$) with Shipley-2 Vocabulary IQ scores. Shipley scores were obtained in the same setting as ILK scores and thus could be confounded with poor effort. Gottfried (2013) reported ILK scores were related to dichotomized M-FAST scores ($\geq$6, <6; AUC = .79) and psychologists' ratings of the probability of feigning (AUC = .73), providing evidence of moderate convergent validity.

Rogers et al. (2017) examined whether 70 inmates with extensive criminal histories had sufficient knowledge to accurately answer all the ILK's items. They found that only 28 of the ILK's 61 items were correctly answered by 95% or more of the inmates. Although the authors found excellent discrimination for simulators on the ILK's total scale and for the modified scales they investigated, there was no indication that incompetent subjects were included in the analysis. Gottfried et al. (2017) also presented diagnostic statistics for lower cutoff scores. However, like the primary control groups in the ILK manual, control subjects were in treatment for an average of 2 months and cannot be assumed to be incompetent to stand trial at the time of testing.

Watson and Kivisto (2017) noted that no subjects in Gottfried and Carbonell (2014) were diagnosed with ID. They examined ILK performance among 32 ID day patients with a mean IQ = 59.8 (*SD* = 17.3). The reported a mean ILK score of 34.0 (SD = 4.7), far below the recommended cutoff score (< 47). Further, they found that no cutoff score was useful in distinguishing presumed honest ID participants from simulators, and reported an AUC of .534.

In sum, the ILK can distinguish feigning examinees from general population inmates and examinees with treated mental illness, but it has not demonstrated low false positives among ID or incompetent defendants. This is a significant limitation, as the primary aspiration for a validity test is to distinguish true from feigned presentations of specific impairment.

ILK SUMMARY

Pros:

- The only published instrument designed to assess feigned ignorance of the court system.
- Correlates well with cognitive PVTs.
- Already widely used by CST examiners.
- Covers a wide range of CST-related topics; has good face validity as an actual CST knowledge test.

Cons:

- No evidence that it can distinguish those who are feigning incompetence from those who truly are impaired absent below-chance performance.

- Not suitable for ID defendants.
- The only published review is critical and recommends against use of publisher's cutoff score.
- Low sensitivity (<.20) if significantly below-chance performance is used as the criterion for failure.

TEST OF MALINGERED INCOMPETENCE (TOMI)

The TOMI (K. Colwell, 2017) is a potential rival to the ILK. It consists of two subtests that assess feigned intellectual limitations and feigned ignorance of the court system. Both subtests are 25 items long and can be interpreted by reference to norms for a competency restoration sample or significantly below-chance responding. The TOMI is available through the Global Institute of Forensic Research. There is no charge for the test materials and no manual, with information typically included in a manual (e.g., error rates) being presented in an on-line training program ($249.00; K. Colwell, personal communication, Nov. 27, 2017).

The TOMI has been studied in both simulation and forensic samples (K. Colwell, L. H. Colwell, Perry, Wasieleski, & Billings, 2008; L. H. Colwell & K. Colwell, 2011). Both subscales show moderate to strong correlations with other PVTs, such as the TOMM and the FIT, and with clinical team decisions. The *Legal Knowledge* subtest outperformed the *General Knowledge* subtest overall, and the former is probably of greater inherent interest. In forensic samples, it showed strong effect sizes with all criteria examined, with Cohen's *d*s from 1.7 to 2.6 and AUCs from .90 to .95. Unfortunately, diagnostic statistics were reported for only a single cutoff score, and the authors seem to anticipate use only as a screening test. The available data suggest it performed very well in this capacity, with the *Legal Knowledge* subtest showing very high sensitivity (98% to 100%) and excellent specificity (85% to 88%). These figures suggest that a higher cutoff score could function as strong collaborative evidence of feigning.

Several limitations are important, however. The TOMI has been researched thus far entirely by its creators. The authors also reported that it should not be used with ID individuals and that such persons are prone to false positive errors. This is a serious limitation, as ignorance of the court system sufficient to lead to incompetence is usually in the context of apparent intellectual deficit. Finally, the forensic samples across both studies included only a small number of identified malingerers, and only seven of these were classified based on both treatment team opinion and TOMM results.

TOMI SUMMARY

Pros:

- Correlates well with widely used PVTs.
- Subtests for assessing feigned general ignorance and CST-related ignorance.

- No cost for the test materials.
- Takes minimal time for the examiner.

Cons:

- Not suitable for ID defendants.
- Has not demonstrated ability to accurately classify defendants who are legitimately incompetent.
- New, not widely known or used in CST exams.
- Lack of a manual could cause or support a *Daubert* challenge.

LESSONS FROM THE PAST AND FUTURE DIRECTIONS

Thus far, instruments that attempt to assess feigned ignorance of the court system have not demonstrated the ability to discriminate feigning from genuine incompetence. This appears to be a challenging issue: Gothard, Rogers, and Sewell (1995) and Rogers et al. (2002) found that multiple detection strategies, including floor effect and performance curve analysis, were ineffective because of low specificity among defendants identified as incompetent.

Although the validity tests reviewed in this chapter focus on knowledge or ignorance of the legal system, the more relevant issue may be the defendant's capacity to learn what he or she doesn't initially know and remember and apply this knowledge. Many defendants will lack knowledge of some aspects of their case or workings of the court system, but as long as they can learn and remember this information, their competency is not in question. Thus, validity tests that assess factual knowledge might assess performance both before and after tutoring, as suggested by Grisso (2005), and distinguish between initial knowledge and the capacity to learn. Test developers could draw on the success of tests like the WMT and the MSVT that involve presenting material to be learned and then testing retention in multiple ways, comparing performance on memory tests of known relative difficulty.

At the time of this writing, instruments to assess feigned ignorance are less developed, powerful, and useful than tests of feigned psychopathology and cognitive impairment. If they are used, they should be supplemented by tests in these other domains, as well as with collateral data. The ATP scales are well supported as screening tests.

7

Means of Combining or Summarizing Data

A thorough CST evaluation can produce a wealth of data suggesting invalid responding. There is no established means to combine the various observations and test scores. Studies of feigning in forensic settings have often relied on one of several criteria: performance on the SIRS, judgment of the treating psychiatrist or the clinical team, and, rarely, formal decision rules such as the Slick criteria.

Each of these criteria has substantial limitations pertaining to feigned incompetency. As noted in Chapter 4, the SIRS and SIRS-2 have imperfect sensitivity and specificity, are weak in detecting feigning of cognitive limitations, and do not assess ignorance of the court system. Reliance on clinical judgment is problematic given the unknown reliability and validity of such judgments. Further, there is a world of difference between a subjective clinical judgment based on an intake interview and a careful opinion based on prolonged contact, external collateral information, validity testing, and 3 months of observation in a forensic setting by a seasoned and well-trained staff. When clinical judgment is invoked as a criterion, it is essential to articulate the data that underlie it, and assessment of inter-rater reliability is crucial. The Slick criteria, although well specified and thorough, are not without problems. They are relevant to CST assessment, however, as a substantial number of pretrial examinees do present with cognitive impairment (see the survey data in Chapter 10, this volume). Finally, examiners should be aware that, at least in neuropsychological assessment, there is evidence that feigning one domain (e.g., cognitive, psychopathology) does not necessarily indicate feigning in another (Van Dyke, Millis, Axelrod, & Hanks, 2013).

THE SLICK CRITERIA FOR MALINGERED NEUROCOGNITIVE DYSFUNCTION

The Slick criteria (Slick et al., 1999) were designed to facilitate reliable encoding of all the data that might be used to judge the validity of an examinee's presentation during a neuropsychological evaluation. This includes PTVs, scores on self-report validity scales, and *marked* inconsistencies among observations, sources, and the known course and presentation of a given condition. Four criteria are specified: (a) the presence of a readily identifiable motive for feigning, (b) performance suggestive of feigning or malingering on cognitive tests, (c) self-report data suggestive of feigning, and (d) observed indicators that are not completely accounted for by a genuine mental condition. Criteria b and c have specific subcriteria. When sufficient criteria are met, the decision rules allow for classification of *possible, probable*, or *definite* malingered neurocognitive deficit. *Significantly below-chance* (SBC; $p < .05$) performance on any measure is necessary and sufficient to assign a designation of *definite* malingering if there is an identified external incentive and the presentation is not fully accounted for by a psychiatric disorder.

The Slick criteria have been widely cited and utilized in the neuropsychology literature, with 1790 citations[1] in Google Scholar as this is written (November 2017). Bianchini, Greve, and Glynn (2005) offered similar criteria for the determination of malingered pain, and G. Young (2014) proposed criteria for malingered PTSD, pain, and cognitive dysfunction.

Several authors have criticized or suggested revisions to the original criteria. Boone (2007b) noted that some patient groups, particularly somatoform patients, may produce below-chance scores. Rogers, Bender, and Johnson (2011) asserted the Slick criteria are biased toward a finding of malingering because the inclusion criteria are permissive (e.g., "the presentation *suggests* feigning/malingering"), but the exclusion criteria are stringent (e. g., "the presentation is not *fully* accounted for by a psychiatric disorder"). They argued that one must not confound the presence of a potential incentive (e.g., escaping the death penalty) with a motive present in the examinee, since the examinee might prefer death over life in prison. They also noted that different validity tests are treated equally, despite wide differences in their sensitivities and diagnostic value. Rogers et al. stated that most of the specific Slick criteria have not been empirically tested, as there has been little research on professional judgments about whether a presentation is inconsistent with collateral sources or the known course of a syndrome. They noted that inconsistencies can arise from a variety of factors other than negative response bias, including misunderstanding, clerical error, differences of perspective, and benign mental error. They concluded the inclusion of such judgments renders the Slick criteria unreliable and urged caution against overinterpretation if the Slick criteria are to be used at all.

Others have argued for either more stringent or more lenient criteria. Kane and Dvoskin (2011) and G. Young (2014) suggested a finding of *definite* malingering be withheld unless an examinee produces scores on *two* forced-choice measures that are SBC, while lesser levels of proof are required to question the validity of an examinee's presentation. Boone (2007b) and Larrabee, Greiffenstein, Greve, and Bianchini (2007) argued that failure on three validated, independent SVTs should be sufficient to warrant a *definite* malingering classification, whereas only below-chance performance justified such certainty in the original Slick criteria. Slick and Sherman (2013) proposed that any combination of test results sufficient to yield a probability of feigning (i.e., PPP), after considering base rate and test results, of ≥95%, suffices. Greve and Bianchini (2005) and Slick and Sherman (2012, 2013) proposed that a single "compelling" or "unambiguously incompatible" inconsistency between an examinee's representations and reliable collateral data is sufficient to conclude *definite malingering*.

Slick and Sherman (2013), discussing revised criteria, allow three *marked* inconsistencies to justify a *probable* malingering determination. However, no number of marked inconsistencies, even combined with suggestive validity test performance, permit a finding of *definite malingering*. Others (Curtis, Greve, Bianchini, & Brennan, 2006; Greve, Bianchini, Love, Brennan, & Heinly, 2006; Heinly, Greve, Bianchini, Love, & Brennan, 2005; Larrabee, 2003) have reported that examinees who qualify for only a *probable* malingering classification on the Slick criteria produced test scores on neuropsychological measures comparable to simulators and examinees receiving a *definite malingering* classification.

Because of the difficulty objectively determining the motivation or reasons for invalid test performance, some have suggested that the term *malingering* be dropped or changed to a more general term, such as *noncredible presentation* (Boone, 2011) or *noncompliance with test instructions* (Slick & Sherman, 2013). Rogers et al. (2010) wrote that test scores can reveal negative response bias or feigning, but because they do not address the motive of the test-taker, they cannot, in isolation, demonstrate malingering.

The Slick criteria were developed for classifying malingered cognitive dysfunction. As such, they are not designed to capture feigned serious mental illness, ignorance about the court system, or false helplessness—all of which may occur as part of a feigned presentation in a competency exam.

QUANTITATIVE ISSUES AND APPROACHES

Several quantitative approaches have been proposed to objectively weigh evidence of feigning, including below-chance performance and estimating the probability of multiple validity test failures. Crawford, Garthwaite, and Betkowska (2009; see also Mossman, 2000, 2001) noted that sensitivity, specificity, and base rate are all sample-based estimates and that confidence intervals should be constructed around each figure, as well as around the posterior odds estimates (the odds that the examinee is feigning after considering the base rate and test results). In the absence of large sample sizes, these confidence intervals are large, and Crawford et al. provided a software program to calculate them.

Below-Chance Performance

SBC performance is the strongest psychometric evidence in the response bias literature. Although many have followed the convention of using a $p \leq .05$ level of statistical significance, some test authors have recommended more lenient standards. Binder et al. (2014) recommended $p \leq .20$ for below-chance results on standardized forced-choice tests *with empirically derived cutting scores that are at or above the level of 50% correct*. Thus, normative information is considered in conjunction with binomial probability. Binder et al. recommended one-tailed testing, as the hypothesis to be tested is inherently directional: One is interested if the examinee's score is SBC, not above. The effect on TOMM cutoffs is significant: The cutoff for $p \leq .05$ (one-tailed) is $\leq$18, while for $p \leq .20$ it is $\leq$21.[2] In addition, the authors recommend combining statistically independent scores on sections of forced-choice tests such as the VSVT, TOMM, and PDRT *when scores in each section are below 50% correct*, to increase the number of items and the power of significance testing. Thus, it would be permissible to combine trials on the TOMM, but not with the Albany Consistency Index, which is scored *across* different trials. One could combine trials on the WMT, MSVT, and NV-MSVT *Immediate Recognition* and *Delayed Recognition* scales, but not the *Inconsistency* scales, which depend on responses in other scales and thus are not independent.[3] The authors distinguish between forced-choice tests with norms, like most PVTs, and those without, such as the Denney and Frederick crime-specific SVT used to assess feigned amnesia, discussed in the next chapter. For such tests, the authors recommend a one-tailed $p \leq .10$ test. I believe this standard is too permissive given the unique context of the crime-specific SVT. Unlike other PVTs, there are no other tests (other than a Guilty Knowledge polygraph) that can directly assist in determining the validity of responses in this domain. Further, such testing occurs in a criminal context, where the risk is not merely to money but to one's liberty and even one's life, and involves a constitutional-level protection (to not to be prosecuted if incompetent). Further, we have limited reliable data on the base rate of feigned amnesia, particularly for that induced by psychosis, mania, or rage, which will largely determine the PPP of a failed test. For this reason, I believe a $\leq .05$ level is more appropriate, and an even more stringent one ($p \leq .02$ or $\leq .01$) could be justified. However, the sensitivity of the technique would predictably suffer. Another option would be to retain the $\leq .05$ criterion but to weigh this below-chance performance as less definitive than for other tests.

Base Rates

The meaning of a test score, even for below-chance performance, is highly dependent on the base rate. In very low base rate conditions, even a highly sensitive and specific test will yield more false alarms than valid hits. About 30% to 40% of neuropsychological referrals show evidence of poor effort (Larrabee, 2003; Mittenberg et al., 2002; but see Ruff, Klopfer, & Blank, 2016), and published professional standards (Bush et al., 2005; Heilbronner et al., 2009) proscribe that validity testing should be routinely performed for nearly all referrals. In CST samples (other than those referred for neuropsychological evaluation), estimates of feigning are lower—closer to 20% to 25%. However, the base rate is most relevant when *every* examinee receives the given test. If a test is given only to defendants who present as having the symptoms or deficits relevant to the test, the base rate becomes IV / (IV + G), where "IV" = invalid and "G" = genuinely incompetent defendants. If we combine the median values from Chapter 1 (also Chapter 10, this volume) for feigning (all types; 20%), for factitious disorder (1%), and for those who were simply uncooperative (5%) in the numerator for *Invalid* presentations, and use the figure from Pirelli, Gottdiener, and Zapf (2011) for median percentage of CST referrals found incompetent (25.3%), we have (.20 + .05 + .01)/((.20 + .05 + .01) + .253)) = .507 = 50.7%.[4] This is nearly an ideal situation for test usage. However, examiners may also choose to assess for response bias in some defendants that report or display serious psychiatric symptoms but that are nonetheless assessed to be competent. This could add perhaps 10% to 20% to the denominator, which would yield base rates of 42.4% and 36.4%, respectively. It could be argued that the base rates should be estimated separately for each type of validity test (psychopathology, PVT, ignorance of the court system, etc.; Frederick, 2011). Even so, when the rate of invalid presentations is compared with the sum of invalid and valid presentations of a given sort, the ratio is likely to be substantial. Low base rates of invalid responding in CST evaluations are only problematic if every referral is tested.

Chaining Probabilities

Larrabee (2003, 2008) showed how to calculate the diagnostic value of a test finding given the base rate of the condition and validity of the tests, the latter as indexed by the *likelihood ratio* (LR). The LR is the ratio of true positives (sensitivity) to false positives (Sens.÷FP) and will vary by the cutoff score. Larrabee (2003, 2008) noted that PVTs are virtually uncorrelated in genuine patient populations so that multiple PVT failures provide largely independent evidence of invalid performance. Thus, one can estimate the odds of failure on multiple validity tests by multiplying their respective false positive rates (e.g., .10 × .10 = .01 for failure on two tests; see Larrabee [2008] for a more precise formula). However, the more powerful approach is to "chain" pretest probability of response bias (the base rate)

Box 7.1

Likelihood ratio: A number that indicates how much more likely it is that a test-taker with the condition of interest (e.g., feigning) will test positive on the test than someone without the condition. The (positive) Likelihood ratio (LR+) = Sensitivity÷False Positive Rate.

---

and tests' LRs, yielding a probability of response bias after consideration of the base rate and tests.[5]

Larrabee's approach is often applied to embedded validity indicators (e.g., RDS), many of which have modest (e.g., .40–.50) sensitivity but high specificity (typically set at .90 or higher, as recommended by Greve & Bianchini, 2004). Given that PVTs show low intercorrelations in honest samples, using multiple PVTs can compensate for their low individual sensitivities. Larrabee (2003) reported that a rule of failing any two out of five embedded validity indicators (one of which was the FBS scale) had a sensitivity of 87.5% and specificity of 94.4% (see also Larrabee, 2014a, 2014b). Victor, Boone, Serpa, Buehler, and Ziegler (2009) reported similar figures (83.8%, 93.9%) for failing two of four validity indicators. Davis and Millis (2014a) wrote: "These research findings provide evidence that classification accuracy improves with consideration of multiple PVTs and that failure on two of four to nine PVTs is the optimal cutting point" (p. 201).

If avoiding false positives is a paramount concern, many authors (Boone, 2007b; Chafetz, 2011; Davis & Millis, 2014a; Larrabee et al., 2007; Larrabee, 2008; Meyers, Volbrecht, Axelrod, & Reinsch-Boothby, 2011; Meyers et al., 2014; Schroeder & Marshall, 2011; Smith et al., 2014; Victor et al., 2009) have reported near-perfect specificity (e.g., 99%) for a cutoff of three failed validity indicators, although sensitivity is typically modest (e.g., 30% to 50%). Further, and of potentially great importance, both Larrabee (2008) and Meyers et al. (2014) concluded that post-test probabilities (which are equivalent to PPP) remained very high even in low base rate (i.e., 10%) conditions. Several authors (Larrabee et al., 2007; Boone, 2007b) have argued that failure of three well validated, relatively uncorrelated PVTs provides evidence statistically equivalent to below-chance performance on a single measure and is sufficient to conclude *definite* malingering if the other Slick criteria are met.

However, these authors and their conclusions have been challenged by others (Berthelson, Mulchan, Odland, Miller, & Mittenberg, 2013; Bilder, Sugar, & Helleman, 2014; Odland, Lammy, Martin, Grote, & Mittenberg, 2015; Silk-Eglit et al., 2015), who argued that there is a substantial correlation between the number of PVTs administered and the number of PVTs failed. Berthelson et al. reported that the mean correlation observed between validity measures in multiple clinical samples was .31, not zero, which affects probability estimates. Bilder et al. added that a wide range of intercorrelations and false positive rates are observed among individual validity tests and that it is inappropriate to generalize from a mean figure to an undefined set of other measures. They added that prior studies reporting low false positive rates removed subjects with IQs below 80 from their analysis (Schroeder & Marshall, 2011) or excluded those who failed PVTs (Victor et al., 2009), thus biasing the sample. Bilder et al. (2014) reported evidence that the number of PVTs failed increases with low educational attainment or cognitive impairment. They concluded:

> The existing empirical data . . . do not support the generalized application of any criteria that fail to consider the number of tests, the specific tests used in

combination, the population in which the validation was conducted, and the design of the validation study. (p. 1222)

Davis and Millis (2014b) disputed Bilder et al.'s characterization of the correlation between the number of PVTs administered and the number failed as "large"; they reported a correlation of .13, with an increased relative risk of 1.16 (16%) for each additional PVT administered. In great contrast, Odland et al. (2015) reported that if one assumes an average correlation between validity tests of .20 to .50, the number of validity tests administered strongly predicts (*r*s = .96 to 1.00) the number of validity tests failed. Odland et al. provided tables for estimating the cumulative false positive rate for multiple validity tests for multiple levels of intercorrelation between them and assuming different levels (85%, 90%, 95%) of specificity for each test. However, Odland et al. postulated a sensitivity of 69% and specificity of 90% for their tests, using the average figure for PVTs from Sollman and Berry (2011). Although this may be a valid average for stand-alone PVTs, embedded PVTs tend to have much lower sensitivities (Miele, Gunner, Lynch, & McCaffrey, 2011; Silk-Eglit et al., 2015).

Frederick (2015a, 2015b) argued that the results from PVTs that are passed should also be included and counted against a finding of negative response bias. He also asserted that the intercorrelation of tests is not relevant, in contrast to most other authors. He reported that for examinees administered 24 embedded validity tests, many honest examinees failed two, three, and as many as five SVTs, while those classified as feigning produced a bell-shaped distribution around 12 failures. Although the curves were virtually non-overlapping, Frederick's findings illustrate the problem with employing large numbers of SVTs.

Clearly, a number of issues regarding chaining are not settled, and the reader should be aware of the controversy and ongoing developments. It might be tempting to rely on the elaborate tables provided in some of the aforementioned articles, but one should recall that these tests and their intercorrelations and diagnostic statistics have been studied primarily in neuropsychological samples, and psychiatric samples might produce quite different results.

VALIDITY CRITERIA IN PSYCHIATRIC SAMPLES

Schroeder and Marshall (2011) reported only 5% of general psychiatric and neuropsychological patients failed two or more embedded PVTs (including Reliable Digit Span and the Dot Counting Test E score), and only 7% of psychotic patients did. However, they excluded patients with IQs below 79.

Although the SIRS has often been considered the gold standard for feigned psychopathology, Rogers et al. (2010), despite emphasizing the low false positive rate of the SIRS-2, stated emphatically, "No single measure should be used for the determination of feigned mental disorders" (p. 39). Still, given that the SIRS is said to measure feigning, it seems unduly conservative to say no set of scores (e.g., eight primary scales in the *definite* feigning range; all SIRS-2 criteria met) are sufficient to conclude that negative response bias has occurred.

Rogers et al. (2010) have suggested that tests like the M-FAST or the MMPI-2 can be used to raise the pretest base rate/probability for the administration of the SIRS-2. The authors suggest that elevations on MMPI-2 validity scales that are one to two *SD*s above an appropriate reference group could be regarded as indicators of *possible* feigning, whereas "extreme elevations . . . near the upper limit of those reported in MMPI studies" (p. 46) indicate *likely* feigning. However, Rogers et al. discouraged sole use of the MMPI-2 on the grounds that F and Fp have large *standard errors of measurements* (*SEM*s) in a large clinical database, as well as variable cutoff scores. They maintain that similar concerns are present for the MMPI-2-RF.

Although they favor Fp-r over other indices, Rogers et al. (2010) note that it has a large *SEM* (11 T points). However, these large *SD*s and resulting *SEM*s may be partially due to not considering invalid responding in the clinical populations. The much more favorable *SEM* figures cited for the SIRS-2's scales (one raw score point) are due to basing the *SEM* estimates on inter-rater reliability rather than on internal consistency (Rubenzer, 2010).

Rogers (Rogers, 1997; Rogers, 2008c; Rogers et al., 2012, 2013, 2015) has championed the use of the *SEM* to create a band of indeterminacy around a cutoff score. Such borderline scores, due to the error of measurement, cannot be said to reliably exceed the cutoff score. Not surprisingly, accuracy of classification is often much

---

Box 7.2

Standard error of measurement (*SEM*): A number that reflects the uncertainty of a score. Most scores in psychology will be influenced by random, error variance. The *SEM* depends on the reliability of the test and the variability of scores in a sample (standard deviation; *SD*). The formula is $SEM = SD * \sqrt{(1 - \text{reliability})}$. Test scores can be reported as the score plus or minus (±) one or two *SEM*s, which creates a *confidence interval* around the score (e.g., 95 ± 2). For a score ± 2 *SEM*s, the confidence interval has a 95% probability of containing the true score (if it could be measured without error and observed). Thus, the *SEM* is similar to the *SD* for the score of a single subject.

Reliability refers to *consistency*. If I give the test to the same people on different occasions, will they score the same (have test-retest reliability)? If the tests is scored by two different examiners, will they get the same scores for the different examinees (inter-rater reliability)? The last form of reliability, internal consistency, focuses on the items making up the test. Assuming the test is designed to assess a particular concept, all the items should be related to that concept and not other concepts. To the extent that they do, to a high degree, the test will have high internal consistency. This is measured by an index called *Cronbach's alpha*, which varies from 0.00 to 1.00. This can be interpreted as the percentage of reliable data in a test, so that a test with an alpha of .80 contains 80% reliable variance, 20% error.

---

lower, often near chance, for borderline scores than those that are more extreme (Rogers et al., 2012, 2013; but see Wooley & Rogers, 2015). The implication of this is that cutoff scores on the MMPI-2 or RF be further adjusted to account for the *SEM*. In the case of Fp, the cutoff would be raised from ≥100 to ≥110. This will no doubt decrease sensitivity and increase specificity, at the expense of yielding inconclusive results in perhaps 20% to 30% of examinees. However, the MMPI has numerous response indicators, and failing multiple indicators, even within the *SEM* of each scale, is likely to produce greater PPP than failing one indicator. To my knowledge, this has yet to be demonstrated.

There are a couple of difficulties in applying Rogers' approach. For most tests, multiple types of reliability statistics are reported. Most often these include internal consistency and test-retest reliability, as inter-rater reliability is irrelevant for self-report or objectively scored tests. Which one should be used to calculate the *SEM*? Rogers et al. (2010) used the inter-rater reliability for the SIRS-2. However, this figure produces much smaller *SEM*s than would use of the internal consistency or test-retest reliability figures. Further, the authors then compared the *SEM*s for the SIRS calculated on inter-rater reliability with those of the MMPI-2 based on internal consistency, resulting in much larger *SEM*s for the MMPI-2. Ideally, *SEM*s should account for all sources of error (internal, inter-rater, and test-retest *un*reliability; Suen, 1990), but none of the test manuals reviewed in this volume report the appropriate statistic, the generalizability coefficient. Further, PVTs seek to document *inconsistency* of performance, not consistency, so high internal consistency would not be expected among feigners.

One means to estimate a usable *SEM* is short interval retesting, on the order of a few days, within the same motivational context. In other words, the examinee should have the same set of incentives on both occasions, and this should be tightly controlled or monitored. Another approach would be to estimate internal consistency and *SEM* separately for honest and feigning examinees. Because self-report validity scale items do not tap genuine symptom clusters, low reliability is expected among honest responders, but higher reliability is anticipated for feigners because they are manifesting the construct the scale measures—exaggerating/feigning. Conversely, there should be little variation of scores among honest responders (who typically obtain very low scores), but high variability is often observed in feigning samples. Thus, two offsetting factors suggest *SEM*s might be different for sincere test-takers and those showing negative response bias. Alternatively, reliability and *SEM*s can be estimated on a combined sample of honest and invalid responders. Relying on such estimates from only one sample risks mispecifying the reliability, *SD*, and *SEM* for the other group.

A few studies have examined incremental validity of psychopathology validity scales across measures. Rogers, Hinds, and Sewell (1996) reported MMPI-A validity scales and SIRS scores showed incremental validity over each other among adolescents. Lewis et al. (2002) reported the SIMS Total Score did not improve prediction of SIRS classification over MMPI-2 validity indicators. Boccaccini et al. (2006) reported PAI NIM and the MMPI-2 F scale both displayed incremental validity over the other. Gaines (2009) found that although the M-FAST Total score was more accurate than the PAI NIM and MAL scales, MAL (and several clinical subscales) added incremental validity in predicting SIRS classifications.

COMBINED USE OF SVTs AND PVTs

Several studies have examined the use of both psychopathology and cognitive validity tests in forensic or CST examinees (Duncan & Ausborn, 2002; D. Green, 2010; D. Green et al., 2012; Hayes, Hale, & Gouvie, 1998; Lewis et al., 2002; Rosenfeld, Green, Pivovarova, Dole, & Zapf, 2010; Schretlen & Arkowitz, 1990; Schretlen, Van Gorp, Wilkins, & Bobholz, 1992). These studies generally support the use of validity tests targeting both feigned psychopathology and cognitive impairment, although Hayes et al. reported the SIRS produced an accuracy rate of 95% alone—in ID examinees subjects no less!

Although several authors in the neuropsychological literature argue that failure of two validity tests (mostly PVTs) warrants strong suspicion of feigning, there have been few studies in psychiatric samples. Rosenfeld et al. (2010) reported 17.2% of psychiatric patients with no apparent incentive to feign failed two validity tests (an abbreviated SIRS, MMPI-2, VIP Verbal, TOMM), and 3.4% failed three. However, the MMPI-2 consistency indices (VRIN and TRIN) were not scored, there was no motivation given for patients to perform well on what must have been a tedious and personally meaningless task, and over half of the control subjects were apparent false positives (T > 106) on the MMPI-2 F scale. D. Green et al. (2012; see also D. Green, 2010) reported that of 16 of 23 patients suspected of feigning by psychiatrists, 8 were classified as genuine on the SIRS, and 8 more fell in one of the two indeterminate classifications. Seven of these 16 patients failed two or more PVTs. Thus 7 out of 23 suspected feigners (30.4%) were classified as such only because of the PVTs administered in addition to the SIRS. D. Green (2010) reported that if any two validity tests were failed, 90.9% of genuine forensic patients would be accurately classified, and half of suspected malingerers (50.0%) and simulators (55.6%) identified. If failure on three measures was required, 25% of both suspected malingerers and simulators were correctly identified, and specificity was 97.7%. The sensitivities may be lower here than in neuropsychiatric samples because Green employed only four validity tests to cover feigning of both psychopathology and cognitive dysfunction, where others used as many as nine PVTs focused on cognitive underperformance.

DEALING WITH CORRELATED MEASURES

A difficulty arises in how to treat results from tests like the MMPI-2 or MMPI-2-RF, which may have quite a few, but highly intercorrelated, fake bad indicators. On the one hand, they cannot reasonably be treated as if they are independent PVTs, as in Larrabee's chaining procedure. On the other hand, the SIRS/SIRS-2 allows for three (highly intercorrelated) scales in the *probable* feigning range to justify a *definite* feigning classification. In the field of risk assessment, Babchishin, Hanson, and Helmus (2012) reported that even highly correlated measures added incrementally to predicting recidivism among sex offenders, and the average of multiple correlated tests performed better than the individual measures.

Millis (2009) advocated the use of logistic regression to optimally weigh and combine continuous variables, including those that are substantially intercorrelated. Using a formula based on the natural logarithm, one can calculate the probability that a particular subject performed invalidly given the data. Millis advised against rigid application of cutoff scores on individual tests, noting that this does not make optimum use of the data. A drawback of Millis's approach is that a standard, previously researched test battery is required. This appears to await the designation of a standard battery and is made less practical by the variety of ways in which a defendant can present invalidly during a CST exam. However, Gaines (2009) reported the successful use of this approach combining scores from the M-FAST and PAI.

CRITERIA FOR FEIGNED INCOMPETENCE TO STAND TRIAL

This author spent considerable time attempting to formulate criteria for feigned incompetence analogous to the Slick criteria. I had hoped to create parallel criteria for feigned cognitive and psychopathology presentations, to include and weigh discrepancies between data sources, and to tentatively incorporate behavioral observations and fact patterns described by Drob et al. (1987), Soliman and Resnick (2010), and Cornell and Hawk (1989). However, there has been little empirical research to guide the weight such observations should be given and many issues on which criteria would be arbitrary, such as the number of *marked* discrepancies necessary to conclude *possible* or *definite* feigning.

A further challenge is that the intercorrelation of validity measures, from the various domains (cognitive, psychopathology, knowledge of the court system), has not been studied in honest clinical populations. The available evidence suggests measures of feigned psychopathology are substantially correlated in clinical groups (PAI NIM and MMPI-2 F, $r = .54$, Morey, 1991; MMPI-2 F and Fp, $rs = 61–.67$, Tellegen & Ben-Porath, 2008). This renders some statistical approaches, such as chaining probabilities, unworkable within the psychopathology domain. This being said, I believe that failure on a SIRS-2, or a PAI, MMPI-2, or RF with either an extreme elevation (at least one *SEM* above the appropriate, validated cutoff score) on an established validity indicator or two scores above validated cutoff scores (Wiggins, Wygant, Hoelzle, & Gervais, 2012), is sufficient to conclude probable exaggerated psychopathology in most cases, unless (a) internal consistency indices are elevated, or (b) the tests are given to a subsample with a low base rate.

Thus, the psychopathology and cognitive domains of exaggeration have different parameters, and those of the feigned ignorance of the court system have yet to be clearly mapped. A unified set of criteria appears currently out of reach. After reviewing the various options and the data currently available, I found no better approach than that presented by Rogers (2008d), who suggested that examiners focus on the strength and confluence of findings, and that indicators of dissimulation be ranked with regard to whether they cannot be accounted for by alternative explanations (e.g., poor cooperation or a characteristic histrionic presentation).

FEIGNING VERSUS UNRELIABLE RESPONDING/LACK OF COOPERATION

It has often been recommended that a finding of malingering should be made only on the basis of very strong evidence, as such a finding may deprive a patient of needed treatment and be very stigmatizing to the court. To this end, cutoff scores for diagnostic (as opposed to screening) validity tests have typically been set to minimize false positive errors at the expense of sensitivity. However, such an approach ignores the competing needs of society and victims, who may see justice evaded or delayed by a defendant who successfully feigns incompetence. While the justice system may also consider false positives more problematic in a CST context because the defendant has an absolute right not to be tried while incompetent, the relative weight of diagnostic errors is a matter of values, and thus beyond the ken and authority of a mental health professional (Melton et al., 2007).

One need not supply a label of malingering to note that the defendant's presentation is invalid or unreliable. A finding of malingering is distinct from, and requires additional judgments about motivation and awareness than, a finding that the data are unreliable. In CST cases, the latter issue is primary: If the defendant is assumed to be motivated and honest, his or her answers to questions about the legal system are assumed to approximate the actual level of comprehension. This is a questionable assumption in a forensic context, where performing badly may prevent or postpone prosecution for criminal charges. Recent research has shown that good effort cannot be assumed, including in children (Kirkwood & Kirk, 2010; Kirkwood et al., 2010; S. L. Wise & Smith, 2011) and voluntary participants in research (An, Zakzanis, & Joordens, 2012; Frederick et al., 1994; Giger & Merten, 2013). There is no reason to presume that defendants facing charges perform to the best of their ability. Legitimate seriously mentally ill patients may be at particular risk for poor engagement and motivation (Dandachi-FitzGerald, Ponds, Peters, & Merckelbach, 2011; Gorissen et al., 2005; Marcopulos et al., 2014; Schroeder & Marshall, 2011). Gorissen et al. were most emphatic:

> Researchers and clinicians should be extremely careful in interpreting neuropsychological test results of psychiatric patients, and schizophrenic patients in particular. One should not blindly assume that they are performing to the best of their ability, even if they seem cooperative. (p. 206)

These perspectives call into question previous conclusions about significant cognitive deficits in schizophrenics (Heinrichs & Zakzanis, 1998).

Several published studies (Fox, 2011; Meyers et al., 2011; Proto et al., 2014; Rienstra et al., 2013) have presented compelling evidence that failure of even a single PVT with good specificity compromises interpretation of other cognitive test scores: Expected correlations between brain injury severity and performance on neuropsychological measures are not observed if poor effort cases are not removed from the sample. Meyers et al. (2011) showed that failure of a single validity test led to strong suppression (Cohen's $d = 1.32$) of cognitive test scores and was associated with a larger decrement than the difference between one and two failed validity tests ($d = .76$). Proto et al. (2014) reported similar findings, although the effect of failing one PVT was smaller (about half a standard deviation) across neuropsychological tests. Further, while the PVTs were largely uncorrelated among examinees who showed no evidence of feigning, they intercorrelated strongly among those that failed one PVT. This could not be explained by cognitive impairment, as all subjects were mTBI patients assessed more than 3 months after the index injury. In the presence of failure of any PVT with a specificity of 90% or better in a sizable ($n \geq 30$), representative sample for the given defendant, data from the defendant should be regarded as of questionable validity within that domain. An exception might be if the test entailed significant demands or tedium that was not present during the interview or other tests.

Similar to the relation between cognitive PVTs and subjective memory complaints, failure on MMPI-2-RF validity scales is associated with significantly higher scores on MMPI-2-RF symptom scales (Demakis, Gervais, & Rohling, 2008; Forbey, Lee, Ben-Porath, Arbisi, & Gartland, 2013; Wiggins et al., 2012), whereas the generalization to collateral self-report instruments, such as the MMPI-2-RF to the PAI, are mixed (Crighton, Tarescavage, Gervais, & Ben-Porath, 2015; Forbey et al., 2013; Wiggins et al., 2012). Nonetheless, a positive finding on any well-validated self-report validity indicator that is appropriate for the examinee is a red flag that data provided by self-report may be unreliable.

INQUIRY INTO INVALID PERFORMANCE

Once it has been determined that negative response bias is present, the examiner may, and according to Rogers et al. (2010), *should*, ascertain the motivation or cause. Frederick (2011) asserted that validity test failures, in the context of a CST evaluation, are usually the result of malingering. In contrast, Drob, Meehan, and Waxman (2009) asserted that lack of cooperation, factitious disorder, and somatoform disorders may be misdiagnosed as malingering by forensic examiners who fear being fooled by a malingerer.

Several strategies can help make this distinction. First, if a person has a factitious or somatoform disorder, one would expect evidence of such before the person ran into legal difficulty, or between such episodes for multiple offenders. Factitious disorder cannot be diagnosed if it is manifested only in the context of external incentives, and claiming a psychiatric disorder while in custody and facing charges has a plethora of such benefits. Second, although somatoform disorder examinees occasionally claim to have unusual symptoms, these are typically somatic, and they usually do not fail PVTs unless involved in litigation (P. Green, 2013). *Lack of cooperation* can be specific to the exam or can manifest in other situations as well. An analysis of the rewards and disincentives for other situations may help clarify the matter, as may talking to persons who have regular contact with the defendant. Finally, one can consider the base rates from Chapter 10 (see also Martin et al., 2015): Feigning (all types) was perceived to be the most common form of invalid responding (M = 24.1%; Mdn = 20%), followed by *lack of cooperation* (M = 8.7%; Mdn = 5%), somatoform disorder (M = 1.9%; Mdn = 1%), and factitious disorder (M = 1.2%; Mdn = 1%). Examiners should be particularly attentive to poor cooperation, as opposed to feigning, in juveniles or young offenders, in defendants who object to the competency referral, and in those with either acute or chronic serious mental illness.

CHAPTER SUMMARY

There are multiple approaches to synthesizing the data and observations from a forensic evaluation, although no standard of practice has emerged. A few principles can be articulated, however. It appears widely agreed that examiners should understand and make use of base rate data, although most authors emphasize the base rate for the entire sample. In contrast, I have argued for the importance of the base rate among those examinees who present as significantly impaired. Examiners should rely on tests that have been successfully cross-validated for the purpose they are being used on subjects similar in demographics and other relevant variables to the examinee (American Psychological Association, 2013). There is broad agreement within the field of forensic psychology on the importance of collateral data but, as of yet, little empirical work on how examiners can make optimal use of it. SBC performance on any measure is strong evidence of negative response bias. Other important points include the following:

- Although SBC performance has traditionally employed a 5% ($p < .05$) criterion, different standards may be employed depending on the test and circumstances.
- Failure of even one validated PVT with good specificity (>90%) in an appropriate comparison sample is sufficient to raise doubt about the validity of other data in the same domain.
- Unless a large number of PVTs are used and the examinee is legitimately impaired, failure of two qualifying PVTs is substantial evidence of negative response bias, and failure of three is very strong evidence.
- Unlike PVTs, self-report and interview-based measures of psychiatric symptom over-reporting tend to be highly intercorrelated and thus may not show the same incremental validity as multiple PVTs.

- Applying a label of *malingering* has implications beyond more general terms such as *feigning* or *negative response bias* and should be used responsibly.
- Focus on the validity of data obtained rather than malingering.

NOTES

1. Based on a search using "Slick criteria malingering."
2. These figures were determined from the Vassar Stats web page and differ somewhat from those reported in Binder et al. (2014).
3. In contrast to some standardized PVTs, Green's MV-MSVT and MSVT contain stimulus probes with nonrandom locations of the correct answers. Binder et al. (2014) suggest a more conservative approach when applying significance testing to tests with nonrandom locations of the answers.
4. Using the mean figure of 27.5% (instead of the median value) from Pirelli, Gottdiener, and Zapf (2011) produces nearly the same result (48.6%). If mean values from Chapter 10 are used here as well, the result is 55.3%. Somatoform disorders were not included in these calculations.
5. The procedure for chaining the base rate and test results is as follows: Establish the base rate, then convert it to the pretest odds using this formula: Pretest odds = BR/(1 − BR). Multiply the pretest odds by the LR of the first test to yield the post-test odds. This can be converted back to a post-test probability of feigning (which is the same as Positive Predictive Power): Post-test probability/PPP = Post-test odds/(Post-test odds + 1.0). This process can be repeated for multiple tests. A spreadsheet to perform these calculations is available from the author.

8

Special Problems and Populations in Feigned Incompetence

Evaluations of CST most often involve defendants with mental illness, and the primary impediments to competence involve confusion and poor reality perception. However, a substantial portion of defendants claim lack of memory for the offense. The survey of experienced CST examiners (Chapter 10, this volume) found an average of 14.6% (*Mdn* = 10%) of CST examinees feigned amnesia for the offense. There is both case law and methodology related to detection of malingering in this area. A related assessment challenge is for defendants who complain of or present with dissociative symptoms.

A second special population consists of defendants who present with intellectual limitations. Such defendants, and those with borderline intellectual functioning, may be particularly tempted to play up their deficits when faced with prosecution. They present a considerable challenge in that most validity tests are not well studied in this population. In some jurisdictions, there is not a presumption of competence once the question has been raised, so the examiner may have to seek out affirmative evidence of competence, not just opine that the defendant did not present validly. To this end, I present some data on IQ scores for different ID groups that provide some guidance.

Finally, adolescents may be referred for CST evaluation in both juvenile and adult criminal courts. The limited research on this population is reviewed and summarized later in this chapter.

CLAIMED AMNESIA FOR THE OFFENSE

Although one might think amnesia for the crime would seriously impair the ability to assist one's attorney, most appellate courts have held otherwise. The case *Wilson v. United States* (1968) held that amnesia does not automatically render a defendant incompetent and suggested that triers of fact consider several factors that might permit the defendant an adequate defense. The *Wilson* decision is widely cited by forensic professionals, but it has not been persuasive with other appellant courts (Bourget & Whitehurst, 2007; Perlin, 2013; Smith & Resnick, 2007).

Tysse (2005) suggested that courts' usual denial of amnesia claims is based on the fear that most such claims are fabricated. It has been reported that 10% to 70% of murder defendants claim amnesia for the crime, with some writers (Bradford & Smith, 1979; Bourget & Whitehurst, 2007; Kopelman, 1995, 2002; Parwatikar, Holcomb, & Menninger, 1985; Pyszora, Barker, & Kopelman, 2003; Pyszora, Fahy, & Kopelman, 2014) suggesting these are valid claims, whereas others argue that most amnesia claims, in the context of criminal charges, are likely feigned (Centor, 1982; Cima, Nijman, Merckelbach, Kremer, & Hollnack, 2004; Frederick, 2011; Marshall, Serran, Marshall, & Fernandez, 2005; Merckelbach & Christiansen, 2007; Ornish, 2001; Peters, van Oorsouw, Jelicic, & Merckelbach, 2013). Merckelbach and Christiansen (2007) noted that when normal participants are asked to play the role of a murderer who is confronted with evidence of guilt in an interrogation, the most frequent strategy is to claim amnesia. Tysse (2005) suggested that the advent of validity tests makes it viable for the courts to reconsider their position on amnesia and competency.

Porter, Woodworth, and Doucette (2007) noted several motives for claiming amnesia, despite the fact it does not provide a solid defense or claim of incompetency: Feigned amnesia may elicit sympathy from family or jury members, create doubt about guilt, and/or diminish perceived blameworthiness. Merckelbach and Christianson (2007) added three more incentives. First, it allows the defendant to invoke the right to remain silent without seeming uncooperative, and even to provide testimony that is helpful to his or her side. Second, such a claim may trigger what the authors dub "a psychiatric expert cascade," leading to psychiatric testimony, at least some of which is likely to be sympathetic. This may lead to reduced charges or more lenient sentencing. Finally, if convicted, the defendant is spared having to discuss his or her crime with social workers and therapists.

Potential Causes of Amnesia

Amnesia for a circumscribed event, such as a crime, falls under the diagnosis of transient global amnesia (TGA). Arena and Rabinstein (2015) defined TGA as "the sudden onset of anterograde amnesia (the inability to encode new memories) . . . sometimes with a retrograde (prior to the injury or insult) component, lasting up to 24 hours, without the compromise of other neurological functions" (p. 264). Thus, such a person might appear completely normal to an outside observer but would not create and store memories. Observable signs in such a person might include repetitive questioning and appearing restless, nervous, or confused. Arena and Rabinstein posited that TGA results from a distortion of memory pathways, but they reported that medical tests are generally not helpful when conducted after the event. They reported TGA is not rare, with an incidence of 3.4 to 10.4 per 100,000 people, with a much higher incidence (23.5 per 100,000) among those over age 50. The authors discussed three types of potential medical causes: (a) vascular (venous flow disturbances, focal arterial ischemia), (b) epilepsy-related, and (c) migraine-related. However, none were deemed to be well validated. The leading hypothesis is that TGA is caused by abnormal venous draining from the temporal lobes, resulting in hypertension in the medial temporal lobes (Arena & Rabinstein, 2015).

Amnesia has traditionally been divided into cases with a clear biological cause, such as head injury, seizures, somnolence, or intoxication, and those with a functional origin, such as fugue state or dissociative disorder. Amnesia from sleepwalking and for some epileptic seizures has a biological basis and is not controversial (Bourget & Whitehurst, 2007; Cartwright, 2004; R. D. Miller, 2003; Siclari et al., 2010), and alcohol use may play a part: Ohayon, Mahowald, Dauvilliers, Krystal, and Leger (2012) reported alcohol abuse/dependence increased the risk for frequent sleepwalking (odds ratio [OR] = 3.5), as did obsessive–compulsive disorder (OR = 3.9) and sleep apnea (OR = 3.7). Alcohol consumption alone is a major factor in claimed amnesia and is discussed further in the following paragraphs.

Mart and Connelly (2010) reviewed the literature on epilepsy and crime or violence and cited a listing of characteristics from Reuber and Mackay (2008) to help distinguish actual and feigned epileptic crimes (see Box 8.1).

Box 8.1

INDICATORS OF GENUINE EPILEPSY

Evidence of Epilepsy

1. History of epileptic seizures prior to offense
2. History of epilepsy-related automatism prior to offense
3. EEG abnormalities supportive of diagnosis

Offense Characteristics

1. No obvious motives
2. No planning or premeditation
3. Apparent senselessness
4. No attempts at concealment
5. Clearly out of character with defendant's usual behavior

Characteristics of Seizure Associated With Offense

1. Abnormal behavior should last minutes rather than hours
2. Observation of typical seizure features
3. Amnesia for occurrence
4. No anterograde amnesia after the resumption of conscious awareness

---

Complex partial seizures have the most relevance to amnesia, as persons may perform stereotyped activities and have no memory of them. Mart and Connelly (2010) noted that postseizure confusion is probably the epilepsy state most often associated with aggression. Claims of sleepwalking or epilepsy-related amnesia should trigger a medical evaluation by specialists in each respective area apart from a forensic psychological assessment.

Excessive alcohol use, depressed mood, hysterical traits, and claims of prior blackouts are reported to be associated with *claims* of crime-related amnesia (Hopwood & Snell, 1933; Kopelman, 1995; Parwatiker, Holcomb, & Menninger, 1985). Many claims of amnesia in criminal cases will specify no cause. There are two potential causes that are commonly given and may be plausible: use of alcohol and drugs immediately preceding the crime and extreme anger.

Use of alcohol is widespread, and a sizable percentage of crimes (estimates range from 30% to 70%), including homicides, are committed under the influence of alcohol (Bradford & Smith, 1979; Evans, Schreiber Compo, & Russano, 2009). There is little doubt that alcohol and sedative drugs, particularly somnolent drugs like Ambien (Daley, McNiel, & Binder, 2011) or alcohol and some drugs used together (Hartzler & Fromme, 2003), can cause blackouts. Alcohol affects the formation of new memories while leaving many other cognitive capacities relatively intact (Pressman & Caudill, 2013). The blood alcohol content (BAC) usually required to produce a blackout tends to be very high (.25–.30%; Hartzler & Fromme, 2003; Perry et al., 2006, although some blackouts have been reported for BAC levels as low as .07% (Hartzler & Fromme, 2003). One might assume that claims of alcohol-induced blackouts should be accompanied by collateral observations of intoxication or consumption. However, several studies have reported that some people, presumably chronic alcoholics, can reach very high BACs (e.g., .30%, and as high as .511%) without showing typical signs of intoxication (Perper, Twerski, & Wienand, 1986; Roberts & Dollard, 2010; Rubenzer, 2011b; Sullivan, Hauptman, & Bronstein, 1987; Urso, Gavaler, & Van Thiel, 1981). Perry et al. reported that at a BAC of .31, there is greater than 50% probability of a blackout. Blackouts are not uncommon among alcoholics and even samples of students. Most are "partial," in that some memories are encoded and recoverable, whereas those with a total lack of recall occur about one third as often (Pressman & Caudil, 2013; White, 2003). Pressman, Mahowald, Schenck, and Cramer Bornemann (2007), noting the frequent use of alcohol during crimes, estimated that amnesia for a crime is roughly 5 million times more likely due to alcohol intoxication than to a sleep disorder.

Hopwood and Snell (1933) reported that claims of amnesia in murder cases usually involved emotionally intense crimes, and the authors concluded that 78% of these claims were bona fide cases of dissociation or repression. Other authors have endorsed this view (Pyszora, Barker, & Kopelman, 2003; Pyszora et al., 2014). Swihart, Yuille, and Porter (1999) coined the term *red-out* for amnesia following intense emotion or stress. Some authors have focused on homicides and distinctions between those that were planned and deliberate versus those that were "reactive" to provocation or extreme stress. Generally, claims of amnesia are more frequent for reactive crimes than for planned ones and appear to be given greater credibility by professionals. However, Porter and Woodworth (2007) cautioned that the murderers in their sample "always" exaggerated the degree of reactivity present in their crime. Van Oorsouw and Merckelbach (2010) suggested that psychopathy should be routinely assessed in the context of an amnesia claim and murder, and that it weighs against the credibility of the claim. They reasoned that given psychopaths' lack of emotional responsiveness, there is no rationale for amnesia due to extreme emotions.

Dissociation has frequently been proposed as the mechanism leading to amnesia in violent crimes. Many (Frederick, 2011; Merckelbach & Christianson, 2007; Peters, van Oorsouw, Jelicic, & Merckelbach, 2013) have asserted that dissociation is overvalued in the professional literature on amnesia (see also Centor, 1982; Marshall et al., 2005; Ornish, 2001). Merckelbach and Christianson (2007) and Peters et al. (2013) argued that red-outs contradict three well-established memory principles: (a) Memory tends to be better for *actions* as opposed to spoken words; (b) memory is better for acts committed by oneself than by someone else; and (c) people tend to have reoccurring thoughts about events they try to suppress. Merckelbach and Christianson point out there is little evidence of dissociative amnesia in groups that have experienced truly terrible events, including concentration camp survivors or eyewitnesses to violent crimes. Woodworth et al. (2009) reported that although homicide perpetrators reported elevated levels of emotion associated with their crimes and claimed impaired memory, they nonetheless produced *more* detailed accounts of their murders than of their own less serious crimes. McNally (2003) wrote, "The notion that the mind protects itself by repression or dissociating memories of trauma rendering them inaccessible to awareness is a piece of psychiatric folklore devoid of convincing empirical support" (p. 157). Boysen and VanBergen (2014), reviewing empirical findings regarding dissociation, concluded that transfer of information among different personalities in patients with dissociative identity disorder (DID), despite subjective claims to the contrary, was the most reliable finding of their review.

A third possible cause for amnesia is psychosis or mania. Although Taylor and Kopelman (1984) noted a high proportion of persons with schizophrenia or psychosis in samples of homicide offenders, I was unable to find any empirical study addressing amnesia for a crime in such groups.

Assessment Options

Before investing much time in investigating the issue, examiners may want to examine case law regarding amnesia in their jurisdiction: Many appeals courts have held amnesia is not a barrier to competency. If a claim of amnesia is made and is relevant to a defendant's competence, such a claim should trigger efforts to substantiate any claimed medical cause (e.g., epilepsy, sleep-walking) through medical records and perhaps specialized medical testing.

There are now a variety of ways to assess the validity of claimed amnesia, although most have significant limitations. PVTs, like the TOMM and the WMT, can reveal implausible performance on memory tasks. However, a discerning defendant claiming amnesia may see these tasks as unrelated to the condition he or she needs to portray. As one defendant who claimed amnesia for the crime explained to me as I attempted to administer the WMT: "It's not that kind of memory." Thus, failure on a cognitive validity test provides evidence of feigning, whereas passing provides little clear information.

Frederick, Carter, and Powell (1995) and Denney (1996) proposed using the forced-choice paradigm to create a memory validity measure specific to the crime. The offense report, and perhaps the crime scene, would be reviewed for salient details that would be noticeable and memorable to the perpetrator. However, they must be items that the defendant professes no memory or knowledge about. The examiner would then create a series of questions, such as, "What weapon was used to threaten the clerk? A gun or a knife?" The test-taker must choose one option, even if it is only a guess. Each item should be equally plausible to a naive subject, and some authors have suggested pretesting items on a substantial number of test subjects to weed out biased items. The process will hopefully lead to at least 25 acceptable items. The defendant's score is then compared with chance, and SBC scores are considered compelling evidence of feigning. Dawes (1995) challenged some of the technique's provisions, but Frederick and Denney (1998) responded with data to show the technique is robust if the average probability of incorrect answers remains close to 50%. This procedure is sometimes referred to as the *crime-specific SVT*.

Frederick et al. (1995) and Denney (1996) each reported successful applications of the crime-specific SVT in three case studies. Subsequent simulation studies have reported sensitivities of 27% to 60% (Jelicic, Merckelbach, & van Bergen, 2004a, 2004b; Giger et al., 2010; Meijer, Smulders, Johnson, & Merckelbach, 2007; Merckelbach, Hauer, & Rassin, 2002; Shaw, Vrij, Mann, Leal, & Hillman, 2014; Verschuere, Meijer, & Crombez, 2008). Some of these authors used significant modifications of the original protocol (Giger et al., 2010; Shaw et al., 2014) or used fewer items than the 25 recommended (Giger et al., 2010; Meijer et al., 2007; Merckelbach et al., 2002; Shaw et al., 2014), in part because some potential items showed endorsement probabilities of <.3 or >.7 in pretesting. These authors tended to observe fewer below-chance scores. Yet, Shaw et al. (2014) reported that the first half of a 12-item crime-specific SVT was more sensitive than the latter half.

The probability of obtaining a below-chance score from a defendant probably decreases with the amount of his or her secondary education in math and science. Coaching may also degrade sensitivity: Giger et al. (2010) reported only 10% of coached simulators were detected, and Verschuere et al. (2008) reported that none of 19 coached simulators scored below chance.

Even if items are carefully selected, the procedure will theoretically yield a 5% false positive rate. Unlike most SVTs, *chance* level performance *is* plausible and expected in honestly responding examinees. Users should also remember Denney's (1996) caution about the procedure's use: Failures are informative, but passing is not. This is because specificity is high (theoretically 95%), but sensitivity is quite a bit lower.

Meijer et al. (2007) reported that a crime-specific SVT produced a Cohen's *d* of .79 in their first study on a mock crime, which was considerably lower than for the Guilty Knowledge (polygraph) Test. However, the SVT achieved a *d* of 1.68 in their second study, in which subjects portrayed amnesia for their personal history. Although the Guilty Knowledge Test is normally directed at providing evidence of guilt, Meijer et al. showed it could also be used, and add incremental validity, to the SVT procedure. However, it does require specialized equipment and expertise.

Self-report measures also can be useful in the assessment of memory complaints. As reported in Chapter 3, the MMPI-2-RF's COG scale includes items that query about memory and cognitive complaints, and COG predicts PVT performance. The Memory Complaints Inventory (P. Green, 2004b) is a 57-item self-report inventory that queries the test-taker about cognitive problems in a variety of areas, including amnesia for crimes. Data on more than 4,700 examinees from two neuropsychology practices (both in Edmonton, Canada) for several neuropsychiatric groups are available, many subclassified by their performance on other validity tests such as the WMT. However, there are no norms for those who have legitimately experienced episodic amnesia for an event or complex behavior. Armistead-Jehle (2010) and colleagues (Armistead-Jehle, Gervais, & Green, 2012) reported the MCI scales were more strongly related to cognitive validity performance than were validity scales on the MMPI-2, including RBS, in clinical and veteran samples from the US Midwest. The primary value of the MCI would seem to be in identifying excessive memory complaints in areas (e.g., memory interferes with work, numerical memory) that would not be expected to be affected by episodic amnesia. As discussed in Chapter 4, the SIMS has an Amnestic Disorders scale, and the Total Score is quite effective at detecting those who fail standard PVTs.

Giger et al. (2010) assessed the performance of seven validity tests or scales in detecting feigned amnesia for a mock crime. Three tests, the Amsterdam Short-Term Memory Test (ASMT; Schagen, Schmand, de Sterke, & Lindeboom, 1997), a variant of the Morel Assessment of Emotional Numbing (MENT; Morel, 1998), and the SIMS Total Score, performed very well (sensitivities = 95%, 80%, and 95%, respectively), even when subjects were cautioned to be believable and told that the examiner might use specialized tests to assess credibility (sensitivities = 70%, 65%, and 65%, respectively). The crime-specific SVT was less sensitive (45%), particularly when subjects were warned about detection methods (10%). This was true of all the other tests other than the modified MENT. The MMPI-2 validity scales, including RBS and FBS, were relatively insensitive (45% and 50%, respectively), especially when subjects were forewarned about avoiding detection (25%, 10%). The most important finding was the effectiveness of a standard cognitive validity test (the ASMT), and another (the MENT-R) with no obvious relationship to amnesia. Although the SIMS Amnestic Disorders scale obtained a very large Cohen's *d* of 4.5 in separating feigned amnesia from normal controls, this figure is questionable for distinguishing real from feigned amnesia. The findings for the other tests examined would seem more robust because the tests are relatively insensitive to psychopathology or mild brain damage. The authors advocate for a multi-method approach to assessing claims of amnesia, including standard PVTs.

Dissociative Defendants

A small subset of defendants who claim amnesia for the offense will present as having a dissociative disorder, the most dramatic being dissociative identity disorder. Other defendants may present with dissociative symptoms but not claim lack of memory for the offense. As with amnesia for a crime, there are strongly contrasting perspectives on DID, with some authors considering the condition as caused by early trauma and manifested by extreme disruptions of consciousness (Dalenberg et al., 2012; Dalenberg et al., 2014; Dorahy et al., 2014; Vissia et al., 2016) and others arguing it is something of a factitious disorder (where the patient feigns symptoms in order to be treated like a patient with the condition) resulting from fantasy proneness, suggestibility, social influences, and iatrogenic effects (Lynn, Lilienfeld, Merckelbach, Giesbrecht, & van der Kloet, 2012; Lynn et al., 2014; Piper, & Merskey, 2004; Spanos, 1996). However, even DID proponents such as Brand, Tursich, Tzall, and Loewenstein (2014) acknowledge that 2% to 14% of patients presenting to a dissociative disorders clinic are factitious. The authors of *Three Faces of Eve* (Thigpen & Cleckley, 1957) reported that most apparent DID cases they had seen since publication of the book were factitious (Thigpen & Cleckley, 1984).

Coons (1991) examined 18 homicide cases in which the defendant claimed amnesia. Nearly all the defendants were male, two thirds were suspected of feigning, and all but 2 were convicted. Coons, who was especially critical of the use of leading questions and hypnosis, noted that two experts in the Kevin Bianchi case seemed to assume from the start the defendant had DID rather than seeking to do an objective forensic evaluation of the issue. Coons offered a number suggestions regarding forensic assessment of DID, including allowing a minimum of 3 to 5 hours for interviewing, preferably over multiple occasions, and stated, "The need for collateral information cannot be overemphasized" (p. 764). He also provided a list of indicators of feigned DID, which included overly dramatic presentation, no evidence of alter personalities apart from the clinical interview, and lack of symptoms of mental illness apart from the claimed dissociation. Coons concluded that a high index of suspicion of malingering is required by any clinician evaluating a homicide defendant alleging DID.

Coons and Milstein (1994) compared 11 factitious or malingering DID patients with 50 DID patients deemed genuine. They reported presumed genuine DID subjects displayed alter personalities with varying moods (particularly depression and anger) and different accents, and that they reported shared co-consciousness. Factitious DID patients were more likely to be described as highly dramatic and to show *pseudologia fantastica*,[1] "high exaggeration," lack of consistent work history, *la belle indifference* (lack of concern about one's presented symptom[s]), persistent lying, and refusal to allow interviews with collaterals. Factitious patients were also described as typically hostile, demanding, and deprecating in demeanor; to present with inconsistent alters and histories; and to lack a prior history of dissociation. The groups did not differ on MMPI profiles, including the F scale.

A. Thomas (2001) generated a list of hypothesized differences between genuine and factitious DID, then conducted chart reviews of 18 factitious cases and 18 matched DID cases. Reporting of results is primarily narrative, and it appears significance testing was not done for most signs reported. However, some signs (e.g., ability to give a coherent life history) were present in all factitious patients and in very few or none of the DID cases. Thomas reported that persons who were given a diagnosis of factitious or malingered DID had a minimum of 8 of the 12 listed characteristics, whereas DID patients had at most 3 of these features. However, coding was performed by the author, who was not blind to the identity or diagnosis of the patients or hypotheses investigated. Thus, replication is badly needed.

Welburn et al. (2003) tested the ability of several tests and observations to discriminate between DID patients (n = 12) and staff members (n = 10) asked to simulate DID. They found the Structured Clinical Interview for DSM-IV Dissociative Disorders (SCID-D; Steinberg, 1993) to achieve 100% classification accuracy, whereas the MMPI-2 F, F-K, and Fb scales failed to discriminate the groups. However, the feigning group scored over 120 on F, and DID subjects averaged about 104. The *eye-roll* sign (Spiegel & Spiegel, 1978),[2] an observation used to assess hypnotizability, was more often elevated in DID subjects (M = 2.92; SD = 1.00) and was not simulated by feigners (M = 1.20; SD = 0.79). The results were significant and yielded a Cohen's d of 1.91.[3] However, the study is limited by the small sample sizes and the fact that simulators were reportedly given only a single page of instructions to prepare for their role.

Labott and Wallach (2008) reviewed several Rorschach-based systems for diagnosing DID and the small empirical literature surrounding them. These systems have not addressed possible feigning, but Labott and Wallach reported in an empirical study that simulators did not elevate their DID-relevant indices over control subjects. Thus, the absence of genuine DID signs in the context of claims or representations of DID could help establish feigning.

Brand and Chasson (2015) compared 53 DID patients with 77 student simulators, some of whom received coaching, on the MMPI-2. F, Fb, and Fp were all found to significantly distinguish the groups; notably, DID subjects did *not* elevate the VRIN consistency scale. DID subjects scored lower on validity scales and most clinical scales than the simulators. Fp was found to be the best single discriminator, although a discriminant function provided a somewhat better classification. Cutoff scores and classification rates are given in Table 8.1.

Rogers, Payne, Correa, Gillard, and Ross (2009) reported on 87 dissociative patients who produced high scores on most of the SIRS's subscales and produced high false positive rates when the test's standard decision rules were applied. However, three scales (*Improbable/Absurd Symptoms, Symptom Combinations, Reported vs. Observed Symptoms*) had very low levels of item endorsement even among dissociative examinees. Rogers et al. created the Trauma Index (TI) by

Table 8.1 Cutoff Scores and Diagnostic Statistics From Brand and Chasson (2015)

Scale	Cutoff Score	Sensitivity	Specificity
F	96.9	.84	.58
	106.6	.79	.75
	116.4	.76	.83
Fb	97.4	.88	.53
	107.2	.80	.70
	117	.70	.77
Fp	85.4	.85	.79
	98.0	.74	.89
	110.5	.66	.96
Ds2	76.5	.80	.53
	84.7	.60	.72
	93.0	.41	.81

NOTE: Figures for sensitivity and specificity in this table are transposed from those in Brand and Chasson (2015), as those authors calculated sensitivity on the accuracy rate for DID patients rather than simulators, and vice versa for specificity. Figures here were transposed to remain consistent with presentation elsewhere in this book, where sensitivity refers to the detection of feigners. Cutoff scores are not in whole numbers as they were based on z scores (−.5, 0, .5) for the honest and simulator samples combined (B. Brand, personal communication, November 28, 2016).

summing scores from these three scales to create an index of exaggeration or feigning among those presenting with dissociative symptoms. A TI score of >6, when combined with the SIRS's other decision rules, produced a sensitivity of 58% with a false positive rate of 9%.

Brand et al. (2014) also examined the SIRS's use with dissociative patients and utilized the TI. They reported the TI alone (without either the SIRS or SIRS-2 classification rules; TI > 6) provided the highest overall diagnostic classification (83.3%), with a sensitivity of 85.7% and a specificity of 79.6%. The SIRS-2 had low sensitivity (32.5%) but excellent specificity (100%) when those classified as *Feigning* were compared with all other SIRS-2 classifications (*Indeterminate, Genuine*). Sensitivity improved considerably (55.8%) if those classified as *Indeterminate-Evaluate* were considered as hits, and specificity remained good (91.8%). The authors concluded:

> In sum, the SIRS combined with the TI and the TI alone provided the best balance of sensitivity and specificity, with similar overall diagnostic power noted for both methods. However, for forensic, rather than clinical purposes, evaluators can be quite confident in concluding that an individual is feigning DID if they score above the SIRS-2 cutoff of Feign/I-E + TI > 6 (*Feigning* or *Indeterminate-Evaluate* classification AND the Trauma Index is greater than 6). (p. 314)

Several methodological issues in the studies by Brand (Brand & Chasson, 2015; Brand et al., 2014) warrant comment. Although DID patients were said not to be involved in disability claims, there is no mention of lawsuits or criminal charges, and it is not stated how it was determined that patients did not have disability claims. Apart from relying on the patient's self-report, it is hard to see how this could have been achieved. A request to the author for clarification did not resolve the question. Quite apart from tangible incentives, a patient may exaggerate for factitious motives or for other undisclosed or even unconscious reasons. The subjects who simulated DID were asked to study the book *Sybil* (Schreiber, 1973) and/or the movie. Although Sybil was one of the most visible DID cases, an exposé (Nathan, 2011) charged that she was manipulated by her psychiatrist for financial gain, and that Sybil's condition was, as skeptics have alleged for DID cases generally, at least partly iatrogenic. Thus, the model for those simulating genuine DID may have actually been a case of factitious DID. Finally, most recent simulator studies include instructions that emphasize that subjects should fake subtly and not get caught. No such instructions were reported in the Brand et al. simulation studies reviewed.

Two studies (Coons & Milstein, 1994; A. Thomas, 2001) reported that among presumed genuine DID patients, there were dramatic indicators of the disorder during interviews, including switching of alters, identity confusion, and inability to provide a coherent life history or important dates. From the perspective of response style assessment, this author wonders if this behavior was typical or manifested only in the presence of DID-interested mental health professionals. The behaviors described are so odd and seemingly impairing that they would seem certain to draw comment from other professionals (teachers, physicians, employers) and to preclude employment or virtually any activity that requires sustained attention and effort. It might be argued that a focus on personal matters in a clinical interview would trigger more dissociative symptoms than daily tasks, but DID subjects *were* able to respond consistently on the MMPI-2 in Brand and Chasson (2015), a task that not only accesses personal experiences but also is long and tedious. As with other behaviors suggestive of mental illness, the examiner should examine whether the DID behaviors occur outside of situations where they can be used to material advantage. One DID defendant examined by the author claimed lack of memory for the alleged offense, as well as others of a similar nature. However, she signed a document in her own name and handwriting at the time of her arrest.

Dissociative patients tend to score high on self-report validity scales and on the SIRS/SIR-2. They often claim to have no memory for information obtained while in an alter personality state, but implicit memory tests show otherwise (Boysen & VanBergen, 2014; Lilienfeld et al., 1999). Further, two studies (Huntjens et al., 2006; Kong, Allen, & Glisky, 2008) reported several dissociative subjects scored significantly below chance on a memory test conducted with a different personality than who participated in the learning phase. Thus, there are ample reasons to question the accuracy of self-reports of memory problems in DID patients.

SECTION SUMMARY

Claimed amnesia for the offense is not uncommon, but in many cases it does not pose a barrier to competence. However, there are circumstances in which inability to remember the crime scene might seriously impair a defendant's ability to assist in his or her defense. This can include cases in which specific intent is an element of the crime, and when there are co-defendants in serious cases such as murder or armed robbery and accountability will be divided. Professional opinions on the legitimacy of crime-related amnesia are sharply divided.

Examiners do have the capacity to assess feigned amnesia through examination of situational factors, collateral data, and testing. Testing will typically be more informative in the case of failure on validity testing than if the defendant passes. Additional important points include the following:

- Alcohol use is a factor in many crimes. Alcohol can lead to amnesia if used in large amounts or combined with depressant or somnolent drugs and can also contribute to sleepwalking.
- Postepileptic confusion is the most likely cause for epilepsy-related amnesia.
- Dissociation as a cause of amnesia is controversial, and there is evidence of implicit memory in persons who deny memory for events.
- A crime-specific SVT/PVT can be created from memorable details surrounding the offense and can provide strong evidence that a person does remember an event or crime.
- Self-report SVTs and standard PVTs can also play a role in assessing credibility of claims of amnesia.
- If a DID defendant presents as too dissociated to participate in the adjudication, collateral data should be gathered to assess if this presentation is consistent across different situations.

INTELLECTUALLY DISABLED DEFENDANTS

As reported in the earlier chapters, many standard validity tests show excessive false positives when used with ID individuals (Dean, Victor, Boone, Philpott, & Hess, 2009), and others may be inappropriate due to reading demands. This literature has been thoroughly reviewed by several authors (C. L. Ray, 2012; Salekin & Doane, 2009; Victor & Boone, 2007).

The TOMM is the best-researched instrument in this area but has produced variable results. A number of studies found that the standard cutoff scores may be appropriate (Farkas, 2008; Gast & Hart, 2010; Love et al., 2014; Simon, 2007), or that even higher ones (≤ 48) can lead to perfect specificity in low IQ examinees (Smith et al., 2014). However, other publications (Graue et al., 2007; Hurley & Deal, 2006; Proto, 2008; Shandera et al., 2010) reported high levels of false positive errors unless cutoff scores were dramatically lowered. C. L. Ray (2012) suggested that TOMM Trial 2 and Retention Trial scores from 31 to 44 are of suspect validity, and those below 30 are cause for strongly suspecting malingering. Examination of one data set on the TOMM (Shandera et al., 2010) shows the great majority of subjects scored above 45, and that the low cutoff scores recommended were largely attributable to three outliers. These findings are summarized in Table 8.2.

Like the TOMM, the literature on the WMT with ID examinees is mixed. Brockhaus and Merten (2004) reported that all but one *institutionalized* ID subject passed the primary effort indicators, and it was subsequently discovered that the one who failed had actually malingered. However, Dean et al. (2009) and Salekin and Doane (2009) charged that because subjects were selected for testability, they were not representative of ID subjects.[4] Shandera et al. (2010) reported not only that substantial numbers of community-living, civilly competent ID subjects failed the WMT's primary effort indicators but also that community volunteers scored much lower than expected. P. Green and Flaro (2015) responded by requesting and analyzing Shandera's data, and they reported that 33% of the WMTs failed had a poor effort profile and that about half of Shandera et al.'s ID

Table 8.2 Studies of the TOMM in ID Examinees

Study	*n* ID	Sample	Criterion	Sensitivity	Specificity
Hurley & Deal (2006)	39	IQs 50–78	<45 T2	—	.59
Graue et al. (2007)	26	Mild ID, own guardian	<45 T2	.80	.69
			<45 RT	.80	.81
			<30 T2	.56	.96
			<30 RT	.60	.96
Simon (2007)	21	IQs 51–69, CST	<45 T2	—	.95
			<45 RT		1.00
Proto (2008)	11	*M* IQ = 61.1 (*SD* = 3.1)	< 45 T2	.68	.64
Farkas (2008)	43	IQs 50–75	<45 T2	.91	.84
Shandera et al. (2010)	24	Mild ID	<45 T2	.40	.88
			<45 RT	.44	.92
			<30 T2	.24	.96
			<30 RT	.20	1.00
Gast & Hart (2010)	13	Adolescent pretrial defendants with an IQ <70	<45 T1	—	.85
			<45 T2	—	1.00
			<45 RT	—	.92
Love et al., 2014	21	*M* IQ = 60.89[a]	<45 T2	—	.95
		SD = 6.8	<45 RT	—	1.00

NOTE: T2 = Trial 2; RT = Retention Trial.

[a]All patients had intellectual disability diagnoses. All but one participant had an FSIQ <70 (one patient had an FSIQ of 73, but still had an intellectual disability diagnosis based on deficits in adaptive functioning, etc.). (D. Glassmire, personal communication, November 14, 2016).

subjects were receiving disability benefits. Several authors (Buddin, Schroeder, Teichner, & Ward, 2012; Gervais et al., 2001) have reported that subjects already receiving disability benefits have similar or even higher failure rates on validity tests than those applying for such benefits. Thus, it appears subjects who are currently receiving disability benefits perform very similarly to those who are seeking it, and a significant portion do not perform to the best of their ability. Finally, P. Green and Flaro noted that Shandera et al. used the oral version of the WMT, which may be more subject to influences from the examiner, and that the community volunteers scored considerably lower on the easiest WMT subtests than did ID subjects in the study by P. Green and Flaro (2015). Green and Flaro concluded that many subjects in Shandera et al. were not motivated to perform well. In contrast, the subjects in the study by P. Green and Flaro (2015) were *highly* motivated: They were parents seeking to regain custody of their children. Among Green and Flaro's parents with an IQ less than 70 ($n = 14$), there was a 14.2% false positive rate, although the authors reported one of these two examinees confessed to not wanting the return of her children, and the other presented other evidence of negative impression management throughout her evaluation.

Among ID children ($M_{age} = 13.7$; $SD = 2.9$; $M_{IQ} = 63.3$; $SD = 6.0$), P. Green and Flaro (2016) reported all but 1 of 19 subjects passed the WMT's primary effort indicators (criterion A), and the one boy who failed had a reading grade level less than 3.0 and produced a *genuine impairment* profile. Thus, the WMT showed 100% specificity in this sample. Average scores between ID and other examinees were not significantly different except for the Free Recall subtest, providing further evidence that IQ was not a significant influence on most of the WMT's scores.

The MSVT was also examined by P. Green and Flaro (2015, 2016), and none of the ID children or adults failed the recognition or consistency tests, which are the primary validity indicators. In addition, Chafetz and Biondolillo (2012) reported no ID examinee with an IQ between 60 and 75 scored below the cutoff on the MSVT recognition or consistency scales.

The NV-MSVT is particularly attractive because of avoidance of reading demands and sensitive internal validity checks, but it has limited data in ID examinees: P. Green and Flaro's (2015) paper had only four ID adult subjects for the NV-MSVT. Among 26 ID children ($M_{age} = 13.2$; $SD = 3.1$; $M_{IQ} = 61.2$; $SD = 67.8$), P. Green and Flaro (2016) reported an apparent 11.5% false positive rate, but 2 of these children had diagnoses of severe oppositional defiant disorder, and all 3 produced a *poor effort* profile and there were additional reasons to question their efforts.

A few other PTVs have been supported in two studies with ID examinés. The Letter Memory Test (Inman et al., 1998) and the Digit Memory Test (Guilmette, Hart, Guiliano, & Leininger, 1994) performed well with ID persons in two studies (Graue et al., 2007; Shandera et al., 2010), albeit with adjusted cutoff scores. A DCT total time score greater than 180 seconds was found to have high specificity in two studies (Hurley & Deal, 2006; Proto, 2008) but to have low sensitivity (18%) by Proto (2008). Virtually all other PVTs/indices have excessive error rates, or a mixed record, in ID samples. As with other defendants, examiners are strongly encouraged to obtain collateral data and to compare performance across situations with different motivational contexts.

Chafetz, Abrahams, and Kohlmaier (2007) reported embedded indicators from a mental status exam and WAIS-III (e.g., not knowing one's age or the name of the current president, failing sample items, coding errors, Ganser responses) were effective in distinguishing valid from invalid presentation in low IQ examinees. Smith et al. (2014) recently reported that a battery of embedded validity indicators performed well in identifying feigning among intellectually impaired (IQ < 75) neuropsychology referrals. However, many of the tests employed are not familiar to non-neuropsychologists. Test indices with supportive findings in two or more studies are presented in Table 8.3.

Tests of adaptive functioning may also be of use in assessing over-reporting impairment by family members. Doane and Salekin (2009) found the Adaptive Behavior Assessment System–2nd Edition (P. Harrison & Oakland, 2003), which is completed by a family member or informant, to be quite vulnerable to exaggeration, whereas exaggeration on the Scales of Independent Behavior–Revised (Bruininks, Woodcock, Weatherman, & Hill, 1996) was easily detected. Thus, the latter may be useful in assessing over-reporting of deficits by family members.

The SIRS has been examined in several studies involving ID examinees. Hayes, Hale, and Gouvier (1998) reported the SIRS performed very well in distinguishing genuine from feigned ID and did so much better than the PVTs examined (FIT, DCT). However, about one third of ID examinees failed the SIRS in two studies (Farkas, 2008; Hurley & Deal, 2006), and Shandera et al. (2010) reported 35% of ID examinees scored >76 on the Total Score scale. Weiss et al. (2011) reported 23.3% of presumed genuine ID subjects failed the SIRS, but only 7% failed the SIRS-2. No studies were found examining the use of the MMPI-2/RF or PAI for assessing feigned psychopathology among ID examinees, whereas the

Table 8.3 Performance Validity Tests for ID Examinees

Test Variable	Criterion	Sensitivity	Specificity	Citations
TOMM T2	<35/60%	.24, .56	.96	Graue et al., 2007;
TOMM RT	<35/60%	.20, .60	.96, 1.00	Shandera et al., 2010
DCT Total Counting Time	>180 sec.	.18	.97, 1.00	Hurley & Deal, 2006; Proto, 2008
WMT	Fail A	—	.86–1.00[a]	Brockhaus & Merten, 2004; P. Green & Flaro, 2015, 2016[a]
MSVT	Fail A	—	.98–1.00	P. Green & Flaro, 2015, 2016; Chafetz & Biondolillo, 2012
Letter Memory Test	<70%	.36, .76	.83, .96	Graue et al., 2007; Shandera et al., 2010
Digit Memory Test	<80%	.40, .72	.96	Graue et al., 2007; Shandera et al., 2010

NOTE: "Fail A" indicates failure of Criterion A for the respective tests, which involve subtests of recognition and consistency.

[a]Shandera et al. (2010) reported much higher false positive rates. See text for discussion.

limited data on the M-FAST (Graue et al., 2007) are not supportive. Thus, among SVTs, the SIRS-2 is recommended for ID defendants, and even it has only a single supportive study and may produce higher false positives for ID examinees than for other diagnostic groups.

Chafetz (2015) attributed the conflicting findings regarding PVTs and ID examinees to several factors: (a) failure to distinguish mild ID from more severe levels, (b) failure to account for hidden incentives, (c) failure to make appropriate accommodations for testing, and (d) failure to adjust cutoff scores. Chafetz asserted that at IQs below 60, even well-motivated ID examinees begin to fail PVTs based on recognition memory, such as the TOMM. He also noted that some studies have included ID subjects who had "hidden" motivations, in that they were obliquely seeking disability or were already receiving disability payments that they were motivated to protect. P. Green and Flaro (2015) made a similar argument, and these issues apply to studies of the SIRS as well. Finally, Chafetz noted that some ID examinees have executive problems when asked, for example, to control a computer using a mouse. In such cases, the examiner should assist. Similarly, if reading limitations are present, the examiner might pronounce words that cannot otherwise be read (Chafetz, 2015; P. Green, 2004a).

If IQ scores are available from school or prior treatment records, there are some data to guide the judgment of competence if performance during the CST exam is not reliable. As shown in Table 8.4, several authors have reported average WAIS IQ scores for ID defendants judged incompetent (weighted $M = 56.9$), competent (63.7), and *ID but not referred for CST examination* (67.0). Unfortunately, the version of WAIS used and standard deviations were not reported, nor were other data that would permit an analysis of accuracy rates for given scores. In addition, there is no indication that the competency judgments that formed the

Table 8.4 AVERAGE IQ SCORES FOR INTELLECTUALLY DISABLED DEFENDANTS

Study	**Incompetent**		**Competent**		**Not Referred for Evaluation**	
	Mean IQ	***n***	**Mean IQ**	***n***	**Mean IQ**	***n***
S. A. Smith & Donmoyer (n.d.)	56.9	102	63.7	234	—	—
Everington & Luckasson (1992)[a]	58	11	59	12	67	46
Everington & Luckasson (1992)[b]	56	20	65	15	—	—
Jurecska, Peterson, & Millkey (2012)	—	—	64.3	44	—	—
Weighted mean/*N*	**56.9**	133	**63.7**	305	**67.0**	46

NOTE: The *weighted mean* is the average of other means, weighted by the sample size. For example, the IQ figure reported for *competent* defendants in Smith and Donmoyer (63.7) counts for much more than the one for the Everington and Luckasson Study 2 (59) because it is based on 234 subjects, the latter on only 12.

[a]CAST-MR Study 2.

[b]CAST-MR Study 3.

criterion included decisional competence, which, if operationalized as ability to expressed reasoned choice among alternatives, is by definition more stringent than a standard that does not include this aspect. Everington and Dunn (1995) reported that IQ correlated .66 with the CAST-MR total score, and that only the third CAST-MR subtest, which questions the defendant about the arrest and surrounding events, had incremental validity in predicting competency status over IQ.

Data are also available regarding IQ scores associated with competency restoration attempts (Table 8.5). ID defendants who are unable to be restored to competence have an average IQ of 55.8, whereas those who are successfully restored have an average IQ of 60.8. Again, standard deviations and data to assess cutoff scores were not available.

From the data presented here, an ID defendant with an IQ of 65 or greater (and no mental illness or unusual cultural deprivation) is likely to be CST under *Dusky*, and an ID defendant with a valid IQ of 55 or less is likely to be incompetent and possibly unrestorable. As IQ rises from 55 to 60, the probability of competence increases to approximately 50%.[5] At 65, competence is likely if there are no other impairments and the defendant is able to knowingly and intelligently waive his or her constitutional rights as required in *Godinez v. Moran* (1993).

In addition, an examiner faced with a defendant who is presenting as intellectually disabled will want to look at other indications of capacity, such as the ability to hold a job, to live independently, and to drive. Driving is particularly of interest because it involves learning a substantial number of traffic laws and operating procedures and applying them in real time. Although specific demands may vary, driving is arguably a more challenging task than competency to proceed. That being said, the examiner should ask about any specific accommodations offered (having the test read to the defendant) in the course of driver training and testing, the investment of time and support by family and others (which may be exceptional), and whether the defendant required multiple tries to get a license. As with other data, the examiner should attempt to corroborate any reports of special accommodations, either with family interviewed separately or, ideally, with the agency issuing the license.

Table 8.5 WAIS IQs of ID Competency Restoration Patients

Study	Unrestored		Restored	
	Mean IQ	*n*	Mean IQ	*n*
Ho (1999)	55.9	204	60.9	63
Bennett (2005/6)	51.91	22	62.85	20
Anderson & Hewitt (2002)	57.54	14[a]	66.91	62[a]
Wall & Christopher (2012)	59.44	11	60.17	7
Weighted mean/*N*	**55.8**	251[a]	**60.8**	152[a]

[a] Values were calculated from percentage figures given in the original report, and some are rounded to the next integer.

Although this book is primarily concerned with the assessment of response bias, CST assessment of ID individuals presents some unique challenges. This was the rationale for the creation of the CAST-MR, which uses a multiple-choice item format to assess the examinee's factual knowledge of the court system. This was prompted by findings that this format allowed better assessment of knowledge among examinees who lacked verbal expressive skills. However, review of the original reference (Sigelman, Winer, & Schoenrock, 1982) finds that the adult subjects in these studies had a mean IQ of 39.8—much lower than is likely to be encountered in CST exams.[6] In addition, although the CAST-MR questions were selected to gauge CST-relevant constructs, there appears to have been no systematic attempt to ensure that the items represented all the major facets of CST. Nonetheless, the multiple-choice format for the first section largely eliminates problems of inter-rater reliability and bias, both significant issues for forensic instruments.

The other two fully standardized CST instruments have serious problems when applied to the ID population. The ECST-R has simplified language and short sentences and provides tutoring if the examinee initially does not know the answer to factual understanding items. In addition, the items were created after a systematic content analysis of the CST construct. A panel of judges and legal scholars rated each of about 60 content areas for importance to the CST concept, and only those that received high average ratings were retained. This process yielded only six items to assess the factual understanding prong, and they query only about the most basic aspects of the adjudication process, such as the roles of the judge, prosecutor, and defense attorney. Thus, the items selected are possibly biased, in that they assess only the very foundational aspects of CST that raters agreed are necessary. In addition, the ECST-R does not directly assess decisional competence, which was not included among the CST facets that judges rated for relevance (R. Rogers, personal communication, May, 2017).[7]

Another problem is the way tutoring is implemented. Grisso (2005) noted that juvenile examinees who are tutored often do not retain their newly acquired knowledge when retested 2 weeks later, and he recommended that retesting after 2 weeks be conducted routinely when tutoring is given. In contrast, an examinee administered the ECST-R is apparently retested immediately, although the manual is not explicit on this matter. Although the examinee is prompted to answer about tutored material in his or her own words, the scoring rules do not distinguish between this and simple parroting.

A judge once questioned me on this matter and provided a perspective I had not considered. She pointed out that although the defendant had been able to retain tutored material a half hour after it had been provided, what assurance did she have that he would retain it 2 to 3 months later if the case was set for trial? Thus, the ECST-R's Factual Understanding scale appears too circumscribed and easy to provide a trustworthy assessment that an ID defendant understands the adjudication process and that the tutored information will be retained outside the immediate interview. Perhaps for the reasons described here, experienced CST examiners (see Chapter 10, this volume) rated the ECST-R as poorly suited for assessing ID defendants.

The MacCAT-CA also has serious problems when applied to ID examinees. Jurecska, Peterson, and Millkey (2012) administered the CAST-MR and MacCAT-CA to 113 ID subjects *who had independently been found competent to stand trial.* Every single subject failed three MacCAT-CA items, and the percentages of subjects falling into the *clinically significant impairment* ranges were very high across the subscales: Understanding, 52.2%; Reasoning, 60.2%; and Appreciation, 84.1%. In short, the MacCAT-CA appears too hard for ID examinees. Even more problematic, scores on the MacCAT-CA and CAST-MR subscales did not intercorrelate significantly. Finally, CST examiners (see Chapter 10, this volume) rated the MacCAT-CA as poorly suited for assessing ID examinees. In contrast, the less structured and standardized Fitness Interview Test–Revised received positive appraisals, despite not incorporating tutoring.

SECTION SUMMARY

Defendants with ID can pose a special challenge to accurate CST assessment. Yet, as with other defendants, a combination of validity testing and collateral data can shed light on both validity of presentation and CST-related capabilities. Examiners cannot assume that the presentation during the exam is genuine, even if it is grossly consistent with expectations based on reported IQ scores or descriptions of collaterals. Most SVTs and PVTs must be used cautiously with ID examinees. Examiners need to be knowledgeable about the data available for ID examinees for a given test and to use adjusted cutoff scores if appropriate. If the subject can read at a grade level of 3.1 or greater on the WRAT-4 and has a past measured IQ of ≥60, the WMT and especially the MSVT are good choices. However, the examiner must remain aware of possible problems with executive or motor functioning that might require assistance or accommodation. Valid IQ scores of 60 suggest an even probability of competence or not. An IQ of 65 suggests competence, absent other impairments, whereas 55 and below suggests incompetence and relatively low chance of restoration.

JUVENILE EXAMINEES

Considerable attention has been paid to assessment of CST in juveniles over the past decade (Fogel et al., 2013), but the literature on negative response bias, particularly within forensic psychology, is sparse. Although there are adolescent versions of the MMPI, MMPI-2-RF, and PAI, as discussed later, stand-alone PVTs do not appear to require modification for use with juveniles.

Juvenile CST examinees may differ from adult examinees in ways other than age. Warren et al. (2009) and Zavodny (2016) estimated the proportion of

Table 8.6 Diagnostic Categories of Juvenile CST Examinees

Condition(s)	Warren et al. (2009)[a]	Zavodny (2016)
Mentally ill only	40.0%	42%
Intellectual disability only	11.2%	27%
Both	27.0%	31%
Neither	21.8%	—

[a] Warren, DuVal, Komarovskaya, Chauhan, Buffington-Vollum, & Ryan (2009).

juvenile CST examinees falling into broad diagnostic categories: 1) mentally ill only, 2) intellectually disabled (only), 3) both mentally ill and intellectual limitations, and 4) neither a psychiatric disorder nor intellectual limitations (Table 8.6). Zavodny reported the diagnoses underlying juvenile incompetence in Florida as follows:

- Intellectual disability
- Attention-deficit/hyperactivity disorder
- Anxiety disorders (especially post-traumatic stress disorder)
- Documented brain injury (neurocognitive disorder)
- Mood disorders (major depressive disorder, bipolar disorder, disruptive mood dysregulation (DMD) disorder, etc.—mostly bipolar and DMD disorders)
- Autism spectrum disorder
- Psychotic disorders (very rare)

Symptom Validity Tests

The MMPI-Adolescent (C. Williams, 1992) is a 478-item inventory suitable for ages 14 to 18. It is sold by Pearson, and a hand-scoring kit, including manual, test booklets, and 50 protocols, costs $777.65. A Q-global (online administration and scoring) starter kit costs $210.00 and includes three administrations. Score-only reports cost $17.15 to $21.55, depending on the platform (Q-global, Q Local, or mail-in), and interpretive reports cost $36.00 to $42.00.

The MMPI-A's validity scales have been assessed in several published studies. The first, by Stein, Graham, and Williams (1995), compared nonclinical simulators to a group of clinical adolescents on a 704-item forerunner of the MMPI-A. However, authors did not report diagnoses of the clinical subjects (more than half were from inpatient substance abuse units), and simulators were merely told to fake bad, with no warning to be believable or incentive to try their best. F and F-K were both found effective, although the raw cutoff scores differed substantially between genders.

Rogers, Hinds, and Sewell (1996) examined performance of the SIRS, MMPI-A, and SIMS among 53 adolescent forensic patients. All subjects took the tests twice, once honest and once when asked to feign schizophrenia, anxiety, or major depression. A financial incentive was offered for good performance. However, examiners in the first phase of the study were not blind to the experimental condition. All the SIRS scales had high specificity (≥94%) using adult norms,[8] and optimized norms for the current sample resulted in substantial reduction in the cutoff score for several scales and considerably increased sensitivity for the SIRS overall decision rule (one scale in the *definite* feigning range, or three in the *probable* range) from 66% to 81%. Of note, no mention is made of how accuracy for negative SIRS findings was defined: Were all subjects who did not meet criteria for feigning classified as "passing"? For the MMPI-A, F > 90 had a sensitivity of only 28% but a specificity of 98%. The authors also examined cutoff scores optimized for the adolescent sample and reported favorable sensitivity and specificity values for all the scales examined (F, F1, F2,[9] Fp, F-K, Ds-r, and more). F-K (>20) produced the highest sensitivity (83%), with specificity held to >90%. The SIMS was found to have good sensitivity (87%) at a cutoff score of >16, with adequate specificity (62%) for a screening test. Raising the cutoff score to >40 resulted in a sensitivity of 49% and specificity of 94%, figures comparable to the SIRS in adult samples.

McGrath et al. (2000) developed an Fp scale similar in concept to the respective scale for the MMPI-2 and found it to have modest incremental validity over the F scale. However, it is not scored by the publisher on either the MMPI-A or the MMPI-A-RF (Archer, Handel, Ben-Porath, & Tellegen, 2016).

Lucio, Durán, Graham, and Ben-Porath (2002) compared 138 Mexican, nonclinical simulators to a similar number of adolescents in psychiatric treatment. Male patients carried diagnoses of substance abuse (36%), antisocial personality disorder (25%), and conduct disorder (14%), where females had more internalizing problems such as major depression (35%) and anxiety. Simulators were offered a CD for the best simulator but apparently were not cautioned to respond plausibly. F and F-K were both effective in distinguishing simulators from genuine psychiatric patients, but quite different cutoffs were appropriate for males and females, with those for females considerably higher. For F, a cutoff score of 34[10] had a sensitivity of 70.1% and specificity of 90.8% for girls, whereas for boys, a cutoff score of 30 had a sensitivity of 71.1% and specificity of 91.5%. For F-K, a cutoff score of 27 for girls produced a sensitivity of 68.9% and specificity of 90.8%. For boys, an F-K cutoff score of 19 yielded a sensitivity of 67.8% and specificity of 89.8%.

The Personality Assessment Inventory–Adolescent (Morey, 2007) is a 264-item version of the adult test suitable for adolescents aged 12 to 18 that takes 30 to 45 minutes to complete and 20 minutes to hand-score. Published by Psychological Assessment Resources, Inc., a hand-scoring specimen kit costs $353.00 and includes a manual and materials for 25 administrations. Computer scoring and interpretation is available for $227.00 for 10 uses or $513.00 for 25. The PAI-A can also be administered by computer for $5.00 per use, scored for $6.00, and an interpretive report generated for $17.00.

Only a couple of studies were located addressing the PAI-A's validity scales, and both suffered from methodological shortcomings: Neither cautioned simulators to be believable or offered an incentive for successful feigning. Meyer, Hong, and Morey (2015) examined performance of the PAI-A by comparing the scores of 98 college students (aged 17 to 18) asked to simulate serious mental illness with 50 matched psychiatric patients from the PAI's clinical sample. They found the newly developed Negative Distortion Scale (discussed in Chapter 3) to provide the best discrimination ($d = 2.76$) among all the validity indices examined, which included not only the Negative Impression Management scale and Malingering Index but also Rogers' Discriminant Function and a similar one developed in Korea (Hong & Kim, 2001). The *Hong Malingering Index* was the second-best-performing variable ($d = 2.51$). NIM also performed very well ($d = 2.40$); the Malingering Index also was effective, but less so ($d = 1.36$). The supportive statistics are probably higher than would be obtained if simulators were warned to avoid detection or would be obtained in a known group study.

Rios and Morey (2013) examined the ability of the PAI-A to distinguish feigned from genuine from simulated ADHD among 17- and 18-year-olds. Half of the simulators were "coached" by watching a 7-minute YouTube video of an interview of someone with ADHD. Surprisingly, the Positive Impression Management scales had the strongest correlation with the criterion (feigning or not) for uncoached simulators, while the Rogers' Discriminant Function did for coached subjects. The Negative Impression Management scale produced moderate effect sizes in both groups ($ds = .75$ and $.98$), whereas the Malingering Index was effective only for uncoached subjects ($ds = .82, .33$, respectively). Although the authors reported some strong differences between groups on clinical scales, the clinical group was not a forensic sample, so their low scores on scales like Antisocial Personality would probably not generalize to criminal justice samples.

Performance Validity Tests

In the only study located that addressed feigning on PVTs in adolescent offenders, Gast and Hart (2010) examined TOMM performance among 107 juvenile offenders aged 12 to 17 with an average IQ of 80.8 ($SD = 10.7$). The subjects were told that positive performance would look good to the court, so they were described as motivated to perform well. The researchers found a very low failure rate (<1%) on Trial 2, and none of the 13 subjects with an IQ less than 70 scored below 45. However, 7.7% of ID examinees did fail the Retention Trial, and although Trial 1 and Trial 2 did not correlate with IQ, the Retention Trial score did ($r = .24$). Nonetheless, the authors concluded the TOMM's adult norms can be used with juvenile offenders with a wide range of intellectual functioning.

DeRight and Carone (2015) recently reviewed the literature from 32 studies on the use of PVTs in children (mean age = 11.5). They concluded that standalone PVTs, specifically the TOMM, WMT, and MSVT, the most studied instruments, can be used with children with adult cutoffs. For the WMT and the MSVT, users were cautioned to ensure adequate reading level and to provide assistance for poor readers, as described in the respective manuals. This entails having the examinee read the words out loud during the first presentation trial and the examiner reading out loud any word the examinee struggles with. Reliable Digit Span was reported to produce excessive false positives. DeRight and Carone wrote:

> As a general rule of thumb, embedded PVTs are much more prone to false positives in children compared to free-standing PVTs . . .. This may occur because most embedded PVTs are based on total quantitative performance from tests that were originally designed as cognitive ability tests whereas free-standing PVTs were not. (p. 14)

However, they identified Chafetz's Symptom Validity Scale (Chafetz, 2008; Chafetz, Abrahams, & Kohlmaier, 2007) as a noteworthy exception.

THE MATERIAL REVIEWED IN THIS SECTION PERMIT A FEW CONCLUSIONS:

- Freestanding PVTs can be used with adolescents using adult norms, whereas embedded PVTs may be prone to false positives, particularly with very young or intellectually limited examinees.
- There is support for use of the MMPI-A's validity scales, particularly F and F-K, with adolescents.
- Girls and boys respond differently on F and F-K, and different cutoff scores should be used.
- There is a single study supporting use of the SIRS and SIMS with adolescents.

NOTES

1. "Pseudologia fantastica is typified by these characteristics: (1) the stories are not entirely improbable and are often built upon a matrix of truth; (2) the stories are enduring; (3) the stories are not told for personal profit per se and have a self-aggrandizing quality; and (4) they are distinct from delusions in that the person when confronted with facts can acknowledge these falsehoods" (King & Ford, 1988, p. 1).
2. "The *Eye-Roll* is a measure of distance, or amount of sclera relative to size and shape of the eye, between the lower border of the iris and the lower eyelid as the participant is gazing upward while slowly closing his/her eyelids. Participants receive a score ranging from 0 (indicating low hypnotic potential) to 4 (high hypnotic potential)" (Welburn et al., 2003, p. 117).
3. Calculated from data presented by Welburn et al. (2003).
4. I asked R. Brockhaus about how she selected subjects for her study. In an email to me in November 2013, she indicated she decided that a subject was deemed "testable" if (a) able to understand enough language to know what "repeating" and "forwards" and "backwards" meant, and (b) able to understand the concept of "missing."

5. From Table 8.4, the average IQ of ID defendants found incompetent is 56.9, and the average ID of defendants found competent is 63.7; 60 is close to the midpoint (60.3) between these distributions.
6. In performing approximately 4000 CST exams in three states, I have very rarely encountered a previously documented IQ below 55, and in one of these, it appeared clearly invalid based on collateral data.
7. Conversely, it could be argued that other instruments' focus on other facets distorts the notion of CST as being essentially a general orientation to one's legal situation.
8. The authors reported diagnostic PPP and NPP, but in the footnote 2 on page 246, the formulas for PPP and sensitivity were interposed, as were those for NPP and specificity. The values reported in the current text for sensitivity and specificity were originally labeled PPP and NPP in Rogers et al. (1996).
9. F1 and F2 are simply the first and second halves of the F scale. Both are 33 items long.
10. The authors do not state whether cutoff scores refer to scores greater than the cited score or equal to or greater.

9

Report Writing and Testimony

One of the first and most oft-repeated pieces of advice I received when I entered the forensic psychology field in the mid-1990s was, "Write short reports." Back then, many CST reports consisted of a single paragraph documenting that the examiner had evaluated the defendant, a diagnosis, and that the defendant was competent to stand trial or not. Melton et al. (1997) recommended that a CST report resemble a two-page letter to the judge, with few or no formal sections such as Personal History, Mental Status, or Testing. However, practitioners from this same time frame indicated that forensic reports should contain specific pieces of information well beyond a diagnosis and recommendation (Borum & Grisso, 1996). Much has already been written on report writing and testimony for forensic psychologists (Brodsky, 1991, 1999; Conroy, 2006; Dvoskin & Guy, 2008; Karson & Nadkarni, 2013; Otto, DeMier, & Boccaccini, 2014) and forensic experts in general (Babitsky, Mangraviti, & Todd, 2000). This chapter will focus on CST reports and testimony and the particular challenges they present.

ASSESSMENT PROCESS

An examiner can take steps during the information-gathering stage that will both benefit the assessment and make report writing more efficient. At some point, the examiner will need to retrieve and communicate the various observations and findings from the assessment and select those that will be written into the report. During the evaluation, I find it helpful to mark or highlight data that bear on the primary opinions that will be needed: Is there a diagnosable mental condition? Does the examinee present as impaired on CST-related capacities? Is the examinee presenting validly? Is the examinee competent or not? I use a word processer to make notes and highlight answers or observations relevant to each question, pro and con, in designated colors. When it comes time to review the data, it is easy to copy items from each color/category onto the clipboard, then paste them as a group into a summary section for further organization.

In following this procedure, the examiner may encounter significant observations and facts early in the examination. The examiner should avoid making any notes that might suggest bias or precipitous decision-making. For example, a defense attorney may ask, "Doctor, isn't it true that you suspected my client of faking from almost the very beginning of the evaluation?" Although there may be good reasons to do so, an affirmative answer will likely be used to argue that the examiner was biased and the evaluation was tainted by confirmation bias—the tendency for people to seek out data and interpret ambiguous data so that they support their original opinion.

REPORT WRITING

Multiple authors have offered guidance regarding the goals and perimeters of a forensic psychology report. Conroy (2006) wrote: "The clinician's first obligation is to the integrity of her or his professional work and findings, not to the individual who was evaluated nor to the attorney's case" (p. 246). Otto et al. (2014) enumerated seven purposes of a forensic report:

- Communicating one's professionalism
- Framing the referral question(s)
- Communicating one's work
- Memorializing the evaluation
- Complying with legal requirements
- Forming and coming to opinions
- Anticipating testimony

Griffith, Stankovic, and Baranoski (2010; see also Karson & Nadkarni, 2013) argued that in the absence of a criterion for accuracy of the CST opinion, the goal of a report should be to persuade the reader to agree with the examiner's opinion, utilizing skillful writing, rhetoric, appeal to authority, and storytelling. Otto et al. (2014) also cited persuasion as a relevant goal but only through means other than emotion or trickery.

Process

Examiners should realistically consider the time and budget for the evaluation and, if needed, preparation and testimony. Many community-based CST exams are poorly compensated, with $300 being a common (and very low) figure that I encountered in my informal research. Given such a budget, and taking into account the time required for travel, checking into a jail, or office expenses, one cannot write a 10-page, letter-perfect professional report, even if one believes this length is desirable. Such a report requires substantial time in several phases, including writing, editing, and proofing. Should the case go to hearing, it will require much more testimony preparation time than for a report half its length. A long report is harder to defend: Some judges believe a witness should be able to answer detailed questions from his or her report from memory. A long report may also present attorneys with more opportunities to engage in confirmation bias and cherry-picking facts to support their position (Karson & Nadkarni, 2013; Otto et al., 2014).

The need to distinguish facts, inferences, and opinions in reports has repeatedly been recommended (Karson & Nadkarni, 2013; Melton et al., 2007; Otto et al., 2014) and appears in the Specialty Guidelines for Forensic Psychologists (American Psychological Association, 2013). The examiner must constantly guard against uncritically accepting representations from any source as a fact. Karson and Nadkarni cautioned that a forensic examiner who reports an examinee's unsubstantiated claim, such as that she was sexually abused by her father, is potentially committing libel against the father. Karson and Nadkarni and Otto et al. suggested the examiner use primarily neutral words, such as "said" and "reported," when citing information from the defendant or collateral sources. In contrast, words like "admitted," "acknowledged," or "claimed" can express belief or doubt in the accuracy of what was reported. Stating that an examinee "didn't know" a given answer presumes lack of knowledge rather than intentional failure or lack of cooperation. Similarly, phrases such as "suffers from" are potentially inaccurate[1] and also convey a clinical mindset that is inappropriate when used in connection with some diagnoses, such as narcissistic or antisocial personality disorder. When citing prior diagnoses from other sources, one can simply report, "Mr. Smith was diagnosed with x, y, and z." If supplying a diagnosis from the present exam, appropriate phraseology would include statements such as "Mr. Smith meets criteria for *DSM-5* diagnoses of x, y, z." The writer should avoid buttressing or being openly skeptical of a witness's account in the reporting of that data.

In addition to reviewing data from the perspective of one's own role (e.g., court-appointed examiner or defense-retained), one should actively consider other viewpoints. Chafetz (2015) suggested imagining a minuscule opposing attorney perched on your shoulder, challenging each sentence as it is written. Karson and Nadkarni (2013) recommended that each proposition in a report be interrogated for its accuracy: What is the evidence for it? Against it? The evidence for an alternative formulation? Several other perspectives might be considered: that of a very knowledgeable and competent forensic examiner working the other side of the case, and that of the judge or jury. If you are experienced, you can probably adopt multiple roles at one time. Those who are less experienced might consciously adopt one role at time. The critical part is representing the other side as a check on confirmation and allegiance bias (the tendency to adopt a viewpoint congenial to the side that retained you; Kahneman, 2011; Neal & Grisso, 2014b).

Content

Heilbrun (2001; see also Conroy, 2006; Karson, 2015; Karson & Nadkarni, 2013) emphasized that an examiner should not report every fact uncovered in an evaluation but should present only material that is both reliable (trustworthy) and relevant to the referral question. Further, the American Psychological Association's ethical code, Section 4.04, *Minimizing Intrusions on Privacy* (a), states: "Psychologists include in written and oral reports and consultations, only information germane to the purpose for which the communication is made." The list of topics that are irrelevant in a CST report is long but would include (in most cases), family constellation and parents' alcohol, drug, and medical history if unremarkable, among many, many other possibilities. Otto et al. (2014) suggested ethnicity might be one such example. In fact, there are only a few broad topics that are relevant to nearly all examinees: psychiatric history, issues of cognitive impairment, current mental status and behavior, validity of presentation, and CST-related capacities. Of course, some defendants will have a relevant medical problem or might be withdrawing from alcohol or drugs. But it could be argued that routinely including an alcohol and drug history is not relevant, is more prejudicial than informative in most cases, and could easily lead to additions to a defendant's probation or sentence. The examiner has been retained to do a CST exam, not a social study.

Probative value is the degree to which a piece of data makes a proposition important to the matter more or less likely. *Prejudicial value* is evidence or data that tend to unfairly dispose the listener because of emotional factors (e.g., gory crime scene photos). Courts often decide whether the probative value of a piece of evidence outweighs its prejudicial value, and the examiner should do so in deciding what to include in a report (Conroy, 2006; Karson & Nadkarni, 2013).

This issue reached a head in the case of *Hirschfeld v. Stone* (2000) and was discussed by Poythress and Feld (2002). In *Hirschfeld*, the plaintiff complained that a forensic hospital violated his privacy rights guaranteed by the Constitution and state law by reporting personal or medical issues to the court that were irrelevant to his competency. Officially, the hospital was required to return only a brief form that stated the hospital's judgment regarding restoration of competency (yes or no). The hospital had taken to attaching the psychologist's CST report to provide the data underlying the opinion. The court reviewed CST-related appellate decisions and concluded as follows:

> Much of the information in the Fitness Report falls within the constitutionally protected zone of privacy. . . .The fact that a criminal defendant is HIV-positive and bisexual, was physically abused 14 years earlier, takes HIV related medication, suffers from hepatitis and diabetes, or has siblings who served time in prison, is not essential information which a court must have before determining that defendant has sufficient ability to consult with his lawyers and to understand the proceedings against him. (pp. 9, 13–14)

Poythress and Feld noted that the decision was binding only in the jurisdiction where it was decided and applies only to information *reported* to the court—it does

Table 9.1 Means of Reducing Bias During Report Writing

- Identify possible sources (positive or negative) of bias toward the defendant or attorneys, allegiance bias
- Double score tests; consider using a checklist to ensure completion of important assessment tasks
- Minimize the role of memory (refer to one's notes, recordings)
- Actively generate alternative conclusions; consider the opposite point of view
- Identify and weigh the most valid sources of data; put aside any material that is more prejudicial than probative
- Identify and use relevant base rates
- Take time to review and question facts and one's reasoning, reliance on heuristics
- Strive for objectivity in reporting facts and opinions
- Audit the report for any statements that the other side might rightly consider unfair

not restrict *collection* of data for use in forming the examiner's opinion. However, examiners should be aware that they are likely to be as susceptible to prejudicial material as anyone else, should avoid unnecessary exposure to it, and should not pass it along. Table 9.1 lists ways in which bias can be minimized during the report-writing process.

Hearsay is another issue in which reliability and probative value should be carefully weighed. Hearsay is information that rests on the accuracy and integrity of someone who is not present to testify directly. Courts generally do not allow hearsay as evidence, as it is deemed unreliable, but the Federal Rules of Evidence permit an expert to rely on it if doing so is usual and customary in that profession. Collateral sources, if not medical or administrative records, are hearsay, and the examiner needs to consider, and should discuss, reasons for considering them trustworthy or not. Although hearsay may be admissible because examiners do often rely on such information, readers should consider the downside of relying on information that courts tend to regard as unreliable.

Borum and Grisso (1996) surveyed both forensic psychologists and psychiatrists. Based on their responses, the authors identified 10 identification and evaluation method elements of a forensic report as essential:[2]

1. Identifying information
2. Identifying referral source
3. Purpose
4. Evaluation location
5. Evaluation date
6. Report date
7. List of sources
8. List of tests/procedures
9. Description of evaluation
10. Description of notification given the examinee

Examiners should also carefully review their jurisdiction's CST statute, as well as the court order if one was issued, for any legally mandated requirements. Some states require that the notification contain specific information or that the report address specified CST-related capacities.

Several studies have examined the content and, often, deficiencies of forensic report content. According to Skeem, Golding, Cohn, and Berge (1998), 47% of reports failed to include documentation that the examinee was notified the exam was not confidential. Multiple writers (Grisso, 2010; Melton et al., 2007; Karson & Nadkarni, 2013; Skeem et al., 1998) have lamented that examiners often fail to articulate the connection between psychiatric symptoms and CST deficits. Grisso (2010) detailed the 30 most common errors and problematic features found in work sample reports submitted as forensic ABPP work samples and offered extensive proscriptions for forensic reports. This article is readily available online at the *Open Access Journal of Forensic Psychology*, as is the one by Witt referenced next. Witt (2010) formulated the most frequent issues identified by Grisso into a 10-item checklist that can be applied to all forensic psychology reports.

Report authors should provide the dates that procedures and interviews were accomplished and the amount of time entailed in interviewing the defendant and collaterals (Otto et al., 2014). Otto et al. further recommended that the examiner document all attempts to access collateral data, whether or not successful.

Tailoring the recommendations of Grisso, Witt, and others (CST checklists from Robinson & Acklin, 2010, and those used in Ohio, Georgia, and Colorado), as well as input from multiple forensic psychologists with extensive CST experience, the following criteria represent what I believe to be best practices for CST reports:

1. a) The identity of the examinee is clearly established (e.g., full name, date of birth, or other data), and b) the examinee is determined to be the person he or she claims to be (e.g., picture identification, jail armband).
2. a) The report is identified as a competency examination, and b) the definition of competency in the jusridiction from which the exam was ordered is articulated. c) The charges or case numbers for which the exam is conducted are provided.
3. a) There is documentation that the defendant was advised of the purpose of the evaluation, the examiner's role, the retaining party, and who would or could receive the report, and b) documentation of the examinee's understanding of this material is provided. c) The date, duration, setting, and any noteworthy circumstances of the evaluation are documented.
4. a) Multiple *and varied* sources of data are used and documented if there is legitimate doubt about competency status and possible negative or positive response bias, or if the defendant is uncooperative.[3] b) Sources sought but not obtained are documented. c) Records are obtained directly from institutions, not through the parties. d) If records are provided by either party (as opposed to directly from the institution) and there are omissions or substantial redactions, this is noted. e) Collateral sources are informed of the purpose of the exam and lack of confidentiality, and this is documented. f) Potential biases of sources are considered and the credibility of sources weighted. g) If social media is utilized, the examinee is notified of this and given an opportunity to respond to the material found.

5. The interview and interviews of collaterals are recorded on audio or audiovisual media.[4]
6. a) Instruments and tests used are appropriate to the examinee and purpose employed, and b) are listed and briefly described without compromising test security. c) Tests are double-scored if hand-scored or double-entered if data are entered for computer scoring, and this is documented. d) Tests are interpreted in light of validity evidence, published critiques, or well-established principles (e.g., significantly below-chance responding).
7. a) The report is sensibly organized, well-written, and objective, measured, and professional in all respects. b) Jargon is eliminated or used sparingly and explained.
8. a) The report (other than identifying information, documentation of notifications, etc.) consists of data clearly relevant to the particular examinee's competency and related, penultimate issues.[5] b) Data and opinions that bear primarily on a different psycholegal issue (e.g., sanity, dangerousness), c) that could compromise the defendant's legal position (e.g., account of the offense, defense strategy), d) that are overly prejudicial or e) unnecessarily intrude on privacy, or f) that are beyond the examiner's expertise are not presented.
9. The examinee's a) mental status, b) symptoms (reported, denied, and observed), c) behavior, and d) demeanor are reported.
10. If the defendant is out on bond or has been in jail for less than 90 days and presents as psychotic or otherwise impaired, the defendant's recent substance use is reported and the possibility of intoxication, substance-induced disorder, or withdrawal is considered.
11. If the defendant is receiving any psychiatric medications, a) these are identified along b) with their reported and/or perceived effectiveness and c) any reported or observed side effects.
12. a) Observations and data are clearly distinguished from inferences and conclusions. b) The foundations of both facts and inferences and conclusions are clearly articulated, including the source of information, and the expressed level of certainty is congruent with the weight of evidence. c) Potentially misleading or inaccurate statements (such as that the examinee put forth good effort in the absence of validity testing) and unexplained inconsistent statements are not present.
13. Alternative hypotheses are considered. In particular, if the examinee presents with significant impairments or presents as normal despite reliable reports of possible serious mental disorder, the validity of presentation is thoroughly and competently assessed using testing, collateral data, or both.
14. a) An assessment of competency-related abilities is conducted that considers the statutory requirements, professional literature and guidelines, referral question(s), and the examinee's presentation, and b) includes the capacity to make rational, informed decisions (e.g.,

whether to go to trial or plea bargain, to testify or remain silent, to represent oneself or rely on a lawyer, or to waive the right to a jury trial (if relevant)).[6] c) Examples of the examinee's answers are provided.

15. Opinions regarding presence of a mental condition and competency congruent with the local statute and professional guidelines are provided.
16. If a mental condition and competency deficits are observed, the connections between the mental condition and deficits are articulated.
17. If the statute or court order requires a statement regarding the time, location, or probability of competency restoration or treatment recommendations, a recommendation based on the examinee's treatment history, substance abuse history, and/or base rates of competency restoration is provided.
18. a) Major limitations of the evaluation are accurately stated, and b) a statement is made regarding the adequacy of the data available for the assessment.

Some of the items may not apply in all cases, and I have attempted to balance thoroughness with regard for practical considerations. For example, although collateral data are desirable in all cases, they are not readily assessible in the settings in which some examiners work, and the time and effort necessary to obtain such data may not be warranted in some cases (e.g., a defendant who is referred because of a history of depression and presents with no current symptoms or CST deficits). Similarly, it could be argued that an extensive assessment of CST-related knowledge is unwarranted if the examinee has no mental condition, displays knowledge of advanced legal topics, or is clearly answering incorrectly on purpose. Recording of the interview and collateral interviews is generally desirable but may not be warranted in settings in which findings are very rarely challenged.

Documenting test use poses some dilemmas. At least one validity test author has recommended limited reporting about use of such tests. P. Green (2004a, 2005, 2008) instructs users of his tests to avoid naming the tests in the report and to provide only general information about the results and interpretive strategy to inhibit dissemination and coaching by attorneys for their future clients. Both Otto et al. (2014) and Karson and Nadkarni (2013) condoned these recommendations if full disclosure is made about these issues in a hearing. However, the examiner should then ask the court to seal the record to prevent dissemination.

A few demographic facts at the beginning of the report, such as the defendant's age, gender, race, and marital status, may help orient the reader to the person who is the subject of the assessment. Even though these variables are low in probative value, they are also low in prejudicial value and intrusion on privacy, and readers may expect to see them. As someone wiser than me once observed, nothing that is more than 10% original will ever be accepted. When innovating, preserve some familiar landmarks.

Although not yet a widespread practice, examiners might consider including a photo of the examinee on the day of the exam to record his or her dress, state of grooming, and appearance. However, the examiner should be alert to attempts to manipulate this piece of evidence. I have had more than one examinee adopt a crazy or "retarded" expression as I took their picture. This can be particularly useful if the expression is very different than on the examinee's driver's license or booking photo.

Because response style is so important yet neglected (Lander & Heilbrun, 2009; McDermott et al., 2013; Zavodny, 2016), I believe CST reports should routinely include a section dedicated to the validity of presentation. In most cases, this will involve reporting of validity test results and the congruence of the examinee's presentation and representations with collateral data, especially data that are less likely to be manipulated (objective sources, observations from natural and different settings). Attorneys and judges should expect to see these issues discussed in nearly every CST report unless the defendant presents with minimal or no impairment or charges are so minor that feigning would be superfluous.

Given that a competency evaluation order rarely contains language to evaluate malingering, as well as the American Psychological Association's ethical code statement on including only relevant information, it could be argued that efforts to assess and report *malingering*, apart from establishing the validity or invalidity of presentation, are inappropriate. A finding of malingering can lead to legal jeopardy in the form of an obstruction of justice charge and, thus, might require a warning about this in the informed consent notification. In addition, the *DSM-5* (American Psychiatric Association, 2013) defines malingering as "the intentional production or *gross* [emphasis added] exaggeration of physical or psychological symptoms, motivated by external incentives" (p. 373). Thus, it sets a high threshold for the degree of exaggeration that must be present and requires a demonstration that the feigning is motivated by external incentives. The latter issue is beyond the data provided by test results (Rogers et al., 2010): Even below-chance performance could be due to negativity and willful noncompliance rather than an intent to be found incompetent.

Forensic experts, particularly if court-appointed or retained by the state, may describe the defendant very differently than other mental health professionals. Faced with an unfavorable opinion, a defense attorney may line up multiple treatment providers and family members to contradict the examiner's conclusions. In such circumstances, judges may resolve the incongruity by simply relying on the majority opinion (Gowensmith, Murrie, & Boccaccini, 2012). If the examiner anticipates such a scenario, education regarding the differences between a forensic and clinical orientation may be needed. Proactively, one might include this in one's report or as boilerplate in a report template.

In a CST exam, there are several important topics that must be addressed, and many that should not be. The essential points of a CST exam can be addressed very concisely, as shown in the following example:

> **Does the examinee have a mental disorder?** No. Mr. X reported a vague history of psychiatric history, but this was not corroborated by his mother and wife, or in his accounts to jail medical staff. Although he reported symptoms of mental illness in the current exam, these were deemed not

credible (see Validity section). Mr. X's intelligence appeared roughly average, and neither Mr. X nor his family reported school failure, special education placement, or limitations in his daily functioning.

Validity of presentation: Mr. X's report of his psychiatric history was inconsistent with his own reports to jail medical staff and reports of his wife and mother. He also scored very high on the Miller Forensic Assessment of Symptoms Test, a structured interview designed to assess feigning of mental disorder.

Competency to proceed: Mr. X displayed a good general understanding of the court system and of his own case, including charges and potential defenses and punishments. He reported a positive relationship with his attorney, showed no evidence of problems communicating, and provided a detailed and organized account of the alleged offense. He approached potential defense decisions, such as whether to take a plea bargain, waive a jury trial, or testify, in a rational and realistic manner.

Recommendation: I recommend that Mr. X be found competent to be adjudicated. He does not have mental illness or defect and did not show any significant deficits in competency-related abilities.

The preceding material is meant as an example of a summary. The data underlying these conclusions would be presented elsewhere. This could also be accomplished in a very brief and efficient manner, in the following form:

> Mr. X has been treated as an outpatient for symptoms of anxiety and depression but has no history of psychiatric disorder that is associated with major disturbances in perception of reality, such as schizophrenia (list sources [e.g., "Mr. X, Mr. X's wife, treatment records from Hospital Y"]).

Because some readers of the report may tend to equate findings of feigning or lack of cooperation with a finding of no mental disorder and competence, these issues should be discussed separately, and the distinction made abundantly clear. For example:

> Mr. Smith has a well-documented intellectual disability that led to significant accommodations in his school environment. While there is little doubt that he has cognitive limitations, there was also compelling evidence that he did not perform to the best of his ability during some portions of the examination. This means that his answers about the court system may not reflect his actual level of understanding. Using school records, his recent employment history, and accounts of collaterals as a guide to what he is capable of, I believe . . .

Format

Karson and Nadkarni (2013) described three basic report types. One familiar to most forensic examiners is the *procedure-by-procedure* approach, in which the findings from each source or test are described separately. This allows the reader to identify the basis for a given conclusion but can result in a lengthy, disjointed report. An *issue-by-issue* report instead groups material by topic area, such as cognitive or social functioning, integrating findings across data sources. Finally, a *point-by-point* report is like the *issue-by-issue* report, but the "points" are defined by the psycholegal referral question, such as competency and/or malingering.

Where multiple data bear on a given issue, they can be ranked and sorted into the most compelling arguments for a given position. For example, a given case might present the following on negative response bias:

- Below-chance performance on the CAST-MR; Mr. X scored significantly worse on this test than he would have by simply guessing at the right answer out of three choices.
- Failure on the Word Memory Test, with a profile that indicates performance inconsistent with the difficulty of the subtests.
- Reported hearing voices for the past 3 years in the present evaluation but did not report this symptom in multiple interviews with the jail medical staff.
- Failure on Test of Memory Malingering Trial 2.
- Scored well above the cutoff for suspected exaggerated psychiatric symptoms on the Miller Forensic Assessment of Symptoms Test.

These results are presented in approximate order of probative value. Of course, acronyms and tests used would have to be explained elsewhere. I am reluctant to state cutoff scores, if they could be easily understood and utilized, as this information could be passed on to future examinees. Data contrary to one's opinion should be disclosed and discussed.

Although the examiner should generally should list facts on both side of an issue, response bias data are inherently asymmetrical: Honest reporting of some symptoms or facts is not probative of honest reporting of others. Similarly, some validity tests have low sensitivity (e.g., 30%) yet high specificity (e.g., 95%). Failing such a test is much more probative than passing. It would be misleading to report passing such a test as evidence of valid responding. Rather, one might write as follows:

> Mr. X passed the Structured Inventory of Reported Symptoms–2. However, this test accurately identifies less than half of examinees who feign during competency exams, so this finding cannot rule out the possibility that Mr. X exaggerated or feigned during the evaluation.

Another possible report format is inspired by the way medical examiners document their work. In an autopsy, the medical examiner dictates observations as the procedure progresses, creating a real-time record of the order in which evidence was reviewed and the examiner's perceptions. In addition to the potential convenience and time-effectiveness of the approach, it allows one to tell the *story* of the evaluation, invites the reader to reason along with the report author (Melton et al., 2007), and includes the examiner as an implicit character in the story (Griffith et al., 2010). Of course, a CST examiner will have to postpone dictating the interview portion and be selective to keep reports to a reasonable length. The "body" of the report could be limited to objective data and observations but could also include tentative interpretations. This helps document the examiner's thought processes in real time—something that otherwise is often lost. Ideally, the reader can participate in the satisfaction of solving the case.

If the examiner has collected much detailed data and chooses to include this information in the report, he or she may be asked detailed questions about these facts during direct examination or cross-examination. This can lead to an awkward scenario, where the witness's memory is tested against his or her written report. Frequently stopping to check what was written can be cumbersome and may reduce the perceived credibility of the witness.[7] To help avoid this scenario, detailed supporting data could be presented in an appendix. This may blunt unrealistic expectations that the examiner will possess total recall of it on the witness stand.

Although the report types have been presented as discrete, they could potentially be combined. For example, one might present a summary similar to the first example, with the body of the report being a *procedure-by-procedure, point-by-point*, or narrative "medical examiner" format. The summary might appear at the end, as is traditional, or at the beginning as an executive summary.

One might also question the desirability of a traditional written, text-only report. Much of the crucial CST data, at least for a defendant who presents validly, consists of his or her answers to questions about the court system. The examiner might take notes, then transcribe or dictate these notes to provide the trier of fact with the actual data of the interview, but this is labor-intensive and lacks the objectivity of audio recording. Technology presents what I think is an attractive alternative: Software such as Microsoft's OneNote allows an examiner to create an interview template, then track one's progress through it during the interview, recording and indexing as topics are addressed. Most important, a user can then play back the recording by clicking the desired topic or link, so a judge could easily pull up the defendant's answer to a question such as "What is the role of the judge?" or the question that elicited the response. Such an approach differs dramatically from the traditional view of testing, where the items are carefully concealed from disclosure in the interest of maintaining test security. If video is also recorded, the trier of fact can view the relevant recording to directly observe the defendant's response to questions, as well as dress, grooming, and demeanor, during the evaluation. Although it is still desirable that the examiner summarize observations, the data underlying these conclusions are preserved and made accessible to review. Of course, this approach requires that the court can receive electronic reports, has software capable of viewing them, and is agreeable to the process. Finally, this approach has the potential to reduce the cost of CST reports because it streamlines reporting of responses to the CST questions.

REPORT WRITING SUMMARY

CST examiners must efficiently document and communicate their work and opinions to the court. To do so, they consider the ethical and scientific bases of their work, but also the needs and perspective of their audience. There is general agreement about the required content of CST reports, but less agreement on the structure and presentation style. The American Psychological Association (2002) ethical code states that reports should contain only data relevant to the assessment issue, and this provides a compelling reason, among the other advantages cited, to write short, focused reports in routine CST cases. Data, such as observations and test results, should be reported objectively and distinguished from the examiner's opinions. The possibility of response bias should be addressed in cases in which impairment is presented, and the connection between psychiatric symptoms and competency deficits made explicit.

TESTIFYING

Whereas report writing allows the examiner much freedom and time for reflection, testimony often does not. Even some of the field's most highly respected figures report finding testimony a challenge (Grisso, 2014), and there are whole books devoted to the topic (Brodsky, 1991, 1999). The very first book I read on the topic, Stan Brodsky's *Testifying in Court: Guidelines and Maxims for the Expert Witness* (1991) is a good place to start. The primary function of an expert witness is to "assist the trier of fact to understand the evidence or to determine a fact in issue" (Federal Rules of Evidence 702; Dvoskin & Guy, 2008, p. 203). Some jurisdictions rarely require expert testimony in CST matters, while others do so almost routinely (see Chapter 10, this volume).

If the examiner is called to testify, it may be wise to meet with the attorney who seeks his or her testimony prior to the court date to discuss how testimony will proceed and to clarify any points of misunderstanding (Conroy, 2006). Conroy argues the examiner should insist on this, as it is his or her reputation that is on the line, and attorneys vary widely in their knowledge of CST-related matters and skill in eliciting testimony. Sometimes attorneys will focus on issues the examiner views as unimportant, and a witness will want to be prepared to answer questions that can be anticipated. However, others have argued that meeting with only one side prior to testimony may create bias and the issue may be raised during cross-examination.

Otto et al. (2014) offered a concise, interesting, and helpful review of empirical data on testifying experts. Kwartner and Boccaccini (2008) concluded experts are effective and persuasive to the extent they show clarity and clinical knowledge, testify on case-specific material, and present with confidence. *Clarity* refers to the ability to communicate effectively to the jury, avoiding jargon, so that jurors understand the substance and reasoning of the testimony, not just the conclusion.

Clinical knowledge was not so clearly defined by Kwartner and Boccaccini, but it may be contrasted with scientific knowledge. Jurors appear more receptive to reports of behavior observations, diagnoses, and anecdotes than to testimony about test scores, reliability statistics, and actuarial predictions. Of course, this preference can be contrary to good scientific practice. *Case-specific* information refers to testifying about the given examinee versus testifying about characteristic of, for example, sex offenders or alcoholics. Finally, *confidence and certainty*, unless carried to an extreme, appear strongly related to perceived witness performance.

Babitsky and Mangraviti (2005) suggested that a witness adopt the role of a wise and patient teacher. Other pointers, from various sources, include the following:

- Treat everyone with respect, even if the attorneys are rude or insulting. Attorneys sometimes act up as a strategy to anger or unbalance the witness or to get the witness to roll in the mud with the advocates. Stay above the fray and be the adult in the room.
- Always tell the truth, and if you make a mistake, correct it on the record as soon as feasible.
- If you don't know the answer to a question, say so (Dvoskin & Guy, 2008). Don't speculate.
- If a question is compound, ambiguous, or convoluted, ask that it be restated: Don't answer a question you don't understand or one that implies something incorrect. Sometimes attorneys will ask a question that just doesn't make sense. This might reflect a lack of knowledge, but it could also be an attempt to get the witness to show impatience or disdain.
- Respond to attacks in a respectful, nondefensive, but firm manner. Don't take them personally.

Experts should avoid becoming personally invested in the case. Dvoskin and Guy (2008) wrote, "The most egregious errors by expert witnesses are almost always attributable to narcissistic needs, including the need to be praised, to make money, to be right, and to win" (p. 203). It is the attorney's job to "win," not the expert's. The expert should be concerned primarily with accurately and clearly communicating his or her findings and opinions to the judge or jury.

Attorneys will sometimes ask a witness if he or she recognizes a given book or person as authoritative on a given topic. This is usually a trap to show that the authority whom the witness has just endorsed as the field's preeminent scholar in fact disagrees with him or her. You can recognize the person or work as a valuable resource but not one to whom all professionals are expected to defer.

Similarly, attorneys will sometimes ask witnesses if they would change their opinion if they were to learn A, B, or C. Often these "facts" are dramatic: "Would it change your mind if you learned that the defendant has been screaming for the last 72 hours and has been given three shots of Haldol by the jail medical staff?" The attorney's goal is often to show bias—that even when presented with jaw-dropping evidence, witnesses are not open to modifying their opinion. Take this as an opportunity to show that you are reasonable in considering evidence from the other side.

If the examiner concludes a defendant showed poor effort, a prosecutor may attempt to equate this with malingering in eliciting testimony. The examiner should consider the evidence and implications of supplying this label and should not simply acquiesce. As discussed earlier, the label of malingering requires a conclusion about motivation, requires gross exaggeration, and potentially imposes legal jeopardy.

Although multiple testifying manuals recommend a witness make eye contact with the jury, Otto et al. (2014) reported that too much attention to the jury (at the expense of eye contact with the attorney asking the question) was perceived negatively. If there is no jury, one can attempt to make eye contact with the judge. However, some judges seem to avoid this, and the seating position of the witness chair relative to the judge can make this awkward. Don't make any heroic efforts.

TESTIMONY SUMMARY

If subpoenaed to testify, the examiner may prepare with the attorney who has summoned him or her, but this may raise questions of bias. During testimony, the examiner should respond truthfully, clearly, and thoughtfully. The examiner's role, at least during direct questioning, will be to explain his or her credentials, the examination process, the primary findings, and the conclusion. Do so humbly, confidently, and in plain language. Cross-examination can be perfunctory or detailed and confrontational, particularly if the examiner concludes negative response bias was present. The examiner should seek to remain emotionally detached from the drama that sometimes unfolds, and should maintain the role of a mature, knowledgeable, and objective adviser to the judge or jury.

NOTES

1. It is often the people who must live and deal with persons with a narcissistic or antisocial personality disorder who suffer, not the person with the diagnosis.
2. The authors also identified essential clinical data and opinion elements.
3. I included exceptions for this criterion because not every CST assessment is difficult or requires extensive collateral data. Some cases are clearly competent or incompetent based on presentation and minimal collateral data.
4. Recording of testing is contraindicated because this may affect test performance and compromise test security.
5. E.g., psychiatric history if any, school or medical data if examinee presents with cognitive impairment, evidence of functional level (living situation, employment), or credibility of examinee or key sources.
6. In many jurisdictions, a mental disorder is a precondition for a finding of incompetence: In the absence of such a condition, competency should not be in question.

A lengthy assessment of competency-related knowledge, such as in the Fitness Interview Test–Revised, does not seem to be an optimal use of one's time in such a case. Similarly, if the defendant is not responding validly, there may be little value in a detailed assessment of purported competency deficits. However, in some cases, these answers can be compared with other data, such as from prior reports or phone calls that may reveal feigning. Also, there is no universal agreement that decisional competence should be addressed as part of a CST assessment: Rogers et al. (2004) argue from a legal analysis that it is not part of the *Dusky* criteria; Grisso (2000) and Zapf and Roesch (2009) argue it should be addressed.

7. In general, it appears jurors and lawyers alike are impressed by witnesses who are confident, including in the correctness of their memories. This confidence is often misplaced. A witness who takes the time to check his or her memory is being conscientious and professional.

10

A Survey of Competency to Stand Trial Examiners

This chapter broadens the scope of topics beyond just assessing negative response bias in CST exams. It reviews CST practices as reported by prior surveys of forensic professionals and diplomates and presents results from a survey conducted by the author. Data from the current survey will be presented on test and collateral data usage, desirable features of CST instruments, and base rates of invalid responding broken down by type.

There have been several prior surveys of forensic psychology practitioners regarding CST evaluations (Archer, Buffington-Vollum, Stredny, & Handel, 2006; Borum & Grisso, 1995; Lally, 2003; Ryba, Cooper, & Zapf, 2003). Borum and Grisso (1995) reported that 42% of psychologist respondents *almost always* used objective personality inventories, predominantly the MMPI/MMPI-2, when conducting CST evaluations. Intellectual tests (not including neuropsychological tests) were reported to be used less frequently, although 25% of psychologists reported using them *almost always*. Lally (2003) reported whether tests were deemed *Recommended*, *Acceptable*, *Equivocal*, or *Unacceptable* for CST evaluations, among other types of assessments, by forensic diplomates of the American Board of Professional Psychology (ABPP). The most highly recommended tests for CST evaluations were the Wechsler Adult Intelligence Scale–III (WAIS-III; Wechsler, 1997), which was recommended by 62% of respondents, and the MacArthur Competence Assessment Tool–Criminal Adjudication (MacCAT-CA; Poythress et al., 1999), which was endorsed by 56% of respondents. Tests deemed *Acceptable* included the Competency Screening Test (Lipsitt, Lelos, & McGarry, 1971), Competency Assessment Instrument (Laboratory of Community Psychiatry, 1973), Minnesota Multiphasic Personality Inventory–2 (MMPI-2; Butcher et al., 1991), and Personality Assessment Inventory (PAI; Morey,

1991). The Georgia Court Competency Test (GCCT; Johnson & Mullett, 1987), Competence Assessment for Defendants with Mental Retardation (CAST-MR; Everington & Luckasson, 1992), and Wechsler Abbreviated Scale of Intelligence (WASI; Wechsler, 1999) were deemed *equivocal*. All projective clinical tests were deemed *unacceptable*. Although Lally (2003) collected data on the frequency with which the tests were used, this was not reported. Finally, the author did not report if *recommended* ratings given pertained to use in every CST exam or for selective use.

Archer et al. (2006) surveyed members of the American Psychology–Law Society (AP-LS) and ABPP forensic diplomates (n = 152) about their use of tests in CST and insanity evaluations (which the authors combined as a single category). The MacCAT-CA was the most frequently used CST measure by a substantial margin, followed by the CAST-MR and Evaluation of Competency to Stand Trial–Revised (ECST-R; Rogers, Tillbrook, & Sewell, 2004). The GCCT lagged behind, and the Interdisciplinary Fitness Interview–Revised (IFI-R; Golding, 1993) and Fitness Interview Test–Revised (FIT-R; Roesch, Zapf, Eaves, & Webster, 1998) were reported to be rarely used.

Neal and Grisso (2014a) contacted psychologist and psychiatrist members of professional organizations in the United States, Canada, Europe, Australia, and New Zealand. Participants were asked to report on their use of collateral data and instruments in their last two forensic evaluations, referring to the actual report for their data. They reported the ECST-R was used in 6.8% of CST exams, the MacCAT-CA in 5.6%, and the Juvenile Adjudicative Competence Interview (JACI; Grisso, 2005) in 5.0%. The WAIS (any version) was used in 11.8% of CST evaluations, the MMPI (any version) in 8.1%, the PAI in 6.2%, and the WRAT in 6.2%.[1] Although testing was not used frequently, collateral data were: Neal and Grisso reported 91.3% of evaluations used justice system records, 90.9% used mental health/medical records, 43.5% used collateral interviews with other professionals, 41.6% used nonprofessional collateral interviews, 28% used additional observations, and 26.7% used educational records.

Several studies queried participants about instruments used to assess feigning. The Structured Inventory of Reported Symptoms (SIRS; Rogers, Bagby, & Dickens, 1992) was the most highly recommended validity test in Lally (2003) and the most widely used in Archer et al. (2006), although the latter authors did not include the MMPI-2 or PAI as options in this category. Neal and Grisso (2014a) reported the Test of Memory Malingering (TOMM; Tombaugh, 1996) was used in 9.9% of CST reports they reviewed, and the Miller Forensic Assessment of Symptoms (M-FAST; H. A. Miller, 2001) was used in 9.3%. The SIRS was not mentioned.

Several distinctions among examiners are of potential interest. Those working in inpatient settings may have greater access to collateral observations and may have more time per case to devote to their assessments. This might lead to greater use of testing than by community examiners, who may be subject to relatively low compensation for CST evaluations, in some places as little as $170 (Gowensmith, Pinals, & Karas, 2015). Such limited compensation would tend to discourage time-consuming tests and seeking of collateral data. Conversely, the lack of readily available collateral data in community evaluations may lead examiners to compensate with greater use of tests. Some prior surveys have distinguished between forensic ABPP respondents and other respondents, and such comparisons can suggest areas where more qualified respondents differ in their practices from others.

Murrie and Boccaccini (2015) showed that the judgments of psychologists on forensic tasks appear to be heavily influenced by who is believed to be the referral source. No survey to date has examined the effect of referral source on judgments of malingering, feigning, or lack of cooperation among CST examiners.

The present survey was conducted to update and expand on previous surveys and to focus on issues most relevant to the current practice of CST assessment. Among the areas queried are the use of forensic assessment instruments (FAIs), forensically relevant instruments (FRIs), and clinical instruments. FAIs are designed to assess a specific psycholegal issue, such as competency to stand trial. FRIs are instruments that target a construct related to forensic assessment, such as malingering. Clinical instruments are those such as the WAIS-IV or MMPI-2. Respondents were asked to rate the importance of different CST instrument qualities, to provide their perceptions of the strengths and weaknesses of the most commonly used CST instruments, and to estimate the frequency of feigning different types of impediments. The effects of practice setting, forensic ABPP status, and referral source on ratings were examined.

METHOD

Participants

Participants were solicited from multiple forensic psychology listservs, including Psylaw-L (PSYLAW-L@listserv.unl.edu), Psychlaw (psychlaw@freelists.org), and Competency_forum (http://tech.groups.yahoo.com/group/competency_forum/). Messages identifying the survey as one addressing CST assessment practices and inviting members to participate were posted twice to each of the listservs named. In addition, some initial respondents asked permission to forward the invitation to co-workers or colleagues involved in CST practice, and this was encouraged. Seventy-three surveys were returned, although two had no usable data. All data were collected from November 6 to 18, 2012.

Because many members of general forensic psychology listservs may not perform competency evaluations, it is not possible to accurately estimate what proportion of competency examiners contacted did participate. However, the Competency_forum listserv, which is devoted to CST issues, had been formed shortly before the survey was announced and drew members from several other forensic psychology listservs. It had about a hundred members at the time of the survey.

Respondents were distributed throughout US geographical regions (Northeast 14.5%; Southeast 26.1%; Midwest 14.5%; Southwest 26.1%; Northwest 17.4%), and only one response from outside the United States was received. Nearly all (97.2%) of participants were doctoral-level psychologists, and no physicians participated. Respondents worked primarily in private practice (47.9%) or state hospitals (39.4%), although court clinics (8.5%) and state forensic offices (7.0%) also provided significant numbers. Board certification (ABPP) in forensic psychology was reported by 22.5% of respondents, and 4.2% of respondents reported having a Doctor of Jurisprudence (JD) degree. Seven percent of respondents reported ABPP board certification in clinical psychology; an additional 4.2% did so for clinical neuropsychology.

Participants were asked to estimate the number of competency evaluations they had completed over the course of their career and in the past year. Respondents' estimates averaged 683.7 CST evaluations in their career (*Mdn* = 300; *SD* = 916.9) and 71.7 such evaluations in the past year (*Mdn* = 45; *SD* = 147.6). They estimated that CST evaluations and resulting testimony constituted 43.5% (*SD* = 34.0) of their practice, and that 77.2% of their CST cases were court-referred, 44.2% were defense-referred, 8.4% were prosecution-referred, and 9.2% were from other sources. Among the "other" referral sources cited were jails (*n* = 3), private hospitals (*n* = 2), a law practice, a probation office, a state prison, and a military hospital. The percentages sum to more than 100% so respondents may have considered some referrals as stemming from more than one entity (e.g., court *and* the prosecution or jail). An estimated 9.8% (*Mdn* = 5; *SD* = 16.7) of CST evaluations resulted in court testimony.

Materials

An online survey was created by the author using Survey Monkey, an online survey service. Questions were generated to reflect parameters of CST assessment practice (test use, use of particular collateral sources), perceived qualities of CST instruments, and the perceived rate of different types of feigning and other invalid presentations, such as factitious disorder. Many questions asked respondents to provide a numerical estimate of, for example, how many CST evaluations they had performed, or the prevalence of feigning a given presentation. Most other questions were posed in 5- or 6-point Likert scale format. The survey was estimated to take about 15 to 30 minutes to complete, depending on how many CST FAIs the respondent chose to judge on psychometric issues and content coverage. Some of the survey questions were expected to be answered by all respondents, but this was not true of questions about individual competence instruments, which required technical knowledge and familiarity with each test. Instruments were chosen for rating based on several factors: publication status, citation in prior surveys, recent research, and frequency of use in competency reports reviewed by this author. Missing data were most frequent for items asking about the Interdisciplinary Fitness Interview–R, which was reported to be the least frequently used CST measure. A number of respondents did not provide answers in different areas of the survey, such as reporting the frequency of use of specific validity instruments or data sources,[2] and in sections inquiring about psychometric qualities of CST instruments.

RESULTS

Instrument Usage

Four CST instruments, the MacCAT-CA, ECST-R, CAST-MR, and CAI, were reported to be used to a nearly equivalent degree. These results are reported in more detail in Table 10.1. In addition to percentages of responses in each category, I also report the *Total Mentions* (TM; percentage of respondents reporting at least occasional use of a measure) and the *Weighted Sum* (WS; sum of $n \times$ numerical weight of ratings: *Never* = 1, *Rarely* = 2, *Sometimes* = 3, etc.). The Juvenile Adjudicative Competence Interview and the Georgia Court Competency Test were not listed by name on the survey, but each was mentioned as a "write-in" by three respondents.

Pertaining to general clinical instruments, respondents reported most often using a mini-mental state exam (either the Folstein MMSE or other similar instrument). This received an average WS rating of 2.89, slightly less than the anchor *sometimes*, which corresponds to a value of 3.0 (Table 10.2). The WAIS (any version) obtained the highest TM ratings. Respondents reported using the PAI slightly more often than any version of the MMPI; the MCMI and Rorschach were rarely used.

Turning to FRIs and measures of feigned psychopathology, categorized as symptom validity tests (SVTs) by Larrabee (2012), the M-FAST was the most frequently used such instrument in this sample (Table 10.3). However, both the SIRS and the SIRS-2 (Rogers, Sewell, & Gilliard, 2010) received high ratings,

Table 10.1 Reported Use of Competency Assessment Instruments

	Usage Rating Totals								
	Never	**Rarely**	**Sometimes**	**Often**	**Almost Always**	**Always**	**TM**	**WS**	***n***
MacCAT-CA	34.0%	30.2%	24.5%	7.5%	3.8%	0.0%	66.0%	2.17	53
ECST-R	38.5%	36.5%	9.6%	5.8%	7.7%	1.9%	61.5%	2.13	52
CAI[a]	64.7%	5.9%	9.8%	3.9%	5.9%	9.8%	35.3%	2.10	51
CAST-MR	41.8%	21.8%	27.3%	5.5%	3.6%	0.0%	58.2%	2.07	55
FIT-R	69.2%	11.5%	3.8%	9.6%	3.8%	1.9%	30.8%	1.73	52
IFI-R	97.9%	2.1%	0.0%	0.0%	0.0%	0.0%	2.1%	1.02	47

NOTE: Figures shown in all but the last two columns are percentages of responses for that instrument in each category. TM = total mentions = percent of respondents who reported sometimes using the instrument; WS = weighted sum: *Never* = 1; *Rarely* = 2; *Sometimes* = 3; *Often* = 4; *Almost always* = 5; *Always* = 6.

[a]Includes modified or augmented versions.

Table 10.2 Use of Clinical Measures in CST Evaluations (Percentages)

Instrument	Usage Rating Totals								
	Never	Rarely	Sometimes	Often	Almost Always	Always	TM	WS	*n*
MMSE	37.0	8.7	17.4	15.2	8.7	13.0	63.0	2.89	46
WAIS (any version)	26.0	30.0	32.0	4.0	6.0	2.0	74.0	2.40	50
PAI	39.2	27.5	19.6	5.9	7.8	0.0	60.8	2.16	51
MMPI (any version)	40.8	26.5	22.4	6.1	4.1	0.0	59.2	2.06	49
MCMI (any version)	76.1	17.4	0.0	4.3	2.2	0.0	23.9	1.39	46
Rorschach (any version)	80.9	12.8	4.3	2.1	0.0	0.0	19.1	1.28	47

Note: For all tests, any version of the test is counted as included. For example, the label "MMPI" includes the original instrument, MMPI-2, and MMPI-2-RF. Figures shown in all but the last two columns are percentages of responses for that instrument. TM = total mentions = percent of respondents who reported sometimes using the instrument; WS = weighted sum: *Never* = 1; *Rarely* = 2; *Sometimes* = 3; *Often* = 4; *Almost always* = 5; *Always* = 6.

which, if combined, surpass the M-FAST. The MMPI-2 was the most frequently used self-report inventory, whereas the ECST-R Atypical Presentation Scales, the MMPI-2-RF (Ben-Porath & Tellegen, 2008), and the Structured Inventory of Malingered Symptomatology (Widows & Smith, 2005) were used less often. The Test of Memory Malingering was rated the most frequently used performance validity test (PVT), followed by the Validity Indicator Profile (Frederick, 1997), the Inventory of Legal Knowledge (ILK; Musick & Otto, 2010), and the Rey 15 Item Test (Rey, 1941). The Word Memory Test (P. Green, 2005), Medical Symptoms Validity Test (P. Green, 2004a), Nonverbal Medical Symptoms Validity Test (P. Green, 2008), and Memory Complaints Inventory (P. Green, 2004b) were all infrequently used in this sample.

Collateral Data Use

Forensic examiners are strongly encouraged to use collateral data (Heilbrun, 2001; Melton et al., 2007; Zapf & Roesch, 2009). Participants in the current study indicated they often accessed police reports, the defendant's criminal history, and psychiatric records. Input from defense attorneys was less frequently utilized. Jail disciplinary records and input from jail personnel were "often" used, but school personnel were rarely contacted. Table 10.4 reports the frequency of use of these and other sources. A substantial number of respondents indicated they make observations of the defendant outside of the interview and speak with probation or parole officers.

Table 10.3 Use of Response Style Measures (Percentages) in CST Evaluations

	Usage Rating Totals (%)								
Instrument	**Never**	**Rarely**	**Sometimes**	**Often**	**Almost Always**	**Always**	**TM**	**WS**	***n***
Psychopathology SVTs									
M-FAST	21.6	13.7	31.4	17.6	15.7	0.0	67.7/78.4	2.92	51
SIRS-2	25.5	10.9	38.2	14.5	5.5	5.5	68.3/74.5	2.80	55
SIRS	22.0	22.0	34.0	12.0	4.0	6.0	65.0/78.0	2.72	50
MMPI-2	31.3	27.1	25.0	8.3	8.3	0.0	55.0/68.8	2.35	48
ECST-R ATP[a]	48.9	21.3	19.1	2.1	6.4	2.1	40.0/51.1	2.02	47
MMPI-2-RF	51.1	17.8	17.8	11.1	0.0	2.2	36.7/48.9	1.98	45
SIMS[c]	56.8	15.9	20.5	4.5	0.0	2.3	31.7/43.2	1.82	44
Cognitive PVTs									
TOMM	5.5	18.2	41.8	27.3	3.6	3.6	86.7/94.5	3.16	55
VIP	46.8	12.8	21.3	8.5	6.4	4.3	41.7/53.2	2.28	47
ILK	46.8	8.5	23.4	17.0	2.1	2.1	41.7/53.2	2.26	47
Rey 15 Item	39.1	26.1	19.6	10.9	2.2	2.2	46.7/60.9	2.17	46
Reliable Digit Span[b]	56.8	22.7	11.4	0.0	4.5	4.5	31.7/43.2	1.86	44
Dot Counting Test[d]	58.1	25.6	11.6	2.3	2.3	0.0	30.0/41.9	1.65	43
WMT[e]	74.4	11.6	11.6	0.0	2.3	0.0	18.3/25.6	1.44	43
MSVT[f]	84.1	2.3	6.8	4.5	2.3	0.0	11.7/15.9	1.39	44
Coin in the Hand[g]	88.4	7.0	0.0	4.7	0.0	0.0	8.3/11.6	1.21	43

(*Continued*)

Table 10.3 CONTINUED

Instrument	Usage Rating Totals (%)								
	Never	**Rarely**	**Sometimes**	**Often**	**Almost Always**	**Always**	**TM**	**WS**	***n***
NV-MSVT[h]	90.7	2.3	4.7	0.0	2.3	0.0	6.7/9.3	1.21	43
Memory Complaints Inventory[i]	90.5	7.1	0.0	2.4	0.0	0.0	6.7/9.5	1.14	42

NOTE: Figures shown in all but that last two columns are percentages of responses for that instrument. TM = total mentions = percent of respondents who reported sometimes using the instrument. The first value in the TM column reported is based on assuming that missing values, when rater provided ratings for other tests, are assumed to be "Never." For all tests, $n = 60$ for this figure. The second figure in this column is the total mentions based only on subjects who provided a rating for that test. WS = weighted sum: *Never* = 1; *Rarely* = 2; *Sometimes* = 3; *Often* = 4; *Almost always* = 5; *Always* = 6.

[a]Atypical Presentation Scales.

[b]Reliable Digit Span; Greiffenstein, Baker, & Gola (1994).

[c]Structured Inventory of Malingered Symptoms (Widows & Smith, 2004).

[d]Rey (1941).

[e]Word Memory Test (P. Green, 2005).

[f]Medical Symptom Validity Test (P. Green, 2004a).

[g]Kapur (1994).

[h]Non-Verbal Medical Symptom Validity Test (P. Green, 2008).

[i]Memory Complaints Inventory (P. Green, 2004b).

Table 10.4 Collateral Sources Used in CST Evaluations (Percentages)

Source	Usage Rating Totals (%)								
	Never	Rarely	Sometimes	Often	Almost Always	Always	TM	WS	*n*
Police reports	1.7	1.7	1.7	10.3	22.4	62.1	98.3	5.36	58
Criminal history	0.0	1.7	3.4	13.6	27.1	54.2	100.0	5.29	59
Psychiatric records	0.0	0.0	8.5	25.4	25.4	40.7	100.0	4.98	59
Defense attorney	3.4	8.5	27.1	16.9	20.3	23.7	96.6	4.14	59
Jail/facility disciplinary records	5.2	8.6	29.3	19.0	15.5	22.4	94.8	3.98	58
Jail/facility medical or psychiatric staff	8.8	15.8	26.3	14.0	12.3	22.8	91.2	3.74	57
Behavioral observations outside of interview	12.3	17.5	21.1	15.8	15.8	17.5	87.7	3.58	57
Police interviews[a]	6.9	13.8	44.8	12.1	5.2	17.2	93.1	3.47	58
Interview treatment providers	10.7	25.0	21.4	16.1	12.5	14.3	89.3	3.38	56
Family members	5.3	19.3	47.4	14.0	5.3	8.8	94.7	3.21	57
Jail/facility security staff	17.5	33.3	26.3	3.5	10.5	8.8	82.5	2.90	58
Probation or parole officer	12.3	29.8	36.8	12.3	5.3	3.5	87.7	2.82	57
Other persons[b]	8.3	16.7	66.7	8.3	0.0	0.0	91.7	2.79	57
School records	49.1	24.6	14.0	3.5	5.3	3.5	50.9	2.75	12[c]
Jail/facility recorded phone calls	36.8	40.4	14.0	5.3	1.8	1.8	63.2	2.02	57
Witnesses (interview)	43.9	33.3	15.8	5.3	1.8	0.0	56.1	2.00	57
Police officers	63.6	27.3	9.1	0.0	0.0	0.0	36.4	1.88	57
School personnel (interview)	41.7	8.3	8.3	8.3	8.3	25.0	58.3	1.45	11[c]

NOTE: Figures shown in all but that last two columns are percentages of responses for that instrument. TM = total mentions; WS = weighted sum: *Never* = 1; *Rarely* = 2; *Sometimes* = 3; *Often* = 4; *Almost always* = 5; *Always* = 6.

[a]Transcripts or recordings of the police interview.

[b]Other persons who had contact with defendant.

[c]These items were inadvertently omitted from the initial survey, which is why the number of responses is lower than other items.

Valued Aspects of CST Instruments

CST instruments are quite varied in their rationale and content. Survey respondents were asked their perception of the importance of various factors in a CST instrument. A 5-point Likert scale was used, anchored by *Not at All* (important) on one end and *Essential* on the other. The results are displayed in Table 10.5. Issues of construct validity were highly valued, although correspondence of instrument subscales to *Dusky* (*Dusky v. United States*, 1960) subcriteria (e.g., factual understanding, rational understanding, ability to assist attorney) was not. Ease of communicating results to the court was rated the third most important attribute. Low value was assigned to the ability to detect feigning, incorporating tutoring, ability to cite individual items (without violating test security), and querying the defendant's account of the offense.

Ratings of CST Instruments on Valued Attributes

Participants were then asked to rate each instrument they felt "quite familiar" with on the attributes listed in the previous section. No participant provided ratings for the IFI-R, and the FIT-R was rated by fewer respondents than the other tests. Thus, apart from use ratings of the tests, participants appeared most familiar with

Table 10.5 RATINGS OF IMPORTANCE FOR VARIOUS CST INSTRUMENT ATTRIBUTES

Attribute	*M*	*SD*	95% CI	*n*
Coverage of *Dusky* criteria	4.36	1.02	[4.09, 4.63]	56
Evidence of construct validity	3.93	1.08	[3.64, 4.42]	56
Ease of communication to court of results	3.91	1.00	[3.64, 4.18]	56
Norms (for intended population)	3.84	1.12	[3.54, 4.14]	56
Coverage of all relevant CST facets	3.82	1.08	[3.53, 4.11]	56
Coverage of decisional competence	3.80	1.13	[3.50, 4.10]	56
Evidence of high inter-rater reliability	3.80	1.05	[3.52, 4.08]	56
Evidence of external validity	3.75	1.08	[3.46, 4.04]	56
Standardized questions and scoring	3.66	1.03	[3.38, 3.94]	56
Ease and flow of administration and scoring	3.63	1.15	[3.32, 3.94]	56
Able to meet *Daubert* criteria	3.46	1.37	[3.09, 3.83]	56
Queries about defendant's own case (as opposed to hypothetical case)	3.44	1.28	[3.09, 3.79]	54
Correspondence of subscales to *Dusky* prongs	3.37	1.17	[3.05, 3.69]	54
Suitable for intellectually limited defendants	3.27	1.16	[2.96, 3.58]	55
Has means of detecting feigning	3.07	1.26	[2.73, 3.41]	56
Incorporates tutoring	2.98	1.21	[2.66, 3.30]	56
Ability to cite individual questions and answers, without violating publisher's test security policy	2.77	1.25	[2.44, 3.10]	56
Asks/assesses defendant's account of offense	2.67	1.37	[2.30, 3.04]	54

NOTE: A 5-point Likert scale was used, anchored by 1= *Not at All* (important) on one end and 5 = *Essential* on the other.

the MacCAT-CA, CAST-MR, ECST-R, and FIT-R, respectively. Table 10.6 reports ratings for each test on the CST instrument criteria. The ECST-R received the most positive ratings overall, as evidenced by the highest mean rating. It was highly rated for construct validity and thorough coverage of the *Dusky* criteria, evidence of high inter-rater reliability, ability to meet *Daubert* admissibility requirements, evidence of external validity, and ease of communicating results to the court.

The MacCAT-CA earned high ratings for its standardization, norms, and incorporating tutoring but was faulted for its limited queries about the defendant's own case, (poor) flow and ease of administration, and the difficulty in citing item stems to a trier of fact. The FIT-R's lack of norms was offset by its broad coverage of CST abilities, ease and flow of administration, and ability to cite individual items and answers without violating test security agreements.

The CAST-MR was rated as the most appropriate FAI for ID defendants, and as the only instrument that requests and scores a defendant's account of the offense, it received high marks in this category. However, it received lower ratings on others, including the breadth of coverage (e.g., decisional competence), evidence of construct validity, and ability to meet *Daubert* criteria. Both of the two other fully standardized instruments, the MacCAT-CA and ECST-R, received low suitability ratings for use with ID defendants. This was despite the ECST-R's explicit emphasis on developing short and simple questions.

Prevalence of Negative Response Bias

Raters were asked to estimate the base rates of various types of feigning and invalid presentations among their CST referrals. The results are displayed in Table 10.7. The most frequently referenced styles of feigning were cognitive (e.g., ignorance of court system, amnesia, intellectual limitations, impaired memory). In addition to feigned psychosis, feigned anxiety and depression were both rated as fairly prevalent, as was disingenuous demeanor (e.g., false helplessness, vulnerability, speech impediment, childlike presentation).

The average estimated base rate for any kind of feigning was 24.1% (Mdn = 20; SD = 19.4). Median values are also reported, as the distributions were often skewed, and the median value may be more representative under such conditions. Factitious disorder was seen as rare among CST referrals (M = 1.2%; Mdn = 1; SD = 2.0), as was somatoform disorder (M = 1.9%, Mdn = 1; SD = 4.0). *Lack of cooperation* without feigning was estimated to occur in 8.7% (Mdn = 5; SD = 8.6) of CST referrals. Participants estimated that an average of 13.8% (Mdn = 5; SD = 17.8) of defendants who were feigning were nonetheless incompetent.

Possible Moderators

Respondents who worked in an inpatient setting were no more or less likely to use clinical tests ($t(53) = -.09$; $p = .928$), validity tests ($t(58) = .36$; $p = .720$), CST

Table 10.6 Ratings of CST Instruments on Criteria in Order of Importance

	MacCAT-CA[a]		ECST-R[b]		FIT-R[c]		CAST-MR[d]	
	M	CI	*M*	CI	*M*	CI	*M*	CI
Coverage of *Dusky* criteria	3.7[h]	[3.25, 4.12]	**4.3**[e,h]	[3.89, 4.63]	**4.3**[e,h]	[3.04, 4.88]	3.0	[2.67, 3.39]
Evidence of construct validity	3.6[h]	[3.30, 3.95]	**4.0**[e,h]	[3.71, 4.38]	3.5	[2.76, 4.24]	2.9	[2.38, 3.34]
Ease of communication to court of results	3.5	[3.17, 3.90]	**4.0**[e]	[3.71, 4.29]	3.9	[3.41, 4.42]	3.7	[3.25, 4.09]
Norms (for intended population)	**3.9**[g,h]	[3.54, 4.21]	**3.9**[g,h]	[3.48, 4.27]	2.1	[1.36, 2.79]	3.3[g]	[2.83, 3.77]
Coverage of all relevant CST facets	3.1[h]	[2.69, 3.44]	3.7[e,h]	[3.20, 4.26]	**4.2**[e,h]	[3.51, 4.80]	2.6	[2.19, 3.01]
Coverage of decisional competence	3.7[f,h]	[3.37, 4.06]	3.1[h]	[2.78, 3.48]	**3.8**[f,h]	[2.98, 4.68]	2.5	[2.09, 2.84]
Evidence of high inter-rater reliability	3.7	[3.32, 3.99]	**3.9**[h]	[3.52, 4.22]	3.3	[2.77, 3.90]	3.2	[2.84, 3.64]
Evidence of external validity	3.5[h]	[3.24, 3.82]	**3.6**[h]	[3.22, 3.91]	3.3[h]	[2.55, 4.12]	2.9	[2.46, 3.27]
Standardized questions and scoring	**4.1**	[3.85, 4.40]	**4.1**	[3.78, 4.40]	3.7	[3.18, 4.21]	**4.1**	[3.80, 4.47]
Ease and flow of administration and scoring	3.5	[3.15, 3.79]	3.8[e]	[3.47, 4.21]	**4.0**[e]	[3.38, 4.61]	3.9[e]	[3.46, 4.34]
Able to meet *Daubert* criteria	3.5[h]	[3.17, 3.83]	**4.1**[e,h]	[3.80, 4.46]	3.7	[2.80, 4.54]	2.8	[2.41, 3.25]
Queries about defendant's own case (as opposed to hypothetical case)	2.3	[1.94, 2.68]	**3.6**[e,h]	[3.09, 4.10]	3.7[e,h]	[2.98, 4.35]	2.7	[2.22, 3.16]
Correspondence of subscales to Dusky prongs	3.2	[2.78, 3.66]	**4.2**[e,h]	[3.76, 4.61]	3.7[e,h]	[2.93, 4.40]	2.8	[2.32, 3.21]

Suitable for intellectually limited defendants	2.0	[1.59, 2.34]	2.1	[1.75, 2.51]	3.1[e,f]	[2.32, 3.84]	**3.9**[e,f,g]	[3.37, 4.36]
Has means of detecting feigning	1.3	[1.09, 1.47]	**3.8**[e,f,g]	[3.31, 4.34]	1.2	[.87, 1.59]	1.9[e,g]	[1.49, 2.24]
Incorporates tutoring	**3.3**[g,h]	[2.85, 3.71]	2.9[h]	[2.38, 3.36]	2.8[h]	[1.91, 3.63]	1.6	[1.25, 1.89]
Ability to cite individual questions and answers, without violating publisher's test security policy	3.0	[2.60, 3.47]	3.2	[2.64, 3.69]	**3.8**[e]	[3.07, 4.62]	3.1	[2.73, 3.51]
Asks/assesses defendant's account of offense	2.0	[1.55, 2.38]	2.7[e]	[2.12, 3.21]	2.9	[1.92, 3.88]	**3.0**[e]	[2.49, 3.51]
Average rating	3.2	[2.96, 3.36]	**3.6**[e,h]	[3.39, 3.81]	3.4[e,h]	[2.95, 3.81]	3.0	[2.72, 3.26]

NOTE: The highest value for each row is highlighted in **bold,** the lowest value is underlined. A 5-point Likert scale was used, anchored by 1 = *Poor/None* on one end and 5 = *Excellent* on the other. Confidence intervals based on Student's *t* distribution.

[a]n = 30–32.

[b]n = 21–25.

[c]n = 12–13.

[d]n = 29–30.

[e]Score is above the confidence interval for the MacCAT-CA.

[f] Score is above the confidence interval for the ECST-R.

[g]Score is above the confidence interval for the FIT-R.

[h]Score is above the confidence interval for the CAST-MR.

Table 10.7 Invalid Responding Rates (Percentages) in CST Evaluations

Presentation	*M*	*Mdn*	*SD*	Low	High	Skew	*n*
Feigned ignorance of the court system	17.2	15	16.2	1	75	2.0	54
Feigned amnesia for offense	14.6	10	12.7	1	60	1.5	55
Feigned or exaggerated intellectual limitations	14.5	10	15.7	0	75	2.4	55
Feigned memory problems (NOT amnesia for offense)	12.8	10	11.8	0	70	2.4	53
Feigned hallucinations	10.5	8	10.2	0	50	2.5	55
Feigned depression	10.2	5	10.8	0	50	1.6	54
Feigned anxiety or PTSD	8.2	5	8.7	0	40	1.5	53
Feigned demeanor[a]	7.5	5	13.9	0	75	4.1	53
Feigned paranoia	6.7	5	6.1	0	25	1.2	53
Feigned/exaggerated medical issues[b]	4.3	2	5.2	0	20	1.6	52
Feigned agitation/mania	2.3	1	3.2	0	18	2.7	52
Feigned disorganized speech	1.7	1	2.4	0	10	1.9	52
Other feigned presentation (not listed above)	1.6	0	3.6	0	15	2.8	26
ANY kind of feigning (all previous styles)	24.1	20	19.4	0	90	1.9	49
Factitious disorder	1.2	1	2.0	0	10	2.6	46
Somatoform or conversion disorder	1.9	1	4.2	0	25	4.3	46
Lack of cooperation *without* malingering, factitious, or somatoform disorder	8.7	5	8.6	0	50	2.5	55
Percentage of those feigning who really ARE incompetent	13.8	5	17.8	0	75	2.0	53
Percentage of those presenting invalidly that are malingering[c]	44.2	40	36.1	0	100	0.3	54

[a]E.g., helplessness, vulnerability, childlike demeanor, speech impediment.

[b]E.g., unneeded cane, wheelchair, oxygen tank.

[c]The actual item read: "What percentage OF THOSE PRESENTING INVALIDLY do you believe are Malingering, specifically to be found incompetent and/or influence their case?"

FAIs ($t(57) = -.95$; $p = .346$), or collateral sources ($t(52.92) = .18$; $p = .860$) than examiners working in other settings. However, they tended to use the MacCAT-CA, MMPI-2-RF, PAI, and WMT less often and reported a lower rate of feigned medical presentation or factitious disorder (Table 10.8).

Given evidence of an allegiance effect in forensic examiners (Murrie & Boccaccini, 2015), it seemed plausible that respondents who were hired primarily by defense attorneys might report lower use of validity tests or lower levels of feigning than court-appointed examiners or those hired by the prosecution. Because respondents reported few referrals came from prosecutors, an index was created to combine the three categories into a single index according to the formula: 3*(% Prosecution referred) + 2*(% Court appointed) + % Defense referrals /

Table 10.8 Significant Differences Between Respondents Working in an Inpatient Setting and Others

	Inpatient Respondents			Community Respondents					
Variable	*M*	*SD*	*n*	*M*	*SD*	*n*	*t*	*p*	*d*
Use of MacCAT	1.65	0.71	23	2.57	1.19	30	−3.46[a]	.001	−0.97
Use of MMPI-2-RF	1.55	0.94	20	2.32	1.35	25	−2.17	.036	−0.67
Use of PAI	1.68	0.78	22	2.52	1.4	29	−2.70[a]	.010	−0.77
Use of WMT	1.15	0.49	20	1.70	1.06	23	−2.21[a]	.035	−0.71
Base rate of feigned medical presentation	2.63%	3.46%	24	5.75%	6.80%	28	−2.32	.025	−0.61
Base rate of factitious disorder	.52%	.75%	21	1.80%	2.45%	25	−2.47[a]	.020	−0.80

Note: All *p* values based on two-tailed *t*-test.

[a]Denotes *t*-test calculated for unequal variance (as observed via *F* test). Items answered on the scale: *Never* = 1; *Rarely* = 2; *Sometimes* = 3; *Often* = 4; *Almost always* = 5; *Always* = 6.

(%Prosecution + %Court + %Defense).[3] Thus, high scores on the index suggest a predominance of prosecution or court referrals, low scores a predominance of defense referrals. Contrary to expectations, there was no relation between the index and validity test use ($r(60) = -.064$; *ns*),[4] and there was no difference in reported use of most validity tests or collateral data sources. Further, respondents with more defense referrals estimated a considerably *higher* level of feigning (all types, $r(43) = -.471$; $p < .001$) than examiners who were more often court-appointed or hired by prosecutors. The difference was particularly striking in the perception of feigned medical conditions ($r(46) = -.562$; $p < .0001$) and feigned demeanor ($r(47) = -.512$; $p < .0001$). Significant correlations of referral source with the type of invalid presentation are shown in Table 10.9. Defense-retained examiners were also more likely to see defendants as uncooperative or presenting

Table 10.9 Significant Correlations of Prosecution/Defense Affiliation

Variable	*r*	*df*	*p*
Feigned hallucinations	−.429	49	.002
Feigned depression	−.351	48	.012
Feigned demeanor	−.512	47	<.001
Feigned medical condition	−.562	46	<.0001
Feigned intellectual disability	−.465	49	<.001
Feigned amnesia for crime	−.388	49	.005
Feigned memory impairment	−.351	47	.013
Any type of feigning	−.471	43	.001
Somatoform presentation	−.333	40	.031
Lack of cooperation (not feigning)	−.292	49	.039
Percent of those feigning who are incompetent	−.286	47	.046

Note: All *p* values based on a nondirectional test.

with a somatoform disorder, to perceive even those defendants they judged to be feigning as being competent, and to use the MacCAT-CA ($r(50) = -.418; p = .003$) and MMPI-2-RF ($r(43) = -.433; p = .004$).

Forensic ABPP status was associated with a number of variables, including greater use of the MacCAT-CA and the MMPI (any form), and greater use of data from defense attorneys and from persons with contact with the defendant beyond school and psychiatric personnel, family, the defense attorney, and jail staff (see Table 10.10). Because the greater reliance on input from defense attorneys might be confounded with referrals, I examined the partial correlation of forensic ABPP status and use of input from the defense attorney, controlling for referral source. The partial correlation remained substantial and significant ($r(57) = .470, p < .001$), suggesting this was a difference in the practice of advanced practitioners and not an artifact of referral source. Forensic ABPPs also were more critical of the CAST-MR and MacCAT-CA on some test criteria but provided higher ratings on some aspects of the ECST-R. However, there was no difference on most variables, including none at all on the perceived desirability of different CST test attributes.

SUMMARY AND IMPLICATIONS

The findings reported here have a number of potential implications for practitioners. First of all, there appears to be no gold standard instrument for the assessment of CST. Consistent with recent findings by Neal and Grisso (2014a) few of respondents reported regularly using any of the three standardized FAIs. My observations and conversations with CST examiners in New Hampshire, Minnesota, Colorado, and South Carolina suggest the most frequently used FAI instrument for assessing CST is a semistructured interview with items culled from sources like the CAI, FIT-R, and others. Although the formal FAIs were not frequently used, many respondents indicated they are employed selectively, presumably when deemed appropriate for an examinee or the particular CST issues of a case.

Use of traditional clinical tests in CST evaluations appears to have declined over the last couple of decades. Borum and Grisso (1995) reported both psychologists and psychiatrists frequently used intellectual and objective personality tests, and Lally (2003) reported the WAIS-III was highly recommended for use in CST exams. In contrast, Neal and Grisso (2014a) reported the WAIS was used in only 11.8% of CST exams in their international sample. In the present survey, *no* clinical test, apart from a mini-mental status exam, was reported to be widely used. Several practice guidelines (Melton et al., 2007; Mossman et al., 2007; Zapf & Roesch, 2009) have questioned the usefulness of traditional clinical testing in CST evaluations, which may help explain why respondents reported using such tests infrequently and, perhaps, selectively. Respondents reported extensive use of collateral data, congruent with the findings of Neal and Grisso.

The relative use of different validity tests was consistent with the prior forensic psychology literature but shows the newly released ILK has been widely adopted

Table 10.10 Significant Differences Between Forensic ABPP Raters and Others

	Forensic ABPP Raters			Other Raters					
Variable	*M*	*SD*	*n*	*M*	*SD*	*n*	*t*	*p*	*d*
Use of MacCAT	2.86	1.17	14	1.92	.98	39	2.90	.005	0.71
MacCAT – Corresponding to *Dusky*	2.69	1.25	13	3.58	1.07	19	−2.15	.040	−0.77
ECST-R incorporates tutoring	3.83	1.33	6	2.53	.87	17	2.74	.012	1.20
ECST-R Evidence. of high inter-rater reliability	4.50	.84	6	3.65	.70	17	2.44	.024	1.10
CAST-MR Comprehensive[a]	2.00	.89	11	2.95	1.08	19	−2.46	.020	−0.97
CAST-MR – Construct validity	2.11	1.45	9	3.21	.98	19	−2.37	.025	−0.91
Use of MMPI (any form)	2.75	.87	12	1.84	1.12	37	2.58	.013	0.91
Input from defense attorney	5.29	1.07	14	3.78	1.36	45	3.78	<.001	1.24
Input from "other" person[b]	3.50	1.09	14	2.56	1.14	43	2.71	.009	0.84

NOTE: All p values based on two-tailed t-tests.

[a]Comprehensive coverage of CST construct.

[b]Input from "other" person with contact with defendant. Prior categories included family members, treatment providers, police, defense attorney, school, and jail staff. Items answered on the scale: *Never* = 1; *Rarely* = 2; *Sometimes* = 3; *Often* = 4; *Almost always* = 5; *Always* = 6.

despite a cautionary review (Rubenzer, 2011a). The WMT, MSVT, and NV-MSVT were not widely used, in contrast to a recent survey (Martin, Schroeder, & Odland, 2015), which found all these tests much more widely used than the VIP among neuropsychologists.

Respondents' estimates of feigning were higher than the 17.4% figure provided by Rogers et al. (1998) but consistent with those provided by Mittenberg et al. (2002). Importantly, the estimated rate of feigning is close to the average base rate of incompetence to stand trial reported by Pirelli, Gottdiener, and Zapf (2011). They reported that across 59 samples, the average rate of defendants found *incompetent* was 27.5% (*Mdn* = 25.3%). This means that if validity tests are administered only to those who present having significant deficits, the base rate of feigning in this subgroup will be close to 50%, which is ideal for testing. A higher base rate will produce higher positive predictive power (PPP) figures at a given score, which translates into greater confidence in findings of invalid responding. However, it also means the ability to rule out malingering (negative predictive power [NPP]) will be reduced.

A wide variety of feigned presentations were reported spanning medical, cognitive, and psychopathology domains, as well as simply acting differently than one's usual demeanor. Such affectations may not be detectable by psychometric tests and provide yet another reason to collect collateral data and observations from different settings and motivational contexts. Respondents reported the most common forms of invalid presentation were ignorance of the court system and feigning of psychiatric symptoms, amnesia, and cognitive limitations. These data suggest that instruments like the SIRS, MMPI, and ECST-R Atypical Presentation scales may miss substantial numbers of feigning defendants because they focus on feigned serious mental illness.

The unexpected finding that defense referrals were associated with higher estimates of invalid responding begs for an explanation. A search for possible moderating variables was conducted, but none were identified. However, a few hypotheses can be made. It is possible that defense referrals occur in part because the first examination, by a state examiner, produced evidence of feigning. If so, examiners who provide second opinions for defense attorneys may actually have a higher base rate of feigning than court-appointed examiners who receive unselected cases. Another possibility is that the defense examiners who responded to the survey were self-conscious about being perceived as biased. Such concerns may have led less conscientious defense examiners to forgo participation, or may have led to those that did participate to bolster their estimates to demonstrate their lack of bias. Working in the other direction, respondents who work in state hospitals are typically court-appointed and may receive a select sample of CST cases in which those who are obviously feigning are identified in community evaluations and not hospitalized, leading to a lower base rate in such settings. Unfortunately, with the current data, there is no way to test these hypotheses. Future researchers may wish to query respondents about how many of their referrals are second opinions and the issues raised in the first exam.

Although some researchers (Drob, Meehan, & Waxman, 2009; Rogers et al., 2010) have warned about the need to distinguish malingering from factitious disorders, the latter was seen as quite uncommon by respondents. *Lack of cooperation*, however, occurred in a substantial minority, and distinguishing between feigning and poor cooperation may be the most common differential "diagnosis" in CST response style assessment. Consulting jail security staff and disciplinary records may help resolve this matter. Factitious disorders should be apparent from the defendant's medical history prior to arrest, which is yet another reason to seek medical and psychiatric records.

LIMITATIONS AND ADVANTAGES OF THE CURRENT SURVEY

Prior surveys have usually targeted forensic practitioners with advanced credentials (e.g., ABPP in forensic psychology) or membership in the American Psychology-Law Society. Such respondents are not representative of all CST practitioners: Some very experienced CST practitioners have not joined professional groups or pursued board certification. The forensic ABPP is a "general" credential, not meant to signify expertise in a particular forensic subfield, so even forensic diplomates may not be particularly knowledgeable or engaged in CST assessment: In the study by Archer et al. (2006), only 17.4% of respondents claimed expertise in CST. In contrast, the present study solicited self-identified CST examiners, and the data they provided (number of evaluations completed, amount of their practice devoted to CST) indicate they were, as a group, both highly experienced and active in CST assessment. It is possible that they are not representative of psychologist CST examiners in some way, in that they were recruited through interest-driven forums, and thus may be more invested in CST-related issues than the average practitioner. However, this could be viewed as an asset rather than a liability.

The present study has several significant limitations related to the issues discussed earlier in this chapter. The sample size is smaller than in some previous surveys (although larger than in Lally, 2003), in part because the current study focused on a subgroup of forensic psychology practitioners—CST examiners. The response rate is unknown given the way respondents were recruited, a limitation shared by two other recent surveys that relied on Internet or email solicitation (McLaughlin & Kan, 2014; Neal & Grisso, 2014). Unfortunately, no comprehensive register of competency examiners exists, so it is unclear how a truly representative pool could be identified. In addition, the response rate for some questions, particularly regarding the FIT-R and IFI-R, was much lower than the full sample size. As discussed previously, the sample of examiners with primarily defense referrals may be atypical, as may be the entire sample, and only psychologist examiners participated. The methodology relies on retrospective reports of behavior and subjective estimates, which probably differ from objective reality. To avoid such errors, Neal and Grisso (2014) asked respondents to pick two of their recent reports and answer the survey questions based on their actual practices in those evaluations. Although this approach has the benefit of objectivity, it sacrifices much of the respondent's experience base. Finally, the ratings of the various CST instruments and their attributes were provided by practicing psychologists. Aside from the respondents having doctoral degrees, no data were collected regarding the basis of their expertise on psychometric issues. It is not certain if a panel of such experts were convened that they would agree closely with the participants in this survey.

An ambiguity in the questionnaire and data was the baseline for making ratings about the use of malingering measures. As pointed out by a reviewer, a respondent might base his or her answer assuming either a sample of all CST examinees or only those for which malingering is perceived to be at issue. This distinction has important implications for practice and interpretation of tests through influence on diagnostic statistics like PPP and NPP. Future survey authors may wish to be more explicit in specifying the parameters of the question.

There have been substantial developments in CST practice over the past 10 years (Fogel, Schiffman, Mumley, Tillbrook, & Grisso, 2013), including the release of new instruments and the explosion of research on cognitive malingering. This chapter provides an overview of CST practices and perceptions of experienced CST practitioners, including the types and base rates of feigning during CST exams, which has not been previously available.

NOTES

1. The authors used the acronyms reported here to refer to, for example, all forms of the MMPI (MMPI-2, MMPI-A, MMPI-2-RF); the WAIS included the WISC as was well as revisions of the original WAIS.
2. Although the response format for all items included the option "Never," some respondents left items blank rather than using this or one of the other options, despite providing ratings for other tests.
3. Some respondents indicated other sources of referrals, but these could not be scaled and thus were not included in the index. Two respondents with a high percentage of such referrals were not included in the subsequent analysis.
4. For this analysis, the frequency of reported use for each validity test was summed across tests.

11

Systemic, Policy, and Research Issues

In this chapter, I discuss the enormous implications of moving from a 30- to 90-day, inpatient assessment of competence to assessment within the community or jail. Along with a change in setting, this trend has brought about time pressure on examiners that can easily degrade the quality of CST exams. This chapter addresses both how examiners can address negative response bias even when working under tight budget constraints and how administrators and lawmakers can facilitate obtaining quality assessments without significantly increasing costs. Next, I address some research issues that, if addressed, could increase the validity and usefulness of future investigations. Before delving into these topics, however, a brief overview of the findings from the preceding chapters may be helpful.

RECAP OF FINDINGS

The primary purpose of a validity test, whether a PVT or an SVT, is to provide reliable evidence of invalid responding. To do so, such tests should be able to distinguish examinees with genuine psychosis, mental retardation or severe cognitive impairment, and ignorance of the court system from those who are feigning presentations of these conditions. With the exception of the SIMS,[1] all the self-report and structured interview SVTs reviewed have demonstrated this fundamental validity. Among PVTs, only the WMT and the MSVT have been shown to reliably distinguish feigned from genuine severe cognitive impairment using standard interpretive rules, although even for them, caution is indicated for examinees with IQs below 60 (Chafetz & Biondolillo, 2012; Chafetz, 2015). The two measures of feigned CST ignorance, the ILK and TOMI, are not suitable for ID examinees—the very group in which legitimate ignorance of the court system is likely to arise. Although significantly below-chance performance on these (or other forced-choice tests) potentially can provide strong evidence of negative response bias, the sensitivity of this approach is low (Greve, Binder, & Bianchini, 2009). Further, care must be exercised to accurately communicate the implication of a passing score so that the reader is not misled (see Chapter 9).

POLICY ISSUES

CST exams are performed under the aegis of jurisdictional statutes and case law, but also the local rules and fee structures. These can have substantial implications for the efficiency of the process and practice.

The seismic shift toward outpatient CST assessment requires a rethinking of the assessment process. Many jurisdictions provide a rather minimal standard fee for CST evaluations, with figures as low $170 for an evaluation by a certified CST examiner (Gowensmith, Pinals, & Karas, 2015). Given that this fee may have to cover travel time and checking into the local jail, it is not surprising that some practitioners do little more than a clinical interview as their assessment.

The problem of feigning or poor cooperation has major implications. First of all, a full evaluation of such a defendant will take more time and effort than for a cooperative defendant. Validity testing will likely be required, and there will be a greater need to access treatment records, jail records, the defense attorney, and other collateral data. To the extent these sources are readily available through the standard local CST process, the efficiency of the exam can be maximized. Conversely, if the examiner has to identify potential sources, obtain and send releases or court orders, and follow up to ensure such materials are delivered in a timely manner, costs will escalate. If the local statutes or case law places the burden on the state to prove competence, the conscientious examiner may need to also seek out affirmative evidence of competence. The time required to do this is difficult to predict. Administrators might consider a two-tier fee schedule to account for the extra time needed when the defendant is not cooperative.

Jurisdictions can facilitate the assessment process in several ways, although a balance of interests analysis will be needed. For example, a judge might include language in the court order that directs all educational, psychiatric, and correctional facilities to release records to the examiner. Such a rule is common for those raising the insanity plea, as a defendant is not allowed to place his or her mental state into issue but withhold evidence regarding it. On the other hand, an insanity plea is an affirmative defense,[2] and the issue of competency may be raised against the defendant's will. States and appeals courts might also consider adding a provision that if feigning is detected, the state no longer bears the burden to prove competency in those jurisdictions where it currently does.

LOCATION OF THE EVALUATION

Although jails are now the most common setting for CST exams (Gowensmith et al., 2015), they are generally undesirable environments for psychological assessments: They are loud, and often there are no rooms properly set up for assessment purposes. In some jails, the examiner might have to use an attorney's booth and speak through security glass. This not only hinders communication but also compromises the standardized administration of tests. In other jails, the defendant may be in full view of other inmates. Further, jails induce several time-consuming elements. Often, the examiner will have to travel to the jail, go through security, and then wait for the defendant to be "pulled" from his or her cell or activity. The process of gaining admission and access to the defendant can easily exceed 30 minutes. Of course, if the examiner is an employee or works at the jail, these problems are much reduced. There are also some additional advantages, including being able to observe the defendant outside of the evaluation interview and easily speak with others who do.

An alternative setting to jail or usual community-based evaluation is assessment at the courthouse. Court clinics are becoming more common and present some distinct potential advantages. Much of the wasted time associated with jail-based assessments can be avoided. For the many defendants who will plead out their cases, a court-based assessment could provide data without the lengthy delay often associated with obtaining a CST evaluation through present systems. Potentially, a defendant with mental illness who wants to plead out his or her case could be seen at court; if the defendant is found competent, the plea could be taken later in that same setting. Quite apart from the efficiency of the process, the competency finding is "fresh" rather than weeks old and does not require prediction of how a defendant will present at some future time and situation.

SECOND OPINIONS

Second-opinion CST exams are sometimes ordered when the first examiner opines the defendant is faking. Some psychologists, hired by the defense, tend to rationalize, discount, or ignore the evidence of response bias in the first evaluation and start their own evaluation "with a blank slate." This practice discards relevant data and suggests bias. If the defendant knows his or her presentation has been questioned, future attempts to feign may be more subtle. Evaluations under such circumstances can be particularly challenging and require heightened expertise in response style assessment and a willingness to investigate. However, defense experts may face resistance, for example, when attempting to access jail records that state or court-appointed experts do not.[3] In such cases, defense experts should seek assistance from the referring attorney. But it is entirely possible the defense attorney may also discourage too much digging around, partly out of concern for what might turn up. If the examiner is unable to access desired sources, it should be clearly stated in his or her report that such materials were requested but not received (Otto et al., 2014) and that any conclusions that can be made are limited by their absence. Results from validity tests conducted in the first evaluation should not be discounted unless there is clear evidence that they were inappropriate for the examinee or administered, scored, or interpreted incorrectly.

If a second opinion is needed in such a case, where courts have discretion, I recommend that only examiners with response style expertise and a reputation for objectivity and thoroughness be considered. A budget adequate to accomplish such an evaluation is needed. This can be difficult to estimate, but a complicated case with many records and sources could require 10 to 20 hours of work or more. Failure to heed these recommendations risks wasting the court's time and limited resources, as well as undercutting the accurate determination of competency. While $2,500 or more for a CST exam may seem steep, this is still far cheaper than a 30- to 60-day inpatient evaluation, which costs approximately $500 per day (Kline, 2016) or nearly $23,000 per patient served (Texas Health and Human Services Commission, 2016).

IMPLICATION FOR EXAMINERS

Examiners who work with a very limited budget or time allotment can still assess the validity of presentation but will have to choose wisely how to best invest their time. Speaking to jail staff can be very time-efficient or not, depending on local conditions. Regarding testing, a number of PVTs require less than 10 minutes of the administrator's time (Table 11.1). In addition, examiners will want to consider scoring time and the total time required to administer the test. Computer administration and automated scoring can save significant amounts of time over hand scoring or data entry. Such methods are also prone to error (Barchard & Pace, 2011) and should be checked through double scoring or data entry. Further, computer administration tends to decrease administration time (Ben-Porath & Tellegen, 2008). Some jails do not allow personal computers to be brought in, but the referring judge can write into the CST order that the examiner be allowed to bring and use his or her own electronic devices necessary into the jail to perform the exam.

The MMPI-2/RF, PAI, Paul Green's tests, and the VIP can be administered and scored via computer, whereas most of those that cannot (the TOMM, M-FAST, ECST-R ATP, and ILK) do not require significant scoring time. However, the SIRS-2 does: The publisher estimates 20 minutes to score, and double scoring it for accuracy would presumably take considerably longer. No computer option is currently available or forthcoming (Psychological Assessment Resources customer service representative, personal communication, December 6, 2016).

The Rey 15 Item Test, Reliable Digit Span, TOMM Trial 1, the MSVT, NV-MSVT, and WMT all require less than 10 minutes of the examiner's time. The latter three tests do require a 10- or 30-minute period between administrations

Table 11.1 Times Required for Validity Tests

Test	Examiner Time (Min.)	Testing Time (Min.)	Time to Complete (Min.)
Rey 15[a]	1	1	1
Reliable Digit Span[a]	2–5	2–5	2–5
MMSE[a]	5–6	5–6	5–6
TOMM T1[b]	6–8	6–8	6–8
M-FAST[b]	6–8	5–7	5–7
ECST-R ATP	6–7	5–6	5–6
MSVT[c]	4	5	15
NV-MSVT[c]	4	7–8	17–18
TOMM T1 and T2[b]	11–14	11–14	11–14
SIMS	1, 6[c]	15	15
VIP Verbal[d]	2	20	22
VIP Nonverbal[d]	2	30	32
TOMM T1, T2, RT[b]	13–17	13–17	28–32
WMT[c]	4	12	42
MMPI-2-RF[d]	1	25[e]–50	26[d]–51
PAI[d]	2	<1 hour	<1 hour
MMPI-2[d]	1	60–90	61–91
SIRS-2[d]	60–65	40–45	40–45

NOTE: *Examiner time* refers to the amount of time the examiner must spend directly involved to administer the test and score it. *The figures cited assume that computer administration and scoring are used if available.* Otherwise, scoring time for some tests can be substantial and even prohibitive. *Testing time* refers to the amount of time the examinee must spend actively completing the test. *Time to complete* refers to the total span of time needed to complete the test, including any distraction periods between subtests. Times provided are estimates based on instructions from the manuals and personal experience, and assume a reasonably cooperative and unimpaired examinee. T1 = Trial 1; T2 = Trial 2; RT = Retention Trial. Time figures reported in the table are based on [a] trial adminstrations, [b] information from the test manual, [c] P. Green (2016), or [d] publisher's claims. [e] The manual indicates testing time is roughly 10 to 15 minutes (less if administered via computer).

of subtests, but this time can be used to administer other nonmemory tests, sign release of information forms, or discuss CST-related topics. The quickest tests of all are the Rey 15 Item Test (1 minute) and the Reliable Digit Span (perhaps 2 to 3 minutes for the pre–WAIS-IV versions before Sequencing was added). However, the quality of the PVTs tends to rise with increased administration time. The choice among very quick psychopathology SVTs is limited to the M-FAST and ECST-R Atypical Presentation scales, both of which take about 5 to 7 minutes. The SIMS takes about 15 minutes for the examinee to complete and 2 to 3 minutes to score.

If one has only 15 minutes of administration time for validity assessment, a typical defendant, and one who is possibly faking both psychiatric and cognitive impairment, I recommend the MSVT, with the M-FAST and Rey 15 Item Test and/or RDS administered during the 10-minute period between MSVT tasks. The NV-MSVT could be substituted for the MSVT, particularly when reading limitations are present, with some advantages. Alternatively, one could administer the TOMM Trial 1, M-FAST, and Rey 15, with some loss of sensitivity and ability to classify actual impairment.

If one is not as limited on the total time span to complete a test, the WMT should be strongly considered, especially for brighter or savvier examinees who present with relatively circumscribed or subtle cognitive deficits. The WMT is more credible as a legitimate memory test (Tan et al., 2002) than many PVTs and includes three useful subtests of memory. Although administration takes about 40 to 45 minutes from beginning to end, 30 minutes of this is a distraction period that can be used for other nonmemory tests or tasks (P. Green, 2016). Apart from the time issues discussed here, the choice of tests should be predicated primarily on their validity for the given purpose and appropriateness for the examinee. Generally speaking, the examiner should choose SVTs and PVTs that the examinee is almost certainly able to pass if motivated to answer honestly and perform to the best of his or her ability.

FUTURE CST RESEARCH

Pirelli, Zapf, and Gottdiener (2011) recently identified CST research needs from their meta-analysis (Pirelli, Gottdiener, & Zapf, 2011) and made 13 specific recommendations. To their recommendations, I would add several more. The use of *presumed genuine* patient groups is an anachronism given Rogers et al.'s (1998) findings that 7.2% of genuine patients were thought to be feigning or exaggerating, and recent findings of poor effort in a variety of samples without apparent incentives. Such subjects will greatly distort cutoff scores and underestimate the diagnostic power of a test. This is particularly a risk when using general clinical norms (e.g., Caldwell's MMPI data set) or, worse, samples at high risk for suboptimal effort (jail treatment groups, mTBI litigants) to set cutoff scores on scales like MMPI-2's Fp scale. Even in the absence of external incentives, some examinees (e.g., borderline or histrionic personalities) may present with exaggerated or overly dramatic complaints that portray more pathology than external observers or objective indicators would suggest. High apparent false positives for PVTs like the VIP and WMT in some patient groups may be accurate classifications of patients who are unmotivated and putting forth limited effort on a task of little personal significance. Examinees should not be presumed to perform with good motivation and effort, and there should be an actual assessment of their response style and external incentives. Depressed, schizophrenic, or ID examinees may underperform on cognitive tasks because of limited motivation. When such subjects fail a test like the TOMM, retesting with a substantial incentive for better performance can help distinguish between limited capacity and poor motivation (P. Green & Flaro, 2003).

One of the limitations encountered in reviews of validity tests, most prominently the SIRS, is the tendency for researchers to investigate their own cutoff scores or decision rules while neglecting the official criteria. One the SIRS's greatest assets was its cross-validated decision rules, but few studies since its early development used the standard criteria, turning instead to discriminant analysis and other approaches that do not directly inform clinical decision-making. Individual authors also tend to be idiosyncratic in deciding which cutoff scores to report diagnostic statistics for, so attempts to combine samples from published data run into many missing values. Finally, the use of a single cutoff score to dichotomize subjects into those who are likely feigning and those who are not artificially limits the test and discards data. Having at least two cutoff scores would be more informative, with one to indicate likely feigning or exaggeration, another to indicate that such distortion is unlikely, and a band of indeterminate values between the two scores, as Rogers has repeatedly suggested.

Most studies to date have viewed feigned incompetence in global terms. Studies that contrast variables, such as IQ scores, between competent and incompetent groups will underestimate the importance of these variables in subgroups such as ID defendants. A validity measure that targets feigned psychopathology would not be expected to discriminate those that limit their feigning to ignorance of the court system. Thus, it would be desirable to first determine what deficits an examinee portrays prior to administration of validity measures. Diagnostic statistics for PVTs, for example, would then be based on those who portray cognitive deficits, not those who limit their presentation to psychiatric symptoms or ignorance of the court system. However, some subjects may fail validity tests even in areas in which they did not initially present impairment. It may be that some validity tests "invite" test-takers to display impairment when the opportunity arises, as the ECST-R ATP scales apparently do. This possibility is also of interest but should be considered separately.

There has been relatively little research in CST settings on what this writer believes are the most promising instruments, the WMT, NV-MSVT, and MSVT. The NV-MSVT, in particular, has very desirable characteristics for CST samples (no reading requirement, excellent internal validity checks, high specificity in cognitively impaired groups, brevity, engagement, and probable low reorganizability as a validity test) but has very limited data in psychiatric samples. Future research should consider investigating one or more of these tests along with the M-FAST.

CONCLUSION

Assessment of response style is crucial to valid determinations of competency to be adjudicated. A variety of validated measures for assessing feigned psychopathology and memory problems are available, and some of these are quite brief and cost-effective. There does not yet appear to be a fully satisfactory instrument for assessing feigned ignorance of the court system, given that such instruments are not validated with ID persons and appear affected by genuine incompetence. Collateral data, particularly those that shed light on the defendant's functioning in different settings and motivational contexts, are essential in many cases to provide evidence of feigned impairment as well as data bearing on functional ability.

Readers are encouraged to become experts at assessing response style within the CST context and to constantly question whether the data they receive and observe are a reliable guide to the defendant's actual abilities, level of functioning, and typical demeanor. Given the development of forensic psychology as a specialty discipline and the centrality of response style assessment to forensic evaluation, it is unacceptable for a doctoral-level CST examiner to be fooled by a defendant with a 10th-grade education and modest resources to prepare for his or her performance—a situation I have seen many times in my career. Failure to thoroughly assess for negative response bias, in the presence of apparent deficits sufficient to compromise competency and absence of credible collateral data to corroborate the presented impairment, is persuasive evidence of an inadequate CST evaluation.

NOTES

1. Having been designed as a screening test, the SIMS has a relative low cutoff score that results in high false positives in psychiatric samples. However, it shows very robust effect sizes, so it does show evidence of ability to discriminate.
2. A defense that must be raised or asserted by the defendant.
3. An issue brought to my attention by Eric Mart, PhD, ABPP.

APPENDIX A

Area Under the Curve Explained

Area under the curve (AUC) is an index derived from Receiver Operator Characteristics (ROC), which was developed to help radar operators distinguish signals (planes or ships) from noise on their screens. The ROC curve is expressed on a chart with two axes. The vertical axis represents accuracy in *detecting the target condition* (e.g., enemy planes for radar operators, feigners for CST examiners): The accuracy goes from 0% in the lower corner to 100% at the top left corner of the chart (see Figure A.1).

The horizontal axis represents false positives: 0% at the left corner, 100% at the right. The straight, dashed line extending from the lower left corner to the upper right corner defines a test with no validity. The sensitivity equals the false positive rate, so the test does not distinguish feigners from honest examinees: They both fail at the same rate at all cutoff scores. An AUC of .50 (50%) indicates no relationship between the variables (a correlation = .00), where one of 1.00 (100%) is the

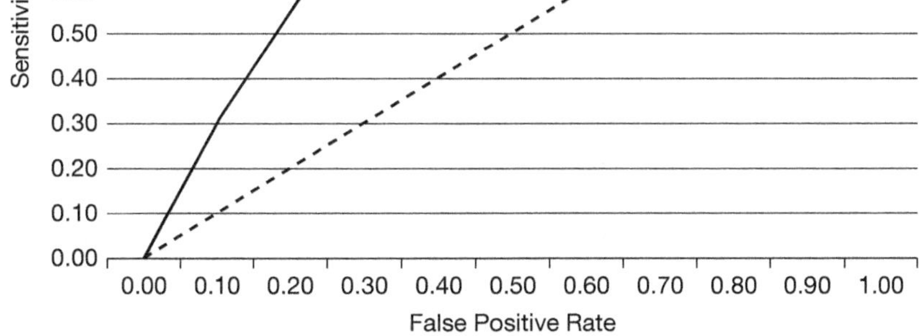

Figure A.1 Example of an ROC Curve

maximum obtainable. At an AUC of 1.00, all subjects, both honest and feigning, are accurately classified.

AUC is a measure of the relationship between a continuous variable, such as scores on a test, and a dichotomous (yes or no; faking or not) variable. The ROC curve in the chart plots the sensitivity and false positive rates of a tests at all possible cutoff points. For example, for the M-FAST, scores range from 0 to 25. Each point would have an associated sensitivity and false positive rate, which are the coordinates for the chart. Thus, rather than giving data for only a single cutoff score, the AUC shows how well the test discriminates all possible cut scores.

The curve shown in Figure A.1 illustrates a test with modest validity. The AUC shown, the area under the heavy curved line, is perhaps 70% of the total chart area. In contrast, an ROC curve for the M-FAST, using the SIRS as the criterion, reaches nearly to the upper-left corner of the chart, and the AUC approaches 95%.

APPENDIX B

Selected Test Indices With Approximately .90 Specificity in Multiple Relevant Studies and Associated Cutoff Scores, Sensitivities, and Citations

Test/Index	Criteria/Cutoff Score	Includes SMI, ID?[a]	Sensitivity	Specificity	Citations
MMPI-2 F[b]	>106	SMI	.67–.78	.76–1.00	Lewis et al., 2002; McCuster et al., 2003; Kucharski & Duncan, 2007
MMPI-2 Fp[b]	>100	SMI	.35–.52	.85–1.00	Lewis et al., 2002; McCuster et al., 2003; Heinze, 2003
MMPI-2 RBS	>17 raw		.13–.50	.88–.99	Gervais et al., 2007; Whitney et al., 2008; Dionysus et al., 2011; Young et al., 2011
MMPI-2-RF F-r	≥120	SMI	.27[c] .64–.89	.88–.92	Sellbom & Bagby, 2010; Sellbom et al., 2011
MMPI-2-RF Fp-r	≥100	SMI	.43[c] .72–.74	.90–.97	Sellbom & Bagby, 2010; Sellbom et al., 2011
PAI NIM	≥110	SMI	.33	.98	Hawes & Boccancini, 2009
PAI MAL	≥4	SMI	.35	.99, 1.00	Hawes & Boccancini, 2009
PAI NDS	≥19	SMI	.64, .79	.90, .97	Mogge et al., 2010; Thomas et al., 2012; Rogers et al., 2013
SIRS	Per manual	SMI	.486	.946	D. Green & Rosenfeld, 2011
SIRS-2	Per manual	SMI, ID	.37 (KG) .325–.75 (Sim)	.93–1.00	D. Green et al., 2013; Brand et al., 2014; Weiss et al., 2011 DeClue, 2011
M-FAST	≥12	SMI	.22–.47[d]	.824–1.00[e]	Miller, 2001; Gaines, 2009 ; Glassmire, Tarascavage et al., 2016; Guy & Miller, 2004

FIT	< 9	SMI	.36	.90[f]	Reznek, 2005; Vickery et al., 2001
RDS	≤6		.30–.35	.96–.97	Schroeder, Twumasi-Ankrah, et al., 2012
TOMM Trial 1	<41		.77	.92	Denning, 2012
TOMMe10	≥2 Errors		.50, .71	.90, .93	Denning, 2012, 2013, 2014; Kulas et al., 2014
TOMM Trial 2	<45	SMI	.654	.938	Sollman & Berry 2011
TOMM Trial 2	<30	ID	.24, .56	.96	Graue et al., 2007; Shandera et al., 2010
TOMM Retention Trial	<45		.48–.50	.971–1.00	Schroeder et al., 2013; Buddin et al., 2014; Kulas et al., 2014
TOMM Retention Trial	<30	ID	.20, .60	.96, 1.00	Graue et al., 2007; Shandera et al., 2010
TOMM ACI	≥10		.71–.77	.853–1.00	Gunner et al., 2012; Schroeder et al., 2013; Buddin et al., 2014; Kulas et al., 2014
WMT	Fail A criteria	ID, SMI	.751	.694	Sollman & Berry, 2011
WMT	with profile analysis	Dem, ID, SMI[g]	—	.86–1.00[h]	Larochette & Harrison, 2012; Martins & Martins, 2010; Eichstaedt et al., 2014; Hampson et al., 2014; P. Green & Flaro (2015, 2016)

(*Continued*)

Test/Index	Criteria/Cutoff Score	Includes SMI, ID?[a]	Sensitivity	Specificity	Citations
MSVT	Without profile analysis	ID, Dem	.90–1.00 Sim	.273–1.00	Merten et al., 2005; Chafetz et al., 2007; Singhal et al., 2009; Blaskewitz et al., 2008; Rudman et al., 2011
MSVT	With profile analysis	ID, Dem[g]	.40–.766[ij]	.94–1.00	Singhal et al., 2009; Bashem et al., 2014; Chafetz & Biondilillo, 2013; Weinborn et al., 2012; Larson et al., 2015; P. Green & Flaro, 2015, 2016; Suesse et al., 2015
NV-MSVT	With profile analysis	ID, Dem	.88, .96 Sim .47–.92 KG	.885, 1.00	Singhal et al., 2009; Henry et al., 2010; Armistead-Jehle & Gervais, 2011; P. Green & Flaro, 2016; Armistead-Jehle & Denney, 2015

NOTE: Figures do not apply to defendants with severe cognitive impairment or serious mental illness unless otherwise noted. Sim = simulator group; KG = known group.

[a]SMI = serious mental illness; ID = intellectually disabled; Dem = dementia.

[b]Cutoff scores reported based only from studies of criminal samples.

[c]Coached subjects.

[d]Based on table from manual (Miller, 2001, p. 12) for clinical sample.

[e]Specificity estimated from the specificity of SIRS's standard criteria reported in D. Green and Rosenfeld (2011), given that nearly all examines with an M-FAST score of >11 failed the SIRS.

[f]Specificity figure does not apply to ID examinees or those with dementia.

[g]Figure is for subjects with a 3.1 or greater reading level on WRAT-4.

[h]This range of figure excludes Eichstaedt et al.'s group of patients with bilateral temporal lobe epilepsy because of its small size ($n = 3$). Further, the subjects who failed in the studies with lower specificities were reported to show other indications of poor effort/validity.

[i]Sensitivity figures include both for failing A criteria and for doing so with an implausible profile.

[j]The highest value cited is from a simulator study. Typical values from actual examinees tended to be much lower, around .45.

GLOSSARY

Area under the curve (AUC): A measure of the relationship between a dichotomous (yes or no; faking or not) variable and another variable such as scores on a test. An AUC of .50 (50%) indicates no relationship between the variables (correlation = .00), whereas one of 1.00 (100%) is the maximum obtainable. It takes into account all possible cutoff scores. See Appendix A for a more thorough explanation.

Base rate: The percentage of examinees in the sample who have the condition of interest (e.g., feigning).

Cohen's *d*, Hedges' *g* (and *d*): Two measures of the size of the difference in scores between two samples. To calculate them, subtract one mean (average score) of sample from the other, then divide the difference by the pooled standard deviation (a measure of variability within each sample).* Generially, Cohen's *d* and Hedge's *g* are referred to as *effect sizes*. Effect sizes larger than 0.8 are generally considered "large," as they indicate a substantial difference in the average score between two samples compared with the variation within each sample (Cohen, 1988), although Rogers (2008b) argued that for forensic practice, a higher standard of $d \geq 1.25$ be required to denote a "large" effect size.

* The *pooled* standard deviation is similar to averaging the standard deviation of the two samples. There appear to be several formulas for calculating it, some of which are complicated. Fortunately, there are several free websites that will allow an uninitiated user to easily calculate effect size indices like Cohen's *d*.

Diagnostic test: A test that, if positive, indicates a high probability the subject has the condition. Thus, a good diagnostic test should have a low false positive rate. Often, however, diagnostic tests also have low or moderate sensitivity.

Internal consistency (alpha coefficient): A measure of the how much the items in a scale share a common core of meaning, ranging from .00 to 1.00 (0-100%). This is a major constraint on how accurate a test or scale can be.

Known group design: A study in which the participants are determined to be honest or feigning through the best available classification procedure. In the literature addressing feigning of psychopathology, the SIRS was often employed as the criterion.

Likelihood ratio: A number that indicates how much more likely it is that a test-taker with the condition of interest (e.g., feigning) will test positive on the test than someone without the condition. The (positive) Likelihood ratio (LR+) = Sensitivity/False Positive Rate.

Negative predictive power (NPP): The probability that an examinee who scores negative (passes) a validity test is indeed performing genuinely. This is the most relevant statistic for an examinee who passes a validity test but requires knowledge of the base rate. NPP equals the probability that the defendant is performing genuinely.

Positive predictive power (PPP): The percentage of examinees who score positive (fail) a validity test who are actually feigning; the accuracy rate for those who fail. This is the most meaningful statistic for an examinee who fails a validity test but requires knowledge of the base rate. PPP gives the probability that an examinee is feigning/not performing validly.

Screening test: Typically a brief test administered to determine if a condition *might* be present. This would then be followed up with a *diagnostic* test, which, if positive, indicates the presence of the condition with high certainty. A screening test should have high sensitivity (identify nearly everyone who has the condition assessed for) but may have a high number of false positive errors.

Significantly below chance (SBC): If a multiple-choice test has four possible answers, an examinee could score approximately 25% correct by guessing, knowing nothing at all about the subject of the test. Of course, if 100 such subjects guess blindly, some would score below 25% correct, and some would score above. But, statistically, very few would score below say, 15%, or above 35%. A score that is statistically below chance is usually defined as occurring in less than 5% ($p < .05$) of test-takers who respond randomly.

Simulation study: Subjects are asked to simulate (fake) a given condition, such as a psychiatric disorder, intellectual disability, or incompetence to stand trial. Usually, a group of genuine clinical subjects also take the same tests and are asked to perform honestly. Scores from the two groups are then compared. Some older studies compared the scores of simulators with those of students or other normal samples, which is a weak and biased study design. Another "design" issue is the presumption that clinical groups do not exaggerate.

The Slick criteria: A set of criteria proposed by Slick, Sherman, and Iverson (1999) to objectively diagnose *malingered* cognitive impairment. They require the presence of an incentive to perform poorly, such as obtaining disability benefits, and either implausible test performance, and/or inconsistencies between the examinee's presentation, self-report, or test scores with other facts or data.

Specificity: The accuracy of a test in classifying persons who do not have the condition of interest, such as faking. Thus, specificity is the accuracy of a malingering test in classifying honest respondents and ranges from 0% to 100% (also written as .00–1.00).

Standard error of measurement (*SEM*): A number that reflects the uncertainty of a score. Most scores in psychology will be influenced by random error variance. The *SEM* depends on the reliability of the test and the variability of scores in a sample (standard deviation; *SD*). The formula is $SEM = SD^{*}\sqrt{(1 - \text{reliability})}$. Test scores can be reported as the score plus or minus ($\pm$) one or two *SEM*s, which creates a *confidence interval* around the score (e.g., 95 ± 2). For a score $\pm$ 2 *SEM*s, the confidence interval has a 95% probability of containing the true score (if it could be measured without error and observed). Thus, the *SEM* is similar to the *SD* for the score of a single subject.

T scores are a type of standard score. The average (mean) score for a sample is 50. A score that is one standard deviation (*SD*) above the average score is 60, and two standard deviations above the average is 70. Similarly, a score one *SD* below the average score is 40, and two *SD*s below the average is 30.

REFERENCES

Akehurst, L., Easton, S., Fuller, E., Drane, G., Kuzmin, K., & Litchfield, S. (2015). An evaluation of a new tool to aid judgements of credibility in the medico-legal setting. *Legal and Criminological Psychology, 22*, 22–46. http://dx.doi:10.1111/lcrp.12079

Allen, L. M., & Green, P. (2002). Equivalence of the computerized and orally administered Word Memory Test effort measures. *WebPsychEmpiricist, Retrieved Nov. 11, 2017.*

Alwes, Y. R., Clark, J. A., Berry, D. T., & Granacher, R. P. (2008). Screening for feigning in a civil forensic setting. *Journal of Clinical and Experimental Neuropsychology, 30*(2), 133–140. http://dx.doi.org/10.1080/13803390701260363

American Psychiatric Association. (2013). *Diagnostic and statistical manual of mental disorders* (5th ed. text rev.). Washington, DC: Author. http://dx.doi.org/10.1176/appi.books.9780890425596

American Psychological Association. (2002). Ethical principles of psychologists and code of conduct. *American Psychologist, 57*(12), 1060–1073.

American Psychological Association. (2013). Specialty guidelines for forensic psychology. *American Psychologist, 68*(1), 7–19. http://dx.doi.org/10.1037/a0029889

An, K., Zakzanis, K., & Joordens, S. (2012). Conducting research with non-clinical healthy undergraduates: Does effort play a role in neuropsychological test performance? *Archives of Clinical Neuropsychology, 27*, 849–857. http://dx.doi.org/10.1093/arclin/acs085

Anderson, S. D., & Hewitt, J. (2002). The effect of competency restoration training on defendants with mental retardation found not competent to proceed. *Law and Human Behavior, 26*(3), 343–351.

Archer, R. P., Buffington-Vollum, J. K., Stredny, R. V., & Handel, R. W. (2006). A survey of psychological test use patterns among forensic psychologists. *Journal of Personality Assessment, 87*(1), 84–94. http://dx.doi.org/10.1207/s15327752jpa8701_07

Archer, R. P., Handel, R. W. Ben-Porath, Y. S., & Tellegen, A. (2016). *The Minnesota Multiphasic Personality Inventory–Adolescent Restructure Form.* Minneapolis, MN: University of Minnesota Press.

Ardolf, B. R., Denney, R. L., & Houston, C. M. (2007). Base rates of negative response bias and malingered neurocognitive dysfunction among criminal defendants referred for neuropsychological evaluation. *Clinical Neuropsychologist, 21*(6), 899–916. http://dx.doi.org/10.1080/13825580600966391

Arena, J. E., & Rabinstein, A. A. (2015). Transient global amnesia. *Mayo Clinic Proceedings, 90*(2), 264–272. http://dx.doi.org/10.1016/j.mayocp.2014.12.001

Arkes, H. R. (1989). Principles in judgment/decision making research pertinent to legal proceedings. *Behavioral Sciences & the Law, 7*, 429–456. http://dx.doi.org/10.1002/bsl.2370070403

Armistead-Jehle, P. (2010). Symptom validity test performance in U.S. veterans referred for evaluation of mild TBI. *Applied Neuropsychology, 17*(1), 52–59. http://dx.doi.org/10.1080/09084280903526182

Armistead-Jehle, P., & Buican, B. (2013). Comparison of select Advanced Clinical Solutions embedded effort measures to the Word Memory Test in the detection of suboptimal effort. *Archives of Clinical Neuropsychology, 28*(3), 297–301. http://dx.doi.org/10.1023/A:1015328505884.

Armistead-Jehle, P., & Denney, R. L. (2015). The detection of feigned impairment using the WMT, MSVT, and NV-MSVT. *Applied Neuropsychology: Adult, 22*(2), 147–155. http://dx.doi.org/10.1080/23279095.2014.880842

Armistead-Jehle, P., & Gervais, R. O. (2011). Sensitivity of the Test of Memory Malingering and the Nonverbal Medical Symptom Validity Test: A replication study. *Applied Neuropsychology, 18*(4), 284–290. http://dx.doi.org/10.1080/09084282.2011.595455

Armistead-Jehle, P., Gervais, R. O., & Green, P. (2012). Memory Complaints Inventory results as a function of symptom validity test performance. *Archives of Clinical Neuropsychology, 27*(1), 101–113. http://dx.doi.org/10.1093/arclin/acr081

Ashendorf, L., Constantinou, M., & McCaffrey, R. J. (2004). The effect of depression and anxiety on the TOMM in community-dwelling older adults. *Archives of Clinical Neuropsychology, 19*, 125–130. http://dx.doi.org/10.1016/S0887-6177(02)00218-4

Axelrod, B. N., & Schutte, C. (2010). Analysis of the dementia profile on the Medical Symptom Validity Test. *Clinical Neuropsychologist, 24*(5), 873–881. http://dx.doi.org/10.1080/13854040903527295

Axelrod, B. N., & Schutte, C. (2011). Concurrent validity of three forced-choice measures of symptom validity. *Applied Neuropsychology, 18*(1), 27–33. http://dx.doi.org/10.1080/09084282.2010.523369

Babchishin, K. M., Hanson, R. K., & Helmus, L. (2012). Even highly correlated measures can add incrementally to predicting recidivism among sex offenders. *Assessment, 19*(4), 442–461. http://dx.doi.org/10.1177/1073191112458312

Babitsky, S., & Mangraviti, J. (2005). *How to become a dangerous expert witness: Advanced techniques and strategies*. Falmouth, MA: SEAK.

Babitsky, S., Mangraviti, J., & Todd, C. J. (2000). *The comprehensive forensic services manual: The essential resources for all experts*. Falmouth, MA: SEAK. http://dx.doi.org/10.1080/019476401750365246

Bacchiochi, J. B., & Bagby, R. M. (2006). Development and validation of the Malingering Discriminant Function Index for the MMPI-2. *Journal of Personality Assessment, 87*(1), 51–61. http://dx.doi.org/10.1207/s15327752jpa8701_04

Back, C., Boone, K. B., Edwards, C., Parks, C., Burgoyne, K., & Silver, B. (1996). The performance of schizophrenics on three cognitive tests of malingering, Rey 15-Item Memory Test, Rey Dot Counting, and Hiscock Forced-Choice Method. *Assessment, 3*(4), 449–457. http://dx.doi.org/10.1177/107319119600300411

Baer, R. A., Wetter, M. W., & Berry, D. T. (1992). Detection of underreporting of psychopathology on the MMPI: A meta-analysis. *Clinical Psychology Review, 12*(5), 509–525.

Barber-Rioja, V., Zottoli, T. M., Kucharski, L. T., & Duncan, S. (2009). The utility of the MMPI-2 Criminal Offender Infrequency (Fc) Scale in the detection of malingering in criminal defendants. *International Journal of Forensic Mental Health*, *8*(1), 16–24. http://dx.doi.org/10.1080/14999010903014689

Barchard, K. A., & Pace, L. A. (2011). Preventing human error: The impact of data entry methods on data accuracy and statistical results. *Computers in Human Behavior*, *27*(5), 1834–1839. http://dx.doi.org/10.1016/j.chb.2011.04.004

Barkemeyer, C. A., & Callon, E. B. (1989). *Malingering Detection Scale*. Baton Rouge, LA: North Street.

Barkemeyer, C. A., Wymer, J. H., Jones, G. N., & Callon, E. B. (2003). The Barkemeyer-Callon-Jones Malingering Detection Scale (MDS): Further validation of an objective measure of malingering behavior. *Archives of Clinical Neuropsychology*, *18*(7), 780.

Bashem, J. R., Rapport, L. J., Miller, J. B., Hanks, R. A., Axelrod, B. N., & Millis, S. R. (2014). Comparisons of five performance validity indices in bona fide and simulated traumatic brain injury. *Clinical Neuropsychologist*, *28*(5), 851–875. http://dx.doi.org/10.1080/13854046.2014.927927

Batt, K., Shores, E. A., & Chekaluk, E. (2008). The effect of distraction on the Word Memory Test and Test of Memory Malingering performance in patients with a severe brain injury. *Journal of the International Neuropsychological Society*, *14*(6), 1074–1080. http://dx.doi.org/10.1017/S135561770808137X

Bauer, L., & McCaffrey, R. J. (2006). Coverage of the Test of Memory Malingering, Victoria Symptom Validity Test, and Word Memory Test on the Internet: Is test security threatened? *Archives of Clinical Neuropsychology*, *21*(1), 121–126. http://dx.doi.org/10.1016/j.acn.2005.06.010

Bauer, L., O'Bryant, S. E., Lynch, J. K., McCaffrey, R. J., & Fisher, J. M. (2007). Examining the Test of Memory Malingering Trial 1 and Word Memory Test immediate recognition as screening tools for insufficient effort. *Assessment*, *14*(3), 215–222. http://dx.doi.org/10.1177/1073191106297617

Benge, J. F., Wisdom, N. M., Collins, R. L., Franks, R., LeMaire, A., & Chen, D. K. (2012). Diagnostic utility of the Structured Inventory of Malingered Symptomatology for identifying psychogenic non-epileptic events. *Epilepsy & Behavior*, *24*(4), 439–444. http://dx.doi.org/10.1016/j.yebeh.2012.05.007.

Bennett, A. D. (2005–6). *The measurement of adjudicative competence: A comparison of three types of competencies in a sample of individuals with mental retardation* (Doctoral dissertation). Available from ProQuest Information and Learning.

Ben-Porath, Y. S., & Tellegen, A. (2008). *Minnesota Multiphasic Personality Inventory–2 Restructured Form: Manual for administration, scoring, and interpretation.* Minneapolis, MN: University of Minnesota Press. http://dx.doi.org/10.1002/9780470479216.corpsy0573

Ben-Porath, Y. S., Greve, K. W., Bianchini, K. J., & Kaufmann, P. M. (2009). The MMPI-2 symptom validity scale (FBS) is an empirically validated measure of overreporting in personal injury litigants and claimants: Reply to Butcher et al. (2008). *Psychological Injury and Law*, *2*(1), 62–85. http://dx.doi.org/10.1007/s12207-009-9037-4

Ben-Porath, Y. S., Greve, K. W., Bianchini, K. J., & Kaufmann, P. M. (2010). The MMPI-2 symptom validity scale (FBS) is an empirically-validated measure of over-reporting in personal injury litigants and claimants: Reply to William et al. (2009). *Psychological Injury and Law*, *3*(1), 77–80. http://dx.doi.org/10.1007/s12207-009-9049-0

Berry, D. T., & Schipper, L. J. (2007). Detection of feigned psychiatric symptoms during forensic neuropsychological examinations. In G. Larrabee (Ed.), *Assessment of neuropsychological deficits* (pp. 226–263). New York, NY: Oxford University Press. http://dx.doi.org/10.1080/23279095.2016.1189426

Berry, D. T., & Schipper, L. J. (2008). Assessment of feigned cognitive impairment using standard neuropsychological tests. In R. Rogers (Ed.), *Clinical assessment of malingering and deception* (3rd ed., pp. 237–273). New York, NY: Guilford. http://dx.doi.org/10.1080/23279095.2016.1189426

Berthelson, L., Mulchan, S. S., Odland, A. P., Miller, L. J., & Mittenberg, W. (2013). False positive diagnosis of malingering due to the use of multiple effort tests. *Brain Injury, 27*(7-8), 909–916. http://dx.doi.org/10.3109/02699052.2013.793400

Bianchini, K. J., Greve, K. W., & Glynn, G. (2005). On the diagnosis of malingered pain-related disability: Lessons from cognitive malingering research. *Spine Journal, 5*, 404–417.

Bianchini, K. J., Greve, K. W., & Love, J. M. (2003). Definite malingered neurocognitive dysfunction in moderate/severe traumatic brain injury. *Clinical Neuropsychologist, 17*(4), 574–580. http://dx.doi.org/10.1076/clin.17.4.574.27946

Bilder, R. M., Sugar, C. A., & Hellemann, G. S. (2014). Cumulative false positive rates given multiple performance validity tests: Commentary on Davis and Millis (2014) and Larrabee (2014). *Clinical Neuropsychologist, 28*(8), 1212–1223. http://dx.doi.org/10.1080/13854046.2014.969774

Binder, L. M., Larrabee, G. J., & Millis, S. R. (2014, November 11). Intent to fail: Significance testing of forced choice test results. *Clinical Neuropsychologist, 28*(8), 1366–1375. Epub. http://dx.doi.org/ 10.1080/13854046.2014.978383

Binks, P. G., Gouvier, W. D., & Waters, W. F. (1997). Malingering detection with the Dot Counting Test. *Archives of Clinical Neuropsychology, 12*(1), 41–46. http://dx.doi.org/10.1080/13854046.2014.978383

Blaskewitz, N., Merten, T., & Kathmann, N. (2008). Performance of children on symptom validity tests: TOMM, MSVT, and FIT. *Archives of Clinical Neuropsychology, 23*(4), 379–391. http://dx.doi.org/10.1016/j.acn.2008.01.008

Boccaccini, M. T., Murrie, D. C., & Duncan, S. A. (2006). Screening for malingering in a criminal-forensic sample with the Personality Assessment Inventory. *Psychological Assessment, 18*(4), 415–423. http://dx.doi.org/10.1037/1040-3590.18.4.415

Bolinger, E., Reese, C., Suhr, J., & Larrabee, G. J. (2014). Susceptibility of the MMPI-2-RF Neurological Complaints and Cognitive Complaints scales to over-reporting in simulated head injury. *Archives of Clinical Neuropsychology, 29*(1), 7–15. http://dx.doi.org/10.1093/arclin/act082

Bonds v. Padlock et al., 2008 U.S. Dist. LEXIS 96098 (E.D. La. 2008).

Bonnie, R. J., & Grisso, T. (2000). Adjudicative competence and youthful offenders. In T. Grisso & R. G. Schwartz (Eds.), *Youth on trial: A developmental perspective on juvenile justice* (pp. 73–103). Chicago, IL: University of Chicago Press. http://dx.doi.org/10.1007/978-1-4419-1695-2_245

Boone, K. B. (2007a). *Feigned cognitive impairment: A neuropsychological perspective.* New York, NY: Guilford.

Boone, K. B. (2007b). A reconsideration of the Slick et al. (1999) criteria for malingered neurocognitive dysfunction. In K. Boone (Ed.), *Feigned cognitive impairment: A neuropsychological perspective* (pp. 29–49). New York, NY: Guilford.

Boone, K. B. (2009). The need for continuous and comprehensive sampling of effort/response bias during neuropsychological examinations. *Clinical Neuropsychologist, 23*(4), 729–741. http://dx.doi.org/10.1080/13854040802427803

Boone, K. B. (2011). Clarification or confusion? A review of Rogers, Bender, and Johnson's A critical analysis of the MND criteria for feigned cognitive impairment: Implications for forensic practice and research. *Psychological Injury and Law, 4*(2), 157–162. http://dx.doi.org/10.1007/s12207-011-9106-3

Boone, K. B. (2013). *Clinical practice of forensic neuropsychology: An evidence-based approach.* New York, NY: Guilford.

Boone, K. B., Lu, P., Back, C., King, C., Lee, A., Philpott, L., . . . & Warner-Chacon, K. (2002). Sensitivity and specificity of the Rey Dot Counting Test in patients with suspect effort and various clinical samples. *Archives of Clinical Neuropsychology, 17*(7), 625–642. http://dx.doi.org/10.1016/S0887-6177(01)00166-4

Boone, K. B., Lu, P., & Herzberg, D. (2002). *The Dot Counting Test.* Los Angeles, CA: Western Psychological Services.

Boone, K. B., Salazar, X., Lu, P., Warner-Chacon, K., & Razani, J. (2002). The Rey 15-Item recognition trial: A technique to enhance sensitivity of the Rey 15-item memorization test. *Journal of Clinical and Experimental Neuropsychology, 24*(5), 561–573. http://dx.doi.org/10.1076/jcen.24.5.561.1004

Borum, R., & Grisso, T. (1995). Psychological test use in criminal forensic evaluations. *Professional Psychology: Research and Practice, 26*(5), 465–473. http://dx.doi.org/10.1037/0735-7028.26.5.465

Borum, R., & Grisso, T. (1996). Establishing standards for criminal forensic reports: An empirical analysis. *Journal of the American Academy of Psychiatry and the Law Online, 24*(3), 297–317.

Borum, R., Otto, R., & Golding, S. (1993). Improved clinical judgment and decision making in forensic evaluation. *Journal of Psychiatry & Law, 21*, 35–76. http://dx.doi.org/10.1177/009318539302100104

Bourg, S., Connor, E. J., & Landis, E. E. (1995). The impact of expertise and sufficient information on psychologists' ability to detect malingering. *Behavioral Sciences and the Law, 13*(4), 505–515.

Bourget, D., & Whitehurst, L. (2007). Amnesia and crime. *Journal of the American Academy of Psychiatry and the Law Online, 35*(4), 469–480.

Boysen, G. A., & VanBergen, A. (2014). Simulation of multiple personalities: A review of research comparing diagnosed and simulated dissociative identity disorder. *Clinical Psychology Review, 34*(1), 14–28. http://dx.doi.org/10.1016/j.cpr.2013.10.008

Bradford, J. M. W., & Smith, S. M. (1979). Amnesia and homicide: The Padola case and a study of thirty cases. *Journal of the American Academy of Psychiatry and the Law Online, 7*(3), 219–231.

Brady, M., Scher, L. M., & Newman, W. (2013). "I just saw Big Bird. He was 100 feet tall!" Malingering in the emergency room: Four instruments can help you make a rapid assessment of a patient feigning symptoms. *Current Psychiatry, 12*(10), 33–38, 40.

Brand, B. L., & Chasson, G. S. (2015). Distinguishing simulated from genuine dissociative identity disorder on the MMPI-2. *Psychological Trauma: Theory, Research, Practice, and Policy, 7*(1), 93–101. http://dx.doi.org/10.1037/a0035181

Brand, B. L., McNary, S. W., Loewenstein, R. J., Kolos, A. C., & Barr, S. R. (2006). Assessment of genuine and simulated dissociative identity disorder on the Structured

Interview of Reported Symptoms. *Journal of Trauma and Dissociation*, *7*(1), 63–85. http://dx.doi.org/10.1300/J229v07n01_06

Brand, B. L., Tursich, M., Tzall, D., & Loewenstein, R. J. (2014). Utility of the SIRS-2 in distinguishing genuine from simulated dissociative identity disorder. *Psychological Trauma: Theory, Research, Practice, and Policy*, *6*(4), 308–317. http://dx.doi.org/10.1037/a0036064

Brockhaus, D. P. R., & Merten, T. (2004). Neuropsychologische diagnostik suboptimalen leistungsverhaltens mit dem Word Memory Test. *Der Nervenarzt*, *75*(9), 882–887.

Brockman v. State, 852 So.2d 330, 333–34 (Fla. 2d DCA 2003).

Brodsky, S. L. (1991). *Testifying in court: Guidelines and maxims for the expert witness.* Washington, DC: American Psychological Association.

Brodsky, S. L. (1999). *The expert expert witness: More maxims and guidelines for testifying in court*. Washington, DC: American Psychological Association.

Bruininks, R. H., Woodcock, R. W., Weatherman, R. F., & Hill, B. K. (1996). *SIB-R: Scales of Independent Behavior–Revised.* Itasca, IL: Riverside.

Buddin, W. H., Jr., Schroeder, R. W., Hargrave, D. D., Von Dran, E. J., Campbell, E. B., Brockman, C. J., . . . & Baade, L. E. (2014). An examination of the frequency of invalid forgetting on the Test of Memory Malingering. *Clinical Neuropsychologist*, 28(3), 525–542. http://dx.doi.org/10.1080/13854046.2014.906658

Buddin W., Jr., Schroeder, R., Teichner, G., & Waid, R. (2012). Patients applying for disability versus patients already receiving disability: Is there a difference in Medical Symptom Validity Test failure rates? *Archives of Clinical Neuropsychology*, *27*(6), 636.

Burchett, D., Dragon, W. R., Smith Holbert, A. M., Tarescavage, A. M., Mattson, C. A., Handel, R. W., & Ben-Porath, Y. S. (2016). "False feigners": Examining the impact of non-content-based invalid responding on the Minnesota Multiphasic Personality Inventory–2 Restructured Form content-based invalid responding indicators. *Psychological Assessment*, *28*(5), 458–470. http://dx.doi.org/10.1037/pas0000205

Burkett, B. G., & Whitley, G. (1998). *Stolen valor: How the Vietnam generation was robbed of its heroes and its history*. Dallas, TX: Verity Press.

Bush, S. S., Heilbronner, R. L., & Ruff, R. M. (2014). Psychological assessment of symptom and performance validity, response bias, and malingering: Official position of the Association for Scientific Advancement in Psychological Injury and Law. *Psychological Injury and Law*, *7*(3) 197–205. http://dx.doi.org/10.1007/s12207-014-9198-7

Bush, S. S., Ruff, R. M., Troster, A., Barth, J., Koffler, S. P., Pliskin, N. H., et al. (2005). NAN position paper: Symptom validity assessment: Practice issues and medical necessity. *Archives of Clinical Neuropsychology*, *20*(4), 419–426. http://dx.doi.org/10.1016/j.acn.2005.02.002

Butcher, J. N., Gass, C. S., Cumella, E., Kally, Z., & Williams, C. L. (2008). Potential for bias in MMPI-2 assessments using the Fake Bad Scale (FBS). *Psychological Injury and Law*, *1*(3), 191–209. http://dx.doi.org/10.1007/s12207-007-9002-z

Butcher, J. N., Graham, J. R., Ben-Porath, Y. S., Tellegen, A., & Dahlstrom, W. G. (1991). *Minnesota Multiphasic Personality Inventory–2 (MMPI-2): Manual for administration and scoring* (Rev. ed.). Minneapolis: University of Minnesota Press.

Carone, D. A. (2008). Children with moderate/severe brain damage/dysfunction outperform adults with mild-to-no brain damage on the Medical Symptom Validity Test. *Brain Injury*, *22*(12), 960–971. http://dx.doi.org/10.1080/02699050802491297

Carone, D. A. (2009). Test review of the Medical Symptom Validity Test. *Applied Neuropsychology, 16*(4), 309–311. http://dx.doi.org/10.1080/09084280903297883

Carone, D. A., & Bush, S. S. (2013). *Mild traumatic brain injury: Symptom validity assessment and malingering.* New York, NY: Springer.

Carone, D. A., Green, P., & Drane, D. L. (2014). Word Memory Test profiles in two cases with surgical removal of the left anterior hippocampus and parahippocampal gyrus. *Applied Neuropsychology: Adult, 21*(2), 155–160. http://dx.doi.org/10.1080/09084282.2012.755533

Cartwright, R. (2004). Sleepwalking violence: A sleep disorder, a legal dilemma, and a psychological challenge. *American Journal of Psychiatry, 161*(7), 1149–1158. http://dx.doi.org/10.1176/appi.ajp.161.7.1149

Centor, A. (1982). Criminals and amnesia: Comment on Bower. *American Psychologist, 7*(2), 240. http://dx.doi.org/10.1037/0003-066X.37.2.240

Chafetz, M. D. (2008). Malingering on the Social Security disability consultative examination: Predictors and base rates. *Clinical Neuropsychologist, 22*(3), 529–546. http://dx.doi.org/10.1080/13854040701346104

Chafetz, M. D. (2010). Symptom validity issues in the psychological consultative examination for Social Security disability. *Clinical Neuropsychologist, 24*(6), 1045–1063. http://dx.doi.org/10.1080/13854046.2010.481637

Chafetz, M. D. (2011). Reducing the probability of false positives in malingering detection of Social Security disability claimants. *Clinical Neuropsychologist, 25*(7), 1239–1252. http://dx.doi.org/10.1080/13854046.2011.586785

Chafetz, M. D. (2012). The A-test: A symptom validity indicator embedded within a mental status examination for Social Security disability. *Applied Neuropsychology, 19*(2), 121–126. http://dx.doi.org/10.1080/09084282.2011.643953

Chafetz, M. (2015). *Intellectual disability: Criminal and civil forensic issues.* New York, NY: Oxford University Press.

Chafetz, M. D., Abrahams, J. P., & Kohlmaier, J. (2007). Malingering on the Social Security disability consultative exam: A new rating scale. *Archives of Clinical Neuropsychology, 22*(1), 1–14. http://dx.doi.org/10.1016/j.acn.2006.10.003

Chafetz, M. D., & Biondolillo, A. (2012). Validity issues in Atkins death cases. *Clinical Neuropsychologist, 26*(8), 1358–1376. http://dx.doi.org/10.1080/13854046.2012.730674

Chafetz, M. D., & Biondolillo, A. M. (2013). Feigning a severe impairment profile. *Archives of Clinical Neuropsychology, 28*(3), 205–212. http://dx.doi.org/10.1093/arclin/act015

Chafetz, M., & Prentkowski, E. (2011). A case of malingering by proxy in a Social Security disability psychological consultative examination. *Applied Neuropsychology, 18*(2), 143–149. http://dx.doi.org/10.1080/09084282.2011.570619

Chafetz, M. D., Prentkowski, E., & Rao, A. (2011). To work or not to work: Motivation (not low IQ) determines symptom validity test findings. *Archives of Clinical Neuropsychology, 26*(4), 306–313. http://dx.doi.org/10.1093/arclin/acr030

Chafetz, M., & Underhill, J. (2013). Estimated costs of malingered disability. *Archives of Clinical Neuropsychology, 28*(7), 633–639. http:dx.doi.org/10.1093/arclin/act038

Chafetz, M. D., Williams, M. A., Ben-Porath, Y. S., Bianchini, K. J., Boone, K. B., Kirkwood, M. W., . . . & Ord, J. S. (2015). Official position of the American Academy of Clinical Neuropsychology Social Security Administration policy on validity testing: Guidance and recommendations for change. *Clinical Neuropsychologist, 29*(6), 723–740. http://dx.doi.org/10.1080/13854046.2015.1099738

Chmielewski, M., Zhu, J., Burchett, D., Bury, A. S., & Bagby, R. M. (2016). The comparative capacity of the Minnesota Multiphasic Personality Inventory–2 (MMPI-2) and MMPI-2 Restructured Form (MMPI-2-RF) validity scales to detect suspected malingering in a disability claimant sample. *Psychological Assessment*. Advance online publication. http://dx.doi.org/10.1037/pas0000328

Cima, M., Nijman, H., Merckelbach, H., Kremer, K., & Hollnack, S. (2004). Claims of crime-related amnesia in forensic patients. *International Journal of Law and Psychiatry, 27*(3), 215–221.

Clegg, C., Fremouw, W., & Mogge, N. (2009). Utility of the Structured Inventory of Malingered Symptomatology (SIMS) and the Assessment of Depression Inventory (ADI) in screening for malingering among outpatients seeking to claim disability. *Journal of Forensic Psychiatry and Psychology, 20*(2), 239–254. http://dx.doi.org/10.1080/14789940802267760

Cochrane, R., Grisso, T., & Frederick, R. (2001). The relationship between criminal charges, diagnoses, and psycholegal opinions among federal pretrial defendants. *Behavioral Sciences and the Law, 19*, 565–565. http://dx.doi.org/10.1002/bsl.454

Cockshell, S. J., & Mathias, J. L. (2012). Test effort in persons with chronic fatigue syndrome when assessed using the Validity Indicator Profile. *Journal of Clinical and Experimental Neuropsychology, 34*(7), 679–687. http://dx.doi.org/10.1080/13803395.2012.668176

Cohen, J. (1988). *Statistical power analysis for behavioral sciences* (2nd ed.). Hillsdale, NJ: Erlbaum.

Colwell, K. (2017). TOMI On Demand Training. Global Institute of Forensic Research. https://www.gifrinc.com/tomi/

Colwell, K., Colwell, L. H., Perry, A. T., Wasieleski, D., & Billings, T. (2008). The Test of Malingered Incompetence (TOMI): A forced-choice instrument for assessing cognitive malingering in competence to stand trial evaluations. *American Journal of Forensic Psychology, 26*(3), 17–42.

Colwell, L., & Colwell, K. (2011). Assessing feigned cognitive impairment in defendants hospitalized for competency restoration: Further validation of the TOMI. *Journal of Forensic Psychology Practice, 11*(4), 293–310. http://dx.doi.org/10.1080/15228932.2011.

Conroy, M. A. (2006). Report writing and testimony. *Applied Psychology in Criminal Justice, 2*(3), 237–260.

Coons, P. M. (1991). Iatrogenesis and malingering of multiple personality disorder in the forensic evaluation of homicide defendants. *Psychiatric Clinics of North America, 14*(3), 757–768.

Coons, P. M., & Milstein, V. (1994). Factitious or malingered multiple personality disorder: Eleven cases. *Dissociation, 7*(2), 81–85.

Cornell, D. G., & Hawk, G. L. (1989). Clinical presentation of malingerers diagnosed by experienced forensic psychologists. *Law and Human Behavior, 13*(4), 375–383. http://dx.doi.org/10.1007/BF01056409

Covert, J. H. (2008). *Neurocognitive variables underlying group performance on a measure of effort: The Medical Symptom Validity Test (MSVT)* (Doctoral dissertation). Denton, TX: University of North Texas.

Crawford, J. R., Garthwaite, P. H., & Betkowska, K. (2009). Bayes' theorem and diagnostic tests in neuropsychology: Interval estimates for post-test probabilities. *Clinical Neuropsychologist*, *23*(4), 624–644. http://dx.doi.org/10.1080/13854040802524229

Crawford v. Washington, 514 U.S. 36 (2004).

Crighton, A. H., Tarescavage, A. M., Gervais, R. O., & Ben-Porath, Y. S. (2015). The generalizability of overreporting across self-report measures: An investigation with the Minnesota Multiphasic Personality Inventory–2–Restructured Form and the Personality Assessment Inventory in a civil disability sample. *Assessment*. Published online before print, December 16, 2015, http://dx.doi.org/10.1177/1073191115621791

Curtis, K. L., Greve, K. W., Bianchini, K. J., & Brennan, A. (2006). California Verbal Learning Test indicators of malingered neurocognitive dysfunction sensitivity and specificity in traumatic brain injury. *Assessment*, *13*(1), 46–61. doi:10.1177/1073191105285210

Dalenberg, C. J., Brand, B. L., Gleaves, D. H., Dorahy, M. J., Loewenstein, R. J., Cardena, E., . . . & Spiegel, D. (2012). Evaluation of the evidence for the trauma and fantasy models of dissociation. *Psychological Bulletin*, *138*(3), 550–588. http://dx.doi.org/10.1037/a0027447

Dalenberg, C. J., Brand, B. L., Loewenstein, R. J., Gleaves, D. H., Dorahy, M. J., Cardeña, E., . . . & Spiegel, D. (2014). Reality versus fantasy: reply to Lynn et al. (2014). *Psychological Bulletin*, *140*(3), 911–920. http://dx.doi.org/10.1037/a0036685

Daley, C., McNiel, D. E., & Binder, R. L. (2011). "I did what?": Zolpidem and the courts. *Journal of the American Academy of Psychiatry and the Law*, *39*(4), 535–542.

Dandachi-FitzGerald, B., Ponds, R. W. H. M., Peters, M. J. V., & Merckelbach, H. (2011). Cognitive underperformance and symptom overreporting in a mixed psychiatric sample. *Clinical Neuropsychologist*, *25*(5), 812–828. http://dx.doi.org/10.1080/13854046.2011.583280

Daubert v. Merrell Dow Pharmaceuticals, Inc., 113 S.Ct. 2786 (1993).

Davis, J. J., & Millis, S. R. (2014a). Examination of performance validity test failure in relation to number of tests administered. *Clinical Neuropsychologist*, *28*(2), 199–214. http://dx.doi.org/10.1080/13854046.2014.884633

Davis, J. J., & Millis, S. R. (2014b). Reply to Commentary by Bilder, Sugar, and Helleman (2014 this issue) on minimizing false positive error with multiple performance validity tests. *Clinical Neuropsychologist*, *28*(8), 1224–1229. http://dx.doi.org/10.1080/13854046.2014.987167

Davis, J. J., Wall, J. R., & Whitney, K. A. (2012). Derivation and clinical validation of consistency indices on the Test of Memory Malingering. *Archives of Clinical Neuropsychology*, *27*(7), 706–715. doi:10.1093/arclin/acs078

Dawes, R. M. (1995, August). Final comments. In R. M. Dawes (Chair), Courtroom testimony: Does our science justify continuing what we do? Symposium conducted at the 103rd Annual Meeting of the American Psychological Association, New York.

Dawes, R. M., & Meehl, P. E. (1966). Mixed group validation: A method for determining the validity of diagnostic signs without using criterion groups. *Psychological Bulletin*, *66*(2), 63–67. http://dx.doi.org/10.1037/h0023584

Dean, A. C., Victor, T. L., Boone, K. B., & Arnold, G. (2008). The relationship of IQ to effort test performance. *Clinical Neuropsychologist*, *22*(4), 705–722. http://dx.doi.org/10.1080/13854040701440493

Dean, A. C., Victor, T. L., Boone, K. B., Philpott, L. M., & Hess, R. A. (2009). Dementia and effort test performance. *Clinical Neuropsychologist, 23*(1), 133–152. http://dx.doi.org/10.1080/13854040701819050

DeClue, G. (2011). Harry Potter and the Structured Interview of Reported Symptoms? *Open Access Journal of Forensic Psychology, 3*, 1–18.

Delain, S. L., Stafford, K. P., & Ben-Porath, Y. S. (2003). Use of the TOMM in a criminal court forensic assessment setting. *Assessment, 10*(4), 370–381. http://dx.doi.org/10.1007/978-0-387-79948-3_216

Demakis, G. J., Gervais, R. O., & Rohling, M. L. (2008). The effect of failure on cognitive and psychological symptom validity tests in litigants with symptoms of posttraumatic stress disorder. *Clinical Neuropsychologist, 22*(5), 879–895. http://dx.doi.org/10.1080/13854040701564482

Denney, R. L. (1996). Symptom validity testing of remote memory in a criminal forensic setting. *Archives of Clinical Neuropsychology, 11*(7), 589–603. http://dx.doi.org/10.1093/arclin/11.7.589

Denney, R. L. (2007). Assessment of malingering in criminal forensic neuropsychological settings. In K. L. Boone (Ed.), *The assessment of feigned cognitive impairment: A neuropsychological perspective* (pp. 428–450). New York, NY: Guilford.

Denning, J. H. (2012). The efficiency and accuracy of the Test of Memory Malingering Trial 1, errors on the first 10 items of the Test of Memory Malingering, and five embedded measures in predicting invalid test performance. *Archives of Clinical Neuropsychology, 27*(4), 417–432. http://dx.doi.org/10.1093/arclin/acs044

Denning, J. H. (2014). The efficiency and accuracy of the Test of Memory Malingering Trial 1, errors on the first 10 items of the Test of Memory Malingering, and five embedded measures in predicting invalid test performance. *Archives of Clinical Neuropsychology, 29*, 729–730. http://dx.doi.org/10.1093/arclin/acs044

DeRight, J., & Carone, D. A. (2015). Assessment of effort in children: A systematic review. *Child Neuropsychology, 21*(1), 1–24. http://dx.doi.org/10.1080/09297049.2013.864383

Dionysus, K. E., Denney, R. L., & Halfaker, D. A. (2011). Detecting negative response bias with the Fake Bad Scale, Response Bias Scale, and Henry-Heilbronner Index of the Minnesota Multiphasic Personality Inventory–2. *Archives of Clinical Neuropsychology, 26*(2), 81–88. http://dx.doi.org/10.1093/arclin/acq096

Doane, B. M., & Salekin, K. L. (2009). Susceptibility of current adaptive behavior measures to feigned deficits. *Law and Human Behavior, 33*(4), 329–343. http://dx.doi.org/10.1007/s10979-008-9157-5

Donders, J., & Kirkwood, M. W. (2013). Symptom validity assessment with special populations. In D. Carone & S. Bush (Eds.), *Mild traumatic brain injury: Symptom validity assessment and malingering* (pp. 399–410). New York, NY: Springer.

Dorathy, M. J., Brand, B. L., Şar, V., Krüger, C., Stavropoulos, P., Martínez-Taboas, A., . . . & Middleton, W. (2014). Dissociative identity disorder: An empirical overview. *Australian and New Zealand Journal of Psychiatry, 48*(5), 402–417. http://dx.doi.org/10.1177/0004867414527523

Dorgan v. O'Connor, 951 N.E. 2d 55 (Mass. App. 2011).

Drob, S. L., & Berger, R. H. (1987). The determination of malingering: A comprehensive clinical-forensic approach. *Journal of Psychiatry and Law, 15*(4), 519–538.

Drob, S. L., Meehan, K. B., & Waxman, S. E. (2009). Clinical and conceptual problems in the attribution of malingering in forensic evaluations. *Journal of the American Academy of Psychiatry and the Law Online, 37*(1), 98–106.

Dror, I. E. (2016). A hierarchy of expert performance. *Journal of Applied Research in Memory & Cognition*, *5*, 121–127. http://dx.doi.org/10.1016/j.jarmac.2016.03.001

Dror, I. E., & Murrie, D. C. (2017). A hierarchy of expert performance applied to forensic psychological assessments. *Psychology, Public Policy, and Law*. Advance online publication. http://dx.doi.org/10.1037/law0000140

Duncan, A. (2005). The impact of cognitive and psychiatric impairment of psychotic disorders on the Test of Memory Malingering. *Assessment*, *12*(2), 123–129. http://dx.doi.org/ 10.1177/1073191105275512

Duncan, S. A., & Ausborn, D. L. (2002). The use of reliable digits to detect malingering in a criminal forensic pretrial population. *Assessment*, *9*(1), 56–61.

Dunlop, T. (2005). Malingering. [Speech to Administrative Law Judges]. Disability Determination Service, Louisiana, USA.

Dusky v. United States, 362 U.S. 402 (1960).

Dvoskin, J., & Guy, L. (2008). On being an expert witness: It's not about you. *Psychiatry, Psychology and Law*, *15*(2), 202–212. doi:10.1080/13218710802014451

Easton, S., Akehurst, L., Satchell, L., & Turtle, S. (2017). An evaluation of an abbreviated version of a checklist to aid judgements of credibility in the medico-legal setting. *Open Access Journal of Forensic Psychology*, *9*, 1–18.

Edens, J. F., Otto, R. K., & Dwyer, T. (1999). Utility of the Structured Inventory of Malingered Symptomatology in identifying persons motivated to malinger psychopathology. *Journal of the American Academy of Psychiatry and the Law*, *27*(3), 387–396.

Edens, J. F., Poythress, N. G., & Watkins-Clay, M. M. (2007). Detection of malingering in psychiatric unit and general population prison inmates: A comparison of the PAI, SIMS, and SIRS. *Journal of Personality Assessment*, *88*(1), 33–42. http://dx.doi.org/10.1080/00223890709336832

Eichstaedt, K. E., Clifton, W. E., Vale, F. L., Benbadis, S. R., Bozorg, A. M., Rodgers-Neame, N. T., & Schoenberg, M. R. (2014). Sensitivity of Green's Word Memory Test Genuine Memory Impairment Profile to temporal pathology: A study in patients with temporal lobe epilepsy. *Clinical Neuropsychologist*, *28*(6), 941–953. http://dx.doi.org/10.1080/13854046.2014.942374

Etherton, J. L., Bianchini, K. J., Greve, K. W., & Ciota, M. A. (2005). Test of Memory Malingering performance is unaffected by laboratory-induced pain: Implications for clinical use. *Archives of Clinical Neuropsychology*, *20*(3), 375–384. http://dx.doi.org/10.1016/j.acn.2004.09.007

Evans, J. R., Schreiber Compo, N., & Russano, M. (2009). Intoxicated witnesses and suspects: Procedures and prevalence according to law enforcement. *Psychology, Public Policy, and Law*, *15*(3), 194–221. http://dx.doi.org/10.1037/a0016837

Everington, C., & Dunn, C. (1995). A second validation study of the Competence Assessment for Standing Trial for Defendants with Mental Retardation (CAST-MR). *Criminal Justice and Behavior*, *22*(1), 44–59.

Everington, C. T., & Luckasson, R. (1992). *Competency Assessment for Standing Trial (CAST-MR)*. Orlando Park, IL: International Diagnostic Systems.

Everington, C., Notario-Smull, H., & Horton, M. L. (2007). Can defendants with mental retardation successfully fake their performance on a test of competence to stand trial? *Behavioral Sciences and the Law*, *25*(4), 545–560. doi:10.1002/bsl.735

Farkas, M. R. (2008). *Ability of malingering measures to differentiate simulated versus genuine mental retardation* (Doctoral dissertation). Fordham University, New York, NY.

Farkas, M. R., Rosenfeld, B., Robbins, R., & van Gorp, W. (2006). Do tests of malingering concur? Concordance among malingering measures. *Behavioral Sciences and the Law, 24*(5), 659–671. http://dx.doi.org/10.1002/bsl.730

Fazio, R. L., Denning, J. H., & Denney, R. L. (2017). TOMM Trial 1 as a performance validity indicator in a criminal forensic sample. *The Clinical Neuropsychologist, 31*(1), 251–267.

Fazio, R. L., Sanders, J. F., & Denney, R. L. (2015). Comparison of performance of the Test of Memory Malingering and Word Memory Test in a criminal forensic sample. *Archives of Clinical Neuropsychology, 30*(4), 293–301. http://dx.doi.org/10.1093/arclin/acv024

Fogel, M. H., Schiffman, W., Mumley, D., Tillbrook, C., & Grisso, T. (2013). Ten year research update (2001–2010): Evaluations for competence to stand trial (adjudicative competence). *Behavioral Sciences and the Law, 31*(2), 165–191. http://dx.doi.org/10.1002/bsl.2051

Folstein, M. F., Folstein, S. E., & McHugh, P. R. (1975). "Mini mental state": A practical method for grading the cognitive state of patients for the clinician. *Journal of Psychiatric Research, 12*(3), 189–198.

Forbey, J. D., Lee, T. T. C., Ben-Porath, Y. S., Arbisi, P. A., & Gartland, D. (2013). Associations between MMPI-2-RF validity scale scores and extra-test measures of personality and psychopathology. *Assessment, 20*(4), 448–461. http://dx.doi.org/10.1177/1073191113478154

Fox, D. D. (2011). Symptom validity test failure indicates invalidity of neuropsychological tests. *Clinical Neuropsychologist, 25*(3), 488–495. http://dx.doi.org/10.1080/13854046.2011.554443

Frederick, R. I. (1997). *Validity Indicator Profile manual.* Minnetonka, MN: NCS Assessments.

Frederick, R. I. (2000a). Mixed group validation: A method to address the limitations of criterion group validation in research on malingering detection. *Behavioral Sciences and the Law, 18*(6), 693–718. http://dx.doi.org/10.1002/bsl.432

Frederick, R. I. (2000b). A personal floor effect strategy to evaluate the validity of performance on memory tests. *Journal of Clinical and Experimental Neuropsychology, 22*(6), 720–730.

Frederick, R. I. (2003). Review of the validity indicator profile. *Journal of Forensic Neuropsychology, 2*(3–4), 125–145. http://dx.doi.org/10.1300/J151v02n03_06

Frederick, R. I. (2011, July). *Clinical assessment of malingering and deception.* American Academy of Forensic Psychology workshop. Portland, OR.

Frederick, R. I. (2015a, April 14). Chaining likelihood ratios. Message posted to electronic mailing list at npsych@neurolist.com, archived at http://www2.npsych.com.

Frederick, R. I. (2015b, April). Test-based evaluation of feigning in clinical forensic assessments. American Academy of Forensic Psychology workshop. Chicago, IL.

Frederick, R. I., & Bowden, S. C. (2009a). Evaluating constructs represented by symptom validity tests in forensic neuropsychological assessment of traumatic brain injury. *Journal of Head Trauma Rehabilitation, 24*(2), 105–122. http://dx.doi.org/10.1097/HTR.0b013e31819b1210

Frederick, R. I., & Bowden, S. C. (2009b). The test validation summary. *Assessment, 16*(3), 215–236. http://dx.doi.org/10.1177/1073191108325005

Frederick, R. I., Carter, M., & Powel, J. (1995). Adapting symptom validity testing to evaluate suspicious complaints of amnesia in medicolegal evaluations. *Bulletin of the American Academy of Psychiatry and the Law, 23*(2), 231–237.

Frederick, R. I., & Crosby, R. D. (2000). Development and validation of the Validity Indicator Profile. *Law and Human Behavior, 24*(1), 59–82. http://dx.doi.org/10.1023/A:1005426803586

Frederick, R. I., Crosby, R. D., & Wynkoop, T. F. (2000). Performance curve classification of invalid responding on the Validity Indicator Profile. *Archives of Clinical Neuropsychology, 15*(4), 281–300. http://dx.doi.org/10.1016/S0887-6177(99)00002-5

Frederick, R. I., DeMier, R. L., & Smith, M. S. (2014). *Examinations of competency to stand trial: Foundations in mental health case law* (2nd ed.). Sarasota, FL: Professional Resource Press.

Frederick, R. I., & Denney, R. L. (1998). Minding your "*ps* and *qs*" when using forced-choice recognition tests. *The Clinical Neuropsychologist, 12*(2), 193–205.

Frederick, R. I., & Foster, H. G. (1991). Multiple measures of malingering on a forced-choice test of cognitive ability. *Psychological Assessment: A Journal of Consulting and Clinical Psychology, 3*(4), 596–602. http://dx.doi.org/10.1037/1040-3590.3.4.596

Frederick, R. I., Sarfaty, S. D., Johnston, J. D., & Powel, J. (1994). Validation of a detector of response bias on a forced-choice test of nonverbal ability. *Neuropsychology, 8*(1), 118–125. http://dx.doi.org/10.1037/0894-4105.8.1.118

Frederick, R. I., & Speed, F. M. (2007). On the interpretation of below-chance responding in forced-choice tests. *Assessment, 14*(1), 3–11. https://doi.org/10.1177/1073191106292009

Freeman, T., Powell, M., & Kimbrell, T. (2008). Measuring symptom exaggeration in veterans with chronic posttraumatic stress disorder. *Psychiatry Research, 158*(3), 374–380. http://dx.doi.org/ 10.1016/j.psychres.2007.04.002.

Friedland, S. I. (1998). Law, science and malingering. *Arizona State Law Journal, 30*, 337–398.

Gaines, M. V. (2009). *An examination of the combined use of the PAI and the M-FAST in detecting malingering among inmates* (Doctoral dissertation). Lubbuck, TX: Texas Tech University. http://dx.doi.org/2346/10347

Gaines, M. V., Giles, C. L., & Morgan, R. D. (2013). The detection of feigning using multiple PAI scale elevations: A new index. *Assessment, 20*(4), 437–447. doi:10.1177/1073191112458146

Gamache, M. (1998). The Validity Indicator Profile: Review of an instrument to assess response style. *American Psychology-Law Society Newsletter, 18*(2), 11–43. http://dx.doi.org/10.1300/J151v02n03_06

Ganellen, R. J. (2008). Rorschach assessment of malingering and defensive response sets. In C. B. Gacono & F. B. Evans (Eds.), *The handbook of forensic Rorschach assessment* (pp. 89–119). Milton Park, UK: Taylor and Francis.

Gass, C. S., & Odland, A. P. (2014). MMPI-2 Symptom Validity (FBS) Scale: Psychometric characteristics and limitations in a Veterans Affairs neuropsychological setting. *Applied Neuropsychology: Adult, 21*(1), 1–8. http://dx.doi.org/10.1080/09084282.2012.715608

Gass, C. S., Williams, C. L., Cumella, E., Butcher, J. N., & Kally, Z. (2010). Ambiguous measures of unknown constructs: The MMPI-2 Fake Bad Scale (aka symptom validity scale, FBS, FBS-r). *Psychological Injury and Law, 3*(1), 81–85. http://dx.doi.org/10.1007/s12207-009-9063-2

Gassen, M. D., Pietz, C. A., Spray, B. J., & Denney, R. L. (2007). Accuracy of Megargee's criminal offender infrequency (Fc) scale in detecting malingering among forensic examinees. *Criminal Justice and Behavior, 34*(4), 493–504. http://dx.doi.org/10.1177/0093854806295859

Gast, J., & Hart, K. J. (2010). The performance of juvenile offenders on the Test of Memory Malingering. *Journal of Forensic Psychology Practice, 10*(1) 53–68. http://dx.doi.org/10.1080/15228930903173062

Gebart-Eaglemont, J. E. (2001). Review of the Validity Indicator Profile. In B. S. Plake and J. C. Impara (Eds.), *The fourteenth mental measurements yearbook*. Lincoln, NE: Buros Institute of Mental Measurements.

Gervais, R. O., Ben-Porath, Y. S., & Wygant, D. B. (2009). Empirical correlates and interpretation of the MMPI-2-RF Cognitive Complaints (COG) scale. *Clinical Neuropsychologist, 23*(6), 996–1015. http://dx.doi.org/10.1080/13854040902748249

Gervais, R. O., Ben-Porath, Y. S., Wygant, D. B., & Green, P. (2007). Development and validation of a Response Bias Scale (RBS) for the MMPI-2. *Assessment, 14*(2), 196–208.

Gervais, R. O., Ben-Porath, Y. S., Wygant, D. B., & Green, P. (2008). Differential sensitivity of the Response Bias Scale (RBS) and MMPI-2 validity scales to memory complaints. *Clinical Neuropsychologist, 22*(6), 1061–1079. http://dx.doi.org/10.1080/13854040701756930

Gervais, R. O., Ben-Porath, Y. S., Wygant, D. B., & Sellbom, M. (2010). Incremental validity of the MMPI-2-RF over-reporting scales and RBS in assessing the veracity of memory complaints. *Archives of Clinical Neuropsychology, 25*(4), 274–284. http://dx.doi.org/10.1093/arclin/acq018

Gervais, R. O., Rohling M. L., Green, P., & Ford, W. (2004). A comparison of WMT, CARB, and TOMM failure rates in non-head injury disability claimants. *Archives of Clinical Neuropsychology, 19*(4), 475–487. http://dx.doi.org/10.1016/j.acn.2003.05.001

Gervais, R. O., Russell, A. S., Green, P, Allen, L. M., Ferrari, R., & Pieschl, S. D. (2001). Effort testing in patients with fibromyalgia and disability incentives. *Journal of Rheumatology, 28*(8), 1892–1899.

Gierok, S. D., Dickson, A. L., & Cole, J. A. (2005). Performance of forensic and non-forensic adult psychiatric inpatients on the Test of Memory Malingering. *Archives of Clinical Neuropsychology, 20*(6), 755–760. http://dx.doi.org/10.1016/j.acn.2005.04.008

Giger, P., & Merten, T. (2013). Swiss population-based reference data for six symptom validity tests. *Clínica y Salud, 24*(3), 153–159. http://dx.doi.org/10.1016/S1130-5274(13)70016-1

Giger, P., Merten, T., Merckelbach, H., & Oswald, M. (2010). Detection of feigned crime-related amnesia: A multi-method approach. *Journal of Forensic Psychology Practice, 10*(5), 440–463. http://dx.doi.org/10.1080/15228932.2010.489875

Glancy, G. D., Ash, P., Bath, E. P., Buchanan, A., Fedoroff, P., Frierson, R. L., . . . & Zonana, H. V. (2015). AAPL Practice Guideline for the Forensic Assessment. *Journal of the American Academy of Psychiatry and the Law, 43*, S3–S53. Retrieved from http://www.jaapl.org/content/43/2_Supplement/S3.full

Glassmire, D. M., Toofanian Ross, P. T., Kinney, D. I., & Nitch, S. R. (2016). Derivation and cross-validation of cutoff scores for patients with schizophrenia spectrum disorders on WAIS-IV Digit Span–based performance validity measures. *Assessment, 23*(3), 292–306. http://dx.doi.org/1073191115587551

Glassmire, D. M., Tarescavage, A. M., & Gottfried, E. D. (2016). Likelihood of obtaining Structured Interview of Reported Symptoms (SIRS) and SIRS-2 elevations among forensic psychiatric inpatients with screening elevations on the Miller Forensic Assessment of Symptoms Test. *Psychological Assessment, 28*(12), 1586–1596. http://dx.doi.org/10.1037/pas0000289

Godinez v. Moran, 509 U.S. 389 (1993).

Goldberg, H. E., Back-Madruga, C., & Boone, B. B. (2007). The impact of psychiatric disorders on cognitive symptom validity test scores. In K. B. Boone (Ed.), *Assessment of feigned cognitive impairment: A neuropsychological perspective* (pp. 281–309). New York, NY: Guilford.

Golding, S. L. (1993). *Interdisciplinary Fitness Interview–Revised*. Available from the author at the University of Utah, Department of Psychology, Salt Lake City, UT 84112.

Goodrich-Hunsaker, N. J., & Hopkins, R. O. (2009). Word Memory Test performance in amnesic patients with hippocampal damage. *Neuropsychology*, *23*(4), 529–534. http://dx.doi.org/10.1037/a0015444

Goodwin, B. E., Sellbom, M., & Arbisi, P. A. (2013). Posttraumatic stress disorder in veterans: The utility of the MMPI-2-RF validity scales in detecting overreported symptoms. *Psychological Assessment*, *25*(3), 671–678. http://dx.doi.org/10.1037/a0032214

Goodwin, D. W., & Rosenthal, R. (1971). Clinical significance of hallucinations in psychiatric disorders: A study of 116 hallucinatory patients. *Archives of General Psychiatry*, *24*(1), 76–80. http://dx.doi.org/10.1001/archpsyc.1971.01750070078011

Gorissen, M., Sanz, J. C., & Schmand, B. (2005). Effort and cognition in schizophrenia patients. *Schizophrenia Research*, *78*(2), 199–208. http://dx.doi.org/10.1016/j.schres.2005.02.016

Gothard, S., Rogers, R., & Sewell, K. W. (1995). Feigning incompetency to stand trial. *Law and Human Behavior*, *19*(4), 363–373. http://dx.doi.org/10.1007/BF01499137

Gothard, S., Viglione, D. J., Meloy, J. R., & Sherman, M. (1995). Detection of malingering in competency to stand trial evaluations. *Law and Human Behavior*, *19*(5), 493–505. http://dx.doi.org/10.1007/BF01499340

Gottfried, E. D. (2013). *Improving the detection of feigned factual knowledge deficits in defendants adjudicated incompetent to proceed* (Doctoral dissertation). Retrieved from The Graduate School at DigiNole Commons, http://dx.doi.org/10.1177/1073191115605631

Gottfried, E., & Carbonell, J. (2014). The role of intelligence on performance on the Inventory of Legal Knowledge (ILK). *Journal of Forensic Psychiatry and Psychology*, *25*(4), 380–396. http://dx.doi.org/10.1080/14789949.2014.920900

Gottfried, E. D., Hudson, B. L., Vitacco, M. J., & Carbonell, J. L. (2017). Improving the detection of feigned knowledge deficits in defendants adjudicated incompetent to stand trial. *Assessment*, *24*(2), 232–243.

Gowensmith, W. N., Murrie, D. C., & Boccaccini, M. T. (2012). Field reliability of competence to stand trial opinions: How often do evaluators agree, and what do judges decide when evaluators disagree?. *Law and Human Behavior*, *36*(2), 130–139. http://psycnet.apa.org/doi/10.1037/h0093958

Gowensmith, W. N., Pinals, D. A., & Karas, A. C. (2015). States' standards for training and certifying evaluators of competency to stand trial. *Journal of Forensic Psychology Practice*, *15*(4), 295–317. http://dx.doi.org/10.1080/15228932.2015.1046798

Graue, L. O., Berry, D. T. R., Clark, J. A., Sollman, M. J., Cardi, M., Hopkins, J., & Werline, D. (2007). Identification of feigned mental retardation using the new generation of malingered detection instruments: Preliminary findings. *Clinical Neuropsychologist*, *21*(6), 921–942. http://dx.doi.org/10.1080/13854040600932137

Green, D. (2010, Janary 1). Utility of cognitive malingering measures in a forensic psychiatric sample. *ETD Collection for Fordham University*. Paper AAI3438475. http://fordham.bepress.com/dissertations/AAI3438475

Green, D., & Rosenfeld, B. (2011). Evaluating the gold standard: A review and meta-analysis of the Structured Interview of Reported Symptoms. *Psychological Assessment, 23*(1), 95–107. http://dx.doi.org/10.1037/a0021149

Green, D., Rosenfeld, B., & Belfi, B. (2013). New and improved? A comparison of the original and revised versions of the Structured Interview of Reported Symptoms. *Assessment, 20*(2), 210–218. http://dx.doi.org/10.1177/1073191112464389

Green, D., Rosenfeld, B., Belfi, B., Rohlehr, L., & Pierson, A. (2012). Use of measures of cognitive effort and feigned psychiatric symptoms with pretrial forensic psychiatric patients. *International Journal of Forensic Mental Health, 11*(3), 181–190. http://dx.doi.org/10.1080/14999013.2012.723665

Green, P. (2004a). *Manual for the Medical Symptom Validity Test for Windows*. Edmonton, Canada: Green's Publishing.

Green, P. (2004b). *Memory Complaints Inventory*. Edmonton, Canada: Green's Publishing.

Green, P. (2005). *Green's Word Memory Test user's manual*. Edmonton, Canada: Green's Publishing.

Green, P. (2007). The pervasive influence of effort on neuropsychological tests. *Physical Medicine and Rehabilitation Clinics of North America, 18*(1), 43–68. http://dx.doi.org/10.1016/j.pmr.2006.11.002

Green, P. (2008). *Manual for the Nonverbal Medical Symptom Validity Test for Windows*. Edmonton, Canada: Green's Publishing.

Green, P. (2010). *The Advanced Interpretation program for the WMT, MSVT & NV-MSVT*. Edmonton, Canada: Green's Publishing.

Green, P. (2011). Comparison between the Test of Memory Malingering (TOMM) and the Nonverbal Medical Symptom Validity Test (NV-MSVT) in adults with disability claims. *Applied Neuropsychology, 18*(1), 18–26.

Green, P. (2012, October 16). Message posted to wmtusers electronic mailing list, archived at http://tech.groups.yahoo.com/group/wmtuser

Green, P. (2013, October 10). Shandera MR data from 2010 study. Message posted to wmtusers electronic mailing list, archived at http://tech.groups.yahoo.com/group/wmtuser

Green, P. (2015a, October 14). Fazio et al COMMENTS. Message posted to wmtusers electronic mailing list, archived at http://tech.groups.yahoo.com/group/wmtuser

Green, P. (2015b, April 17). An old chestnut that keeps floating to the top of the pond. Message posted to wmtusers electronic mailing list, archived at http://tech.groups.yahoo.com/group/wmtuser

Green, P. (2015c, May 14). WMT TOMM and criminals. Message posted to wmtusers electronic mailing list, archived at http://tech.groups.yahoo.com/group/wmtuser

Green, P. (2016, December 18). Message posted to wmtusers electronic mailing list, archived at http://tech.groups.yahoo.com/group/wmtuser

Green, P., Berendt, J., Mandel, A., & Allen, L. M. (2000). Relative sensitivity of the Word Memory Test and Test of Memory Malingering in 144 disability claimants. *Archives of Clinical Neuropsychology, 15*(8), 841.

Green, P., & Flaro, L. (2003). Word Memory Test performance in children. *Child Neuropsychology, 9*, 189–207. http://dx.doi.org//10.1076/chin.9.3.189.16460

Green, P., & Flaro, L. (2015). Results from three performance validity tests (PVTs) in adults with intellectual deficits. *Applied Neuropsychology: Adult, 22*(4), 293–303. http://dx.doi.org/10.1080/23279095.2014.925903

Green, P., & Flaro, L. (2016). Results from three performance validity tests in children with intellectual disability. *Applied Neuropsychology: Child, 5*(1), 25–34. http://dx.doi.org/10.1080/21622965.2014.935378

Green, P., Flaro, L., Brockhaus, R., & Montijo, J. (2012). Performance on the WMT, MSVT, and NV-MSVT in children with developmental disabilities and in adults with mild traumatic brain injury. In C. R. Reynolds & A. M. Horton, Jr. (Eds.), *Detection of malingering during head injury litigation* (pp. 201–219). New York, NY: Springer.

Green, P., Flaro, L., & Courtney, J. (2009). Examining false positives on the Word Memory Test in adults with mild traumatic brain injury. *Brain Injury, 23*(9), 741–750. http://dx.doi.org/10.1080/02699050903133962

Green, P., & Merten, T. (2013). Noncredible explanations for noncredible performance on symptom validity test. In D. Carone & S. Bush (Eds.), *Mild traumatic brain injury: Symptom validity assessment and malingering* (pp. 73–100). New York, NY: Springer.

Green, P., Montijo, J., & Brockhaus, R. (2011). High specificity of the Word Memory Test and Medical Symptom Validity Test in groups with severe verbal memory impairment. *Applied Neuropsychology, 18*(2), 86–94. http://dx.doi.org/10.1080/09084282.2010.523389

Green, P., Rohling, M. L., Lees-Haley, P. R., & Allen, L. M. A. (2001). Effort has a greater effect on test scores than severe brain injury in compensation claimants. *Brain Injury, 15*(12), 1045–1060. http://dx.doi.org/10.1080/02699050110088254

Greene, R. L. (2000). *The MMPI-2: An interpretive manual.* Boston: Allyn and Bacon.

Greene, R. L. (2008). Malingering and defensiveness on the MMPI-2. In R. Rogers (Ed.), *Clinical assessment of malingering and deception* (3rd ed., pp. 159–181). New York, NY: Guilford.

Greiffenstein, M. F., Baker, W. J., & Gola, T. (1994). Validation of malingered amnesia measures with a large clinical sample. *Psychological Assessment, 6*(3), 218–224.

Greiffenstein, M. F., Fox, D., & Lees-Haley, P. R. (2007). The MMPI-2 Fake Bad Scale in detection of noncredible brain injury claims. In K. B. Boone (Ed.), *Assessment of feigned cognitive impairment: A neuropsychological perspective* (pp. 210–235). New York, NY: Guilford.

Greiffenstein, M. F., Greve, K. W., Bianchini, K. J., & Baker, W. J. (2008). Test of Memory Malingering and Word Memory Test: A new comparison of failure concordance rates. *Archives of Clinical Neuropsychology, 23*(7), 801–807. http://dx.doi.org/10.1016/j.acn.2008.07.005

Greve, K. W., & Bianchini, K. J. (2004). Setting empirical cut-offs on psychometric indicators of negative response bias: A methodological commentary with recommendations. *Archives of Clinical Neuropsychology, 19*(4), 533–541. http://dx.doi.org/10.1016/j.acn.2003.08.002

Greve, K. W., & Bianchini, K. J. (2006). Should the Retention trial of the Test of Memory Malingering be optional? *Archives of Clinical Neuropsychology, 21*(1), 117–119. http://dx.doi.org/10.1016/j.acn.2005.06.009

Greve, K. W., Bianchini, K. J., & Brewer, S. T. (2013). The assessment of performance and self-report validity in persons claiming pain-related disability. *Clinical Neuropsychologist, 27*(1), 108–137. http://dx.doi.org/10.1080/13854046.2012.739646

Greve, K. W., Bianchini, K. J., Love, J. M., Brennan, A., & Heinly, M. T. (2006). Sensitivity and specificity of MMPI-2 validity scales and indicators to malingered neurocognitive dysfunction in traumatic brain injury. *Clinical Neuropsychologist, 20*(3), 491–512.

Greve, K. W., Binder, L. M., & Bianchini, K. J. (2009). Rates of below-chance performance in forced-choice symptom validity tests. *Clinical Neuropsychologist, 23*(3), 534–544. http://dx.doi.org/10.1080/13854040802232690

Greve, K. W., Ord, J., Curtis, K. L., Bianchini, K. J., & Brennan, A. (2008). Detecting malingering in traumatic brain injury and chronic pain: A comparison of three forced-choice symptom validity tests. *Clinical Neuropsychologist, 22*(5), 896–918. http://dx.doi.org/10.1080/13854040701565208

Griffith, E. E., Stankovic, A., & Baranoski, M. (2010). Conceptualizing the forensic psychiatry report as performative narrative. *Journal of the American Academy of Psychiatry and Law, 38*(1), 32–42.

Grisso, T. (1988). *Competency to stand trial evaluations: A manual for practice.* Sarasota, FL: Professional Resource Exchange.

Grisso, T. (2000). *The ability to make relevant decisions: Implications for competence to stand trial evaluations.* Worcester, MA: Law and Psychiatry Program, University of Massachusetts Medical School. Retrieved from https:// www.umassmed.edu/globalassets/forensic-training/documents/cst_decision_ability.pdf

Grisso, T. (2003). *Evaluating competencies* (2nd ed.). New York, NY: Kluwer Academic/Plenum.

Grisso, T. (2005). *Evaluating juveniles' adjudicative competence: A guide for clinical practice.* Sarasota, FL: Professional Resource Press/Professional Resource Exchange.

Grisso, T. (2010). Guidance for improving forensic reports: A review of common errors. *Open Access Journal of Forensic Psychology, 2,* 102–115.

Grisso, T. (2014). *Forward* to Otto, R. K., DeMier, R., & Boccaccini, M. (2014). *Forensic reports and testimony: A guide to effective communication for psychologists and psychiatrists.* Hoboken, NJ: Wiley.

Grossi, L. M., Green, D., Einzig, S., & Belfi, B. (2016, August 8). Evaluation of the Response Bias Scale and Improbable Failure Scale in assessing feigned cognitive impairment. *Psychological Assessment.* Advance online publication. http://dx.doi.org/10.1037/pas0000364

Gu, W., Reddy, H. B., Green, D., Belfi, B., & Einzig, S. (2016, April 4). Inconsistent responding in a criminal forensic setting: An evaluation of the VRIN-r and TRIN-r scales of the MMPI-2-RF. *Journal of Personality Assessment,* 1–11. Published online. http://dx.doi.org/10.1080/00223891.2016.1149483

Guarnera, L., & Murrie, D. C. (2017). Field reliability of adjudicative competence and legal sanity opinions: A systematic review and metaanalysis. *Psychological Assessment, 29,* 795–818. http://dx.doi.org/10.1037/pas0000388

Guilmette, T. J., Hart, K. J., Guiliano, A. J., & Leininger, B. E. (1994). Detecting simulated memory impairment: Comparison of the Rey Fifteen-Item Test and the Hiscock forced-choice procedure. *Clinical Neuropsychologist, 8*(3), 283–294. http://dx.doi.org/10.1080/13854049408404135

Gunner, J. H., Miele, A. S., Lynch, J. K., & McCaffrey, R. J. (2012). The Albany Consistency Index for the Test of Memory Malingering. *Archives of Clinical Neuropsychology, 27*(1), 1–9. http://dx.doi.org/10.1093/arclin/acr089

Guriel-Tennant, J., & Fremouw, W. (2006). Impact of trauma history and coaching on malingering of posttraumatic stress disorder using the PAI, TSI, and M-FAST*. *Journal of Forensic Psychiatry & Psychology, 17*(4), 577–592. http://dx.doi.org/10.1080/14789940600895838

Guy, L. S., Kwartner, P. P., & Miller, H. A. (2006). Investigating the M-FAST: Psychometric properties and utility to detect diagnostic specific malingering. *Behavioral Sciences and the Law, 24*(5), 687–702. http://dx.doi.org/10.1002/bsl.706

Guy, L. S., & Miller, H. A. (2004). Screening for malingered psychopathology in a correctional setting: Utility of the Miller-Forensic Assessment of Symptoms Test (M-FAST). *Criminal Justice and Behavior, 31*(6), 695–716. http://dx.doi.org/10.1177/0093854804268754

Haggerty, K. A., Frazier, T. W., Busch, R. M., & Naugle, R. I. (2007). Relationships among Victoria Symptom Validity Test indices and Personality Assessment Inventory validity scales in a large clinical sample. *Clinical Neuropsychologist, 21*(6), 917–928. http://dx.doi.org/10.1080/13854040600899724

Hale, M. (1736). *Historia placitorum coronae. The history of the pleas of the crown*. Edited by Sollom Emlyn. 2 vols. London, 1736. Reprint. Classical English Law Texts. London, UK: Professional Books, 1971.

Hampson, N. E., Kemp, S., Coughlan, A. K., Moulin, C. J., & Bhakta, B. B. (2014). Effort test performance in clinical acute brain injury, community brain injury, and epilepsy populations. *Applied Neuropsychology: Adult, 21*(3), 183–194. http://dx.doi.org/10.1080/09084282.2013.787425

Harp, J. P., Jasinski, L. J., Shandera-Ochsner, A. L., Mason, L. H., & Berry, D. T. (2011). Detection of malingered ADHD using the MMPI-2-RF. *Psychological Injury and Law, 4*(1), 32–43. http://dx.doi.org/10.1007/s12207-011-9100-9

Harrison, C. (2008). *Assessing malingered responding: Concurrent validation of a forced-choice test using ink blot stimuli for the identification of malingered responses* (Unpublished doctoral dissertation). Oxford, MS: University of Mississippi.

Harrison, P., & Oakland, T. (2003). *Adaptive Behavior Assessment System (ABAS-II)*. San Antonio, TX: Psychological Corporation.

Hartman, D. E. (2002). The unexamined lie is a lie worth fibbing: Neuropsychological malingering and the Word Memory Test. *Archives of Clinical Neuropsychology, 17*(7), 709–714. http://dx.doi.org/10.1016/S0887-6177(01)00172-X

Hartmann, E., & Hartmann, T. (2014). The impact of exposure to Internet-based information about the Rorschach and the MMPI-2 on psychiatric outpatients' ability to simulate mentally healthy test performance. *Journal of Personality Assessment, 96*(4), 432–444.

Hartzler, B., & Fromme, K. (2003). Fragmentary and en bloc blackouts: Similarity and distinction among episodes of alcohol-induced memory loss. *Journal of Studies on Alcohol, 64*(4), 547–550. http://dx.doi.org/10.15288/jsa.2003.64.547

Haskett, J. (1995). *Tehachapi Malingering Scale manual*. Research Revision No. 5, Modesto, CA: Logocraft.

Hawes, S., & Boccaccini, M. (2009). Detection of overreporting of psychopathology on the Personality Assessment Inventory: A meta-analytic review. *Psychological Assessment, 21*(1), 112–124. http://dx.doi.org/10.1037/a0015036

Hayes, J. S., Hale, D. B., & Gouvier, W. D. (1998). Malingering detection in a mentally retarded forensic population. *Applied Neuropsychology, 5*(1), 33–36. http://dx.doi.org/10.1207/s15324826an0501_4

Heilbronner, R. L., Sweet, J. J., Morgan, J. E., Larrabee, G. J., Millis, S. R., & Conference Participants. (2009). American Academy of Clinical Neuropsychology Consensus Conference Statement on the neuropsychological assessment of effort, response bias, and malingering. *Clinical Neuropsychologist, 23*(7), 1093–1129. http://dx.doi.org/10.1080/13854040903155063

Heilbrun, K. (2001). *Principles of forensic mental health assessment.* New York, NY: Kluwer Academic/Plenum.

Heinly, M. T., Greve, K. W., Bianchini, K. J., Love, J. M., & Brennan, A. (2005). WAIS digit span–based indicators of malingered neurocognitive dysfunction classification accuracy in traumatic brain injury. *Assessment, 12*(4), 429–444. doi:10.1177/1073191105281099

Heinrichs, R. V., & Zakzanis, K. K. (1998). Neurocognitive deficit in schizophrenia: A quantitative review of the evidence. *Neuropsychology, 12*, 426–445. http://dx.doi.org/10.1037/0894-4105.12.3.426

Heinze, M. C. (2003). Developing sensitivity to distortion: Utility of psychological tests in differentiating malingering and psychopathology in criminal defendants. *Journal of Forensic Psychiatry and Psychology, 14*(1), 151–177. http://dx.doi.org/10.1080/1478994031000077961

Heinze, M. C., & Purisch, A. D. (2001). Beneath the mask: Use of psychological tests to detect and subtype malingering in criminal defendants. *Journal of Forensic Psychology Practice, 1*(4), 23–51. http://dx.doi.org/10.1300/J158v01n04_02

Henry, G. K., Heilbronner, R. L., Algina, J., & Kaya, Y. (2013). Derivation of the MMPI-2-RF Henry-Heilbronner Index-r (HHI-r) scale. *Clinical Neuropsychologist, 27*(3), 509–515. http://dx.doi.org/10.1080/13854046.2012.739644

Henry, G. K., Heilbronner, R. L., Mittenberg, W., & Enders, C. (2006). The Henry-Heilbronner Index: A 15-item empirically derived MMPI-2 subscale for identifying probable malingering in personal injury litigants and disability claimants. *Clinical Neuropsychologist, 20*(4), 786–797. http://dx.doi.org/10.1080/13854040500287749

Henry, M., Merten, T., Wolf, S. A., & Harth, S. (2010). Nonverbal Medical Symptom Validity Test performance of elderly healthy adults and clinical neurology patients. *Journal of Clinical and Experimental Neuropsychology, 32*(1), 19–27. http://dx.doi.org/10.1080/13803390902791653.

Hickenbottom v. Delaware, L. & W. R. Co., 122 N.Y. 91 (1890).

Hickling, E. J., Blanchard, E. B., Mundy, E., & Galovski, T. E. (2002). Detection of malingered MVA related posttraumatic stress disorder: An investigation of the ability to detect professional actors by experienced clinicians, psychological tests and psychophysiological assessment. *Journal of Forensic Psychology Practice, 2*(1), 33–53.

Hill, D. (2009). *Detecting malingering in correctional settings: A comparison of several psychological tests* (Doctoral dissertation). Forrest Grove, OR: Pacific University. Retrieved from http://commons.pacificu.edu/spp/114

Hilsabeck, R. C., Gordon, S. N., Hietpas-Wilson, T., & Zartman, A. L. (2011). Use of Trial 1 of the Test of Memory Malingering (TOMM) as a screening measure of effort: Suggested discontinuation rules. *Clinical Neuropsychologist, 25*(7), 1228–1238. http://dx.doi.org/10.1080/13854046.2011.589409

Hirschfeld v. Stone, 99 Civ. 11693 (WHP) (2000); 193 F.D.R.175 (S.D.N.Y. 2000).

Hiscock, M., & Hiscock, C. (1989). Refining the forced-choice method for the detection of malingering. *Journal of Clinical and Experimental Neuropsychology, 11*(6), 967–974. http://dx.doi.org/10.1080/01688638908400949

Ho, T. (1999). Examination of racial disparity in competency to stand trial between white and African American retarded defendants. *Journal of Black Studies, 29*(6), 771–789. http://dx.doi.org/10.1177/002193479902900602

Hodge v. West, 153 F. 3d 1356 (Fed. Cir. 1998).

Hoge, S. K., Bonnie, R., Poythress, N. G., & Monahan, J. (1999). *MacArthur Competence Assessment Tool–Criminal Adjudication*. Odessa, FL: Psychological Assessment Resources. http://dx.doi.org/10.1023/A:1024826312495

Hong, S. H., & Kim, Y. H. (2001). Detection of random response and impression management in the PAI: II. Detection indices. *Korean Journal of Clinical Psychology, 20*, 751–761.

Hopwood, J. S., & Snell, H. K. (1933). Amnesia in relation to crime. *Journal of Mental Science, 79*, 27–41.

Hoskins, L. L., Binder, L. M., Chaytor, N. S., Williamson, D. J., & Drane, D. L. (2010). Comparison of oral and computerized versions of the word memory test. *Archives of Clinical Neuropsychology, 25*(7), 591–600. https://doi.org/10.1093/arclin/acq060

Howe, L. L., Anderson, A. M., Kaufman, D. A., Sachs, B. C., & Loring, D. W. (2007). Characterization of the Medical Symptom Validity Test in evaluation of clinically referred memory disorders clinic patients. *Archives of Clinical Neuropsychology, 22*(6), 753–761. http://dx.doi.org/10.1016/j.acn.2007.06.003

Howe, L. L., & Loring, D. W. (2009). Classification accuracy and predictive ability of the Medical Symptom Validity Test's dementia profile and general memory impairment profile. *The Clinical Neuropsychologist, 23*(2), 329–342. http://dx.doi.org/10.1080/13854040801945060

Hubbard, K. L. (2007). *Feigning cognitive deficits among psychiatric inpatients: Validation of three measures of cognitive malingering*. ProQuest.

Hunt, S., Root, J. C., & Bascetta, B. L. (2014). Effort testing in schizophrenia and schizoaffective disorder: Validity Indicator Profile and Test of Memory Malingering performance characteristics. *Archives of Clinical Neuropsychology, 29*(2), 164–172. http://dx.doi.org/10.1093/arclin/act069.

Huntjens, R. J. C., Peters, M. L., Woertman, L., Bovenschen, L. M., Martin, R. C., & Postma, A. (2006). Inter-identity amnesia in dissociative identity disorder: A simulated memory impairment? *Psychological Medicine, 36*(6), 857–863. http://dx.doi.org/10.1017/S0033291706007100

Hurley, K. E., & Deal, W. P. (2006). Assessment instruments measuring malingering used with individuals who have mental retardation: Potential problems and issues. *Mental Retardation, 44*(2), 112–119. http://dx.doi.org/10.1352/0047-6765(2006)44[112:AIMMUW]2.0.CO;2

Ingram, P. B., & Ternes, M. S. (2016). The detection of content-based invalid responding: A meta-analysis of the MMPI-2-Restructured Form's (MMPI-2-RF) over-reporting validity scales. *Clinical Neuropsychologist, 30*(4), 473–496. http://dx.doi.org/10.1080/13854046.2016.1187769

Inman, T. H., Vickery, C. D., Berry, D. T. R., Lamb, D., Edwards, C., & Smith, G. T. (1998). Development and initial validation of a new procedure for evaluating adequacy of effort during neuropsychological testing: The Letter Memory Test. *Psychological Assessment, 10*(2), 128–139. http://dx.doi.org/10.1037/1040-3590.10.2.128

Ivens, S. H. (2001). Review of the Validity Indicator Profile. In B. S. Plake & J. C. Impara (Eds.), *The fourteenth mental measurements yearbook*. Lincoln, NE: Buros Institute of Mental Measurements.

Iverson, G. L. (2006). Ethical issues associated with the assessment of exaggeration, poor effort, and malingering. *Applied Neuropsychology, 13*(2), 77–90. http://dx.doi.org/10.1207/s15324826an1302_3

Iverson, G. L., Franzen, M. D., & Hammond, J. A. (1995). Examination of inmates' ability to malingering on the MMPI-2. *Psychological Assessment*, *7*(1), 118–121. http://dx.doi.org/10.1037/1040-3590.7.1.118

Iverson, G., Franzen, M., & McCracken, L. (1991). Evaluation of an objective assessment technique for the detection of malingered memory deficits. *Law and Human Behavior*, *15*(6), 667–676. http://dx.doi.org/10.1007/BF01065859

Iverson, G. L., Franzen, M. D., & McCracken, L. M. (1994). Application of a forced-choice memory procedure designed to detect experimental malingering. *Archives of Clinical Neuropsychology*, *9*(5), 437–450. http://dx.doi.org/10.1093/arclin/9.5.437

Jackson, R. L., Rogers, R., & Sewell, K. W. (2005). Forensic applications of the Miller Forensic Assessment of Symptoms Test (M-FAST): Screening for feigned disorders in competency to stand trial evaluations. *Law and Human Behavior*, *29*(2), 199–210. http://dx.doi.org/10.1007/s10979-005-2193-5

Jasinski, L. J., Berry, D. T. R., Shandera, A. L., & Clark, J. A. (2011). Use of the Wechsler Adult Intelligence Scale Digit Span subtest for malingering detection: A meta-analytic review. *Journal of Clinical and Experimental Neuropsychology*, *33*(3), 300–314. http://dx.doi.org/10.1080/13803395.2010.516743

Jasinski, L. J., Harp, J. P., Berry, D. T., Shandera-Ochsner, A. L., Mason, L. H., & Ranseen, J. D. (2011). Using symptom validity tests to detect malingered ADHD in college students. *Clinical Neuropsychologist*, *25*(8), 1415–1428. http://dx.doi.org/10.1080/13854046.2011.630024

Jelicic, M., Ceunen, E., Peters, M. J., & Merckelbach, H. (2011). Detecting coached feigning using the Test of Memory Malingering (TOMM) and the Structured Inventory of Malingered Symptomatology (SIMS). *Journal of Clinical Psychology*, *67*(9), 850–855. http://dx.doi.org/10.1002/jclp.20805

Jelicic, M., Hessels, A., & Merckelbach, H. (2006). Detection of feigned psychosis with the Structured Inventory of Malingered Symptomatology (SIMS): A study of coached and uncoached simulators. *Journal of Psychopathology and Behavioral Assessment*, *28*(1), 19–22. http://dx.doi.org/10.1007/s10862-006-4535-0

Jelicic, M., Merckelbach, H., Candel, I., & Geraerts, E. (2007). Detection of feigned cognitive dysfunction using special malinger tests: A simulation study in naïve and coached malingerers. *International Journal of Neuroscience*, *117*(8), 1185–1192. http://dx.doi.org/10.1080/00207450600934697

Jelicic, M., Merckelbach, H., & van Bergen, S. (2004a). Symptom validity testing of feigned amnesia for a mock crime. *Archives of Clinical Neuropsychology*, *19*(4), 525–531. http://dx.doi.org/10.1016/j.acn.2003.07.004

Jelicic, M., Merckelbach, H., & van Bergen, S. (2004b). Symptom validity testing of feigned crime-related amnesia: A simulation study. *Journal of Credibility Assessment and Witness Psychology*, *5*, 1–8.

Jelicic, M., Peters, M. J., Leckie, V., & Merckelbach, H. (2007). Basic knowledge of psychopathology does not undermine the efficacy of the Structured Inventory of Malingered Symptomatology (SIMS) to detect feigned psychosis. *Netherlands Journal of Psychology*, *63*(3), 98–101.

Jewsbury, P. A., & Bowden, S. C. (2013). Considerations underlying the use of mixed group validation. *Psychological Assessment*, *25*(1), 204–215. http://dx.doi.org/10.1037/a0030063

Johnson, W. G., & Mullett, N. (1987). Georgia Court Competency Test–R. In M. Hersen & A. S. Bellack (Eds.). *Dictionary of behavioral assessment techniques* (p. 234). New York, NY: Pergamon Press.

Jones, A. (2013). Test of Memory Malingering: Cutoff scores for psychometrically defined malingering groups in a military sample. *Clinical Neuropsychologist, 27*(6), 1043–1059. http://dx.doi.org/10.1080/13854046.2013.804949.

Jones, A., & Ingram, M. V. (2011). A comparison of selected MMPI-2 and MMPI-2-RF validity scales in assessing effort on cognitive tests in a military sample. *Clinical Neuropsychologist, 25*(7), 1207–1227. http://dx.doi.org/10.1080/13854046.2011.600726

Jones, A., Ingram, M. V., & Ben-Porath, Y. S. (2012). Scores on the MMPI-2-RF scales as a function of increasing levels of failure on cognitive symptom validity tests in a military sample. *Clinical Neuropsychologist, 26*(5), 790–815. http://dx.doi.org/10.1080/13854046.2012.693202

Jurecska, D. E., Peterson, M. A, & Millkey, A. (2012). Comparative study of the MacCAT-CA and CAST-MR for individuals with intellectual disabilities. *American Journal of Forensic Psychology, 30*(2), 67–83.

Kahneman, D. (2011). *Thinking, fast and slow*. New York, NY: Farrar, Straus and Giroux.

Kane, A. W., & Dvoskin, J. A. (2011). *Evaluation for personal injury claims*. New York, NY: Oxford University Press.

Kapur, N. (1994). The coin-in-the-hand test: A new "bed-side" test for the detection of malingering in patients with suspected memory disorder. *Journal of Neurology, Neurosurgery, and Psychiatry, 57*(3), 385–386.

Karr, J. E., Areshenkoff, C. N., & Garcia-Barrera, M. A. (2014). The neuropsychological outcomes of concussion: A systematic review of meta-analyses on the cognitive sequelae of mild traumatic brain injury. *Neuropsychology, 28*(3), 321–336. http://dx.doi.org/10.1037/neu0000037

Karson, M. (2015). What can the rules of evidence teach us about writing forensic reports? *Psychological Injury and Law, 8*(1), 1–10. https://link.springer.com/article/10.1007/s12207-015-9213-7"\l

Karson, M., & Nadkarni, L. (2013). *Principles of forensic report writing*. Washington, DC: American Psychological Association.

Keesler, M. E., McClung, K., Meredith-Duliba, T., Williams, K., & Swirsky-Sacchetti, T. (2017). Red flags in the clinical interview may forecast invalid neuropsychological testing. *The Clinical Neuropsychologist, 31*(3), 619–631.

Keiski, M. A., Shore, D. L., Hamilton, J. M., & Malec, J. F. (2014). Simulation of traumatic brain injury symptoms on the Personality Assessment Inventory: An analogue study. *Assessment, 22*(2), 233–247. http://dx.doi.org/1073191114539380.

Kentucky v. McGorman, 489 S.W.3d 731 (2016).

King, B. H., & Ford, C. V. (1988). Pseudologia fantastica. *Acta Psychiatrica Scandinavica, 77*(1), 1–6. http://dx.doi.org/10.1111/j.1600-0447.1988.tb05068.x.

Kirkwood, M. W., Connery, A. K., Kirk, J. W., & Baker, D. A. (2014). Detecting performance invalidity in children: Not quite as easy as A, B, C, 1, 2, 3 but automatized sequences appears promising. *Child Neuropsychology, 20*(2), 245–252. https://doi.org/10.1080/09297049.2012.759553

Kirkwood, M. W., & Kirk, J. W. (2010). The base rate of suboptimal effort in a pediatric mild TBI sample: Performance on the Medical Symptom Validity Test. *Clinical Neuropsychologist, 24*(5), 860–872. http://dx.doi.org/10.1080/13854040903527287

Kirkwood, M. W., Kirk, J. W., Blaha, R. Z., & Wilson, P. (2010). Noncredible effort during pediatric neuropsychological exam: A case series and literature review. *Child Neuropsychology, 16*(6), 604–618. http://dx.doi.org/10.1080/09297049.2010.495059

Kline, J. (October 21). Cost of commitment. Message posted to Psylaw-L electronic mailing list. Archived at http://listserv.unl.edu/cgi-bin/wa?A0=psylaw-l

Kobelt, A., Göbber, J., Bassler, M., & Petermann, F. (2012). Beschwerdenvalidität im Rahmen stationärer psychosomatischer Rehabilitation. *Rehabilitation, 51*, 349–355. http://dx.doi.org/10.1055/s-0032-1323686

Kong, L. L., Allen, J. J. B., & Glisky, E. L. (2008). Interidentity memory transfer in dissociative identity disorder. *Journal of Abnormal Psychology, 117*, 686–692. http://dx.doi.org/10.1037/0021-843X.117.3.686

Kopelman, M. D. (1995). The assessment of psychogenic amnesia. In A. D. Baddeley, B. A. Wilson, & F. N. Watts (Eds.), *Handbook of memory disorders* (pp. 427–448). West-Sussex, UK: Wiley.

Kopelman, M. D. (2002). Disorders of memory. *Brain, 125*(10), 2152–2190. http://dx.doi.org/10.1093/brain/awf229

Krafka, C., Dunn, M. A., Johnson, M. T., Cecil, J. S., & Miletich, D. (2002). Judge and attorney experiences, practices, and concerns regarding expert testimony in federal civil trials. *Psychology, Public Policy, and Law, 8*, 309–332. http://dx.doi.org/10.1037/1076-8971.8.3.309

Kucharski, L. T., & Duncan, S. (2007). Differentiation of mentally ill criminal defendants from malingerers on the MMPI-2 and PAI. *American Journal of Forensic Psychology, 25*(3), 21–24.

Kucharski, L. T., Johnsen, D., & Procell, S. (2004). The utility of the infrequency psychopathology F(p) and infrequency psychopathology revised scales in the detection of malingering. *American Journal of Forensic Psychology, 22*(1), 33–39.

Kucharski, T. L., Ryan, W., Vogt, J., & Goodloe, E. (1998). Clinical symptom presentation in suspected malingerers: An empirical investigation. *Journal of the American Academy of Psychiatry and the Law, 26*(4), 579–585.

Kucharski, L. T., Toomey, J. P., Fila, K., & Duncan, S. (2007). Detection of malingering of psychiatric disorder with the Personality Assessment Inventory: An investigation of criminal defendants. *Journal of Personality Assessment, 88*(1), 25–32. http://dx.doi.org/10.1080/00223890709336831

Kukucka, J., Kassin, S. M., Zapf, P. A., & Dror, I. E. (in press). Cognitive bias and blindness: A global survey of forensic science examiners. *Journal of Applied Research in Memory & Cognition.*

Kulas, J. F., Axelrod, B. N., & Rinaldi, A. R. (2014). Cross-validation of supplemental Test of Memory Malingering scores as performance validity measures. *Psychological Injury and Law, 7*(3), 236–244. http://dx.doi.org/10.1007/s12207-014-9200-4

Kwartner, P. P., & Boccaccini, M. T. (2008). Testifying in court: Evidence-based recommendations for expert-witness testimony. In R. Jackson (Ed.), *Learning forensic assessment* (pp. 565–588). Abingdon, UK: Routledge.

Labott, S. M., & Wallach, H. R. (2002). Malingering dissociative identity disorder: Objective and projective assessment. *Psychological Reports, 90*(2), 525–538. http://dx.doi.org/10.2466/pr0.2002.90.2.525

Lally, S. J. (2003). What tests are acceptable for use in forensic evaluations? A survey of experts. *Professional Psychology: Research and Practice*, *34*(5), 491–498. http://dx.doi.org/10.1037/0735-7028.34.5.491

Lander, T. D., & Heilbrun, K. (2009). The content and quality of forensic mental health assessment: Validation of a principles-based approach. *International Journal of Forensic Mental Health*, *8*(2), 115–121. http://dx.doi.org/10.1080/14999010903199324

Lange, R. T., Pancholi, S., Bhagwat, A., Anderson-Barnes, V., & French, L. M. (2012). Influence of poor effort on neuropsychological test performance in US military personnel following mild traumatic brain injury. *Journal of Clinical and Experimental Neuropsychology*, *34*(5), 453–466. http://dx.doi.org/10.1080/13803395.2011.648175

Larochette, A., & Harrison, A. (2012). Word Memory Test performance in Canadian adolescents with learning disabilities: A preliminary study. *Applied Neuropsychology: Child*, *1*(1), 38–47. http://dx.doi.org/10.1080/21622965.2012.665777

Larøi, F., Sommer, I. E., Blom, J. D., Fernyhough, C., Ffytche, D. H., Hugdahl, K., . . . & Slotema, C. W. (2012). The characteristic features of auditory verbal hallucinations in clinical and nonclinical groups: state-of-the-art overview and future directions. *Schizophrenia Bulletin*, *38*(4), 724-733. doi:10.1093/schbul/sbs061

Larrabee, G. J. (2003). Detection of malingering using atypical performance patterns on standard neuropsychological tests. *Clinical Neuropsychologist*, *17*(3), 410–425. http://dx.doi.org/10.1076/clin.17.3.410.18089

Larrabee, G. J. (2007). *Assessment of malingered neuropsychological deficits*. New York, NY: Oxford University Press.

Larrabee, G. J. (2008). Aggregation across multiple indicators improves the detection of malingering: Relationship to likelihood ratios. *Clinical Neuropsychologist*, *22*(4), 666–679. http://dx.doi.org/10.1080/13854040701494987

Larrabee, G. J. (2012). Performance validity and symptom validity in neuropsychological assessment. *Journal of the International Neuropsychological Society*, *18*(4), 625–630. https://doi.org/10.1017/S1355617712000240

Larrabee, G. J. (2014a). False-positive rates associated with the use of multiple performance and symptom validity tests. *Archives of Clinical Neuropsychology*, *29*(4), 364–373. http://dx.doi.org/10.1093/arclin/acu019

Larrabee, G. J. (2014b). Cumulative false positive rates given multiple performance validity tests: Commentary on Davis and Millis (2014) and Larrabee (2014). *Clinical Neuropsychologist*, *28*(8), 1230–1242. http://dx.doi.org/10.1080/13854046.2014.988754

Larrabee, G. J., Greiffenstein, M. F., Greve, K. W., & Bianchini, K. J. (2007). Refining diagnostic criteria for malingering. In G. Larrabee (Ed.), *Assessment of malingered neuropsychological deficits* (pp. 334–371). New York, NY: Oxford University Press.

Larson, J. C. G., Flaro, L., Peterson, R. L., Connery, A. K., Baker, D. A., & Kirkwood, M. W. (2015). The Medical Symptom Validity Test measures effort not ability in children: A comparison between mild TBI and fetal alcohol spectrum disorder samples. *Archives of Clinical Neuropsychology*, *30*(3), 192–199. http://dx.doi.org/10.1093/arclin/acv012

Lee, T. T., Graham, J. R., Sellbom, M., & Gervais, R. O. (2012). Examining the potential for gender bias in the prediction of symptom validity test failure by MMPI-2 symptom validity scale scores. *Psychological Assessment*, *24*(3), 618–627. http://dx.doi.org/10.1037/a0026458

Lees-Haley, P. R., Dunn, J. T., & Betz, B. P. (1999, Fall). Test review: The Victoria Symptom Validity Test. *American Psychology-Law Society Newsletter, 19(3)*, 12–16.

Lees-Haley, P. R., English, L. T., & Glenn, W. J. (1991). A Fake Bad Scale on the MMPI-2 for personal injury claimants. *Psychological Reports, 68*(1), 203–210. http://dx.doi.org/10.2466/pr0.1991.68.1.203

Lewis, J. L., Simcox, A. M., & Berry, D. T. (2002). Screening for feigned psychiatric symptoms in a forensic sample by using the MMPI-2 and the Structured Inventory of Malingered Symptomatology. *Psychological Assessment, 14*(2), 170–176. http://dx.doi.org/10.1037/1040-3590.14.2.170

Lewis v. State, 889 So. 2d 623 (Ala. Ct. Crim. App. 2003).

Lezak, M. D. (1983/1995). *Neuropsychological assessment*. New York, NY: Oxford University Press.

Lilienfeld, S. O., Kirsch, I., Sarbin, T. R., Lynn, S. J., Chaves, J. F., Ganaway, G. K., et al. (1999). Dissociative identity disorder and the sociocognitive model: Recalling the lessons of the past. *Psychological Bulletin, 125*(5), 507–523. http://dx.doi.org/10.1037/0033-2909.125.5.507

Lipsitt, P., Lelos, D., & McGarry, A. L. (1971). Competency for trial: A screening instrument. *American Journal of Psychiatry, 128*(1), 105–109. http://dx.doi.org/10.1176/ajp.128.1.105

Loring, D. W., Marino, S. E., Drane, D. L., Parfitt, D., Finney, G. R., & Meador, K. J. (2011). Lorazepam effects on Word Memory Test performance: A randomized, double-blind, placebo-controlled, crossover trial. *Clinical Neuropsychologist, 25*(5), 799–811. http://dx.doi.org/10.1080/13854046.2011.583279

Lockhart, J. J., & Satya-Murti, S. (2017). Diagnosing crime and diagnosing disease: bias reduction strategies in the forensic and clinical sciences. *Journal of Forensic Sciences, 62*(6), 1534–1541. DOI: 10.1111/1556-4029.13453

Love, C. M., Glassmire, D. M., Zanolini, S. J., & Wolf, A. (2014). Specificity and false positive rates of the Test of Memory Malingering, Rey 15-Item Test, and Rey Word Recognition Test among forensic inpatients with intellectual disabilities. *Assessment, 21*(5), 618–627. http://dx.doi.org/1073191114528028

Lucio, E., Durán, C., Graham, J. R., & Ben-Porath, Y. S. (2002). Identifying faking bad on the Minnesota Multiphasic Personality Inventory–Adolescent with Mexican adolescents. *Assessment, 9*(1), 62–69.

Lynn, S. J., Lilienfeld, S. O., Merckelbach, H., Giesbrecht, T., & van der Kloet, D. (2012). Dissociation and dissociative disorders challenging conventional wisdom. *Current Directions in Psychological Science, 21*(1), 48–53. http://dx.doi.org/10.1177/0963721411429457

Lynn, S. J., Lilienfeld, S. O., Merckelbach, H., Giesbrecht, T., McNally, R. J., Loftus, E. F., . . . & Malaktaris, A. (2014). The trauma model of dissociation: Inconvenient truths and stubborn fictions. Comment on Dalenberg et al. (2012). *Psychological Bulletin, 140*(3), 896–910. http://dx.doi.org/10.1037/a0035570

Maggio v. Fulford, 462 U.S. 111, 103 S.Ct. 2261 (1983).

Maldonado, J. R., & Spiegel, D. (2001). Conversion disorder. In K. A. Phillips (Ed.), *Somatoform and factitious disorders* (pp. 95–128). Washington, DC: American Psychiatric Publishing.

Marcopulos, B. A., Caillouet, B. A., Bailey, C. M., Tussey, C., Kent, J. A., & Frederick, R. (2014). Clinical decision making in response to performance validity test failure in a psychiatric setting. *Clinical Neuropsychologist, 28*(4), 633–652. http://dx.doi.org/10.1080/13854046.2014.896416

Marshall, P., & Happe, M. (2007). The performance of individuals with mental retardation on cognitive tests assessing effort and motivation. *Clinical Neuropsychologist, 21*(5), 826–840. http://dx.doi.org/10.1080/13854040600801001

Marshall, W. L., Serran, G., Marshall, L. E., & Fernandez, Y. M. (2005). Recovering memories of the offense in "amnesic" sexual offenders. *Sexual Abuse, 17*(1), 31–38.

Mart, E. G., & Connelly, A. W. (2010). An unusual case of epileptic postictal violence: Implications for criminal responsibility. *Open Access Journal of Forensic Psychology, 2*, 49–58.

Martin, P. K., Schroeder, R. W., & Odland, A. P. (2015). Neuropsychologists' validity testing beliefs and practices: A survey of North American professionals. *Clinical Neuropsychologist, 29*(16), 1–36. http://dx.doi.org/10.1080/13854046.2015.1087597

Martins, M., & Martins, I. P. (2010). Memory malingering: Evaluating WMT criteria. *Applied Neuropsychology, 17*(3), 177–182. http://dx.doi.org/10.1080/09084281003715709

Mason, L. H., Shandera-Ochsner, A. L., Williamson, K. D., Harp, J. P., Edmundson, M., Berry, D. T., & High, W. M., Jr. (2013). Accuracy of MMPI-2-RF validity scales for identifying feigned PTSD symptoms, random responding, and genuine PTSD. *Journal of Personality Assessment, 95*(6), 585–593. http://dx.doi.org/10.1080/00223891.2013.819512

McCarthy-Jones, S., & Resnick, P. J. (2014). Listening to voices: The use of phenomenology to differentiate malingered from genuine auditory verbal hallucinations. *International Journal of Law and Psychiatry, 37*(2), 183–189. http://dx.doi.org/10.1016/j.ijlp.2013.11.004

McCarthy-Jones, S., Trauer, T., Mackinnon, A., Sims, E., Thomas, N., & Copolov, D. L. (2014). A new phenomenological survey of auditory hallucinations: Evidence for subtypes and implications for theory and practice. *Schizophrenia Bulletin, 40*(1), 231–235. Http://dx.doi.org/10.1093/schbul/sbs156

McCusker, P. J., Moran, M. J., Serfass, L., & Peterson, K. H. (2003). Comparability of the MMPI-2 F(p) and F scales and the SIRS in clinical use with suspected malingerers. *International Journal of Offender Therapy and Comparative Criminology, 47*(5), 585–596.

McDermott, B. E., Dualan, I. V., & Scott, C. L. (2013). Malingering in the correctional system: Does incentive affect prevalence? *International Journal of Law and Psychiatry, 36*(3–4), 287–292. http://dx.doi.org/10.1016/j.ijlp.2013.04.013

McDermott, B. E., & Sokolov, G. (2009). Malingering in a correctional setting: The use of the Structured Interview of Reported Symptoms in a jail sample. *Behavioral Sciences and the Law, 27*(5), 753–765. http://dx.doi.org/10.1002/bsl.892

McGrath, R. E., Pogge, D. L., Stein, L. A. R., Graham, J. R., Zaccario, M., & Piacentini, T. (2000). Development of an infrequency-psychopathology scale for the MMPI-A: The Fp-A scale. *Journal of Personality Assessment, 74*(2), 282–295. http://dx.doi.org/10.1207/S15327752JPA7402_8

McLaughlin, J. L., & Kan, L. Y. (2014). Test usage in four common types of forensic mental health assessment. *Professional Psychology: Research and Practice, 45*(2), 128–135. http://dx.doi.org/10.1037/a0036318

McNally, R. J. (2003). *Remembering trauma*. Cambridge, MA: Harvard University Press.

McNulty, J. L., Forbey, J. D., Graham, J. R., Ben-Porath, Y. S., Black, M. S., Anderson, S. V., & Burlew, A. K. (2003). MMPI-2 validity scale characteristics in a correctional sample. *Assessment, 10*(3), 288–298. http://dx.doi.org/10.1177/1073191103255623

Megargee, E. I. (2004, May). *Development and initial validation of an MMPI-2 infrequency scale (Fc) for use with criminal offenders*. Paper presented at the 39th Annual Symposium on Recent Developments on the MMPI-2/MMPI-A, Minneapolis, MN.

Meijer, E. H., Smulders, F. R. Y., Johnson, J. E., & Merckelbach, H. L. (2007). Combining skin conductance and forced choice in the detection of concealed information. *Psychophysiology, 44*(5), 814–822. http://dx.doi.org/10.1111/j.1469-8986.2007.00543.x

Melton, G., Petrila, J., Poythress, N., & Slobogin, C. (1997). *Psychological evaluations for the courts: A handbook for mental health professionals and lawyers* (2nd ed.). New York, NY: Guilford.

Melton, G., Petrila, J., Poythress, N., & Slobogin, C. (2007). *Psychological evaluations for the courts: A handbook for mental health professionals and lawyers* (3rd ed.). New York, NY: Guilford.

Merckelbach, H., & Christianson, S. A. (2007). Amnesia for homicides as a form of malingering. In S. A. Christianson (Ed.), *Offenders' memories of violent crimes* (pp. 165–190). Chichester, UK: Wiley. http://dx.doi.org/10.1002/9780470713082.ch7

Merckelbach, H., Hauer, B., & Rassin, E. (2002). Symptom validity testing of feigned dissociative amnesia: A simulation study. *Psychology, Crime & Law, 8*(4), 311–318. http://dx.doi.org/10.1080/10683160208401822

Merckelbach, H., Smeets, T., & Jelicic, M. (2009). Experimental simulation: Type of malingering scenario makes a difference. *Journal of Forensic Psychiatry and Psychology, 20*(3), 378–386. http://dx.doi.org/10.1080/14789940802456686

Merckelbach, H., & Smith, G. P. (2003). Diagnostic accuracy of the Structured Inventory of Malingered Symptomatology (SIMS) in detecting instructed malingering. *Archives of Clinical Neuropsychology, 18*(2), 145–152. http://dx.doi.org/10.1016/S0887-6177(01)00191-3

Merten, T., Bossink, L., & Schmand, B. (2007). On the limits of effort testing: Symptom validity tests and severity of neurocognitive symptoms in nonlitigant patients. *Journal of Clinical and Experimental Neuropsychology, 29*(3), 308–318. http://dx.doi.org/10.1080/13803390600693607

Merten, T., Green, P., Henry, M., Blaskewitz, N., & Brockhaus, R. (2005). Analog validation of German-language symptom validity tests and the influence of coaching. *Archives of Clinical Neuropsychology, 20*(6), 719–726. http://dx.doi.org/10.1016/j.acn.2005.04.004

Merten, T., & Merckelbach, H. (2013). Symptom validity testing in somatoform and dissociative disorders: A critical review. *Psychological Injury and Law, 6*(2), 122–137. doi:10.1007/s12207-013-9155-x

Messer, J. M., & Fremouw, W. J. (2007). Detecting malingered posttraumatic stress disorder using the Morel Emotional Numbing Test–Revised (MENT-R) and the Miller Forensic Assessment of Symptoms Test (M-FAST). *Journal of Forensic Psychology Practice, 7*(3), 33–57. http://dx.doi.org/10.1300/J158v07n03_02

Meyer, J. K., Hong, S. H., & Morey, L. C. (2015). Evaluating the validity indices of the Personality Assessment Inventory–Adolescent Version. *Assessment, 22*(4), 490–496. http://dx.doi.org/10.1177/1073191114550478

Meyers, J. E. (2007). Malingering mild traumatic brain injury: Behavioral approaches used by both malingering actors and probable malingerers. In K. Boone (Ed.), Assessment of feigned cognitive impairment (pp. 239–258). New York: Guilford Press.

Meyers, J. E., Miller, R. M., Haws, N. A., Murphy-Tafiti, J. L., Curtis, T. D., Rupp, Z. W., . . . & Thompson, L. M. (2014). An adaptation of the MMPI-2 Meyers Index for the MMPI-2-RF. *Applied Neuropsychology: Adult*, *21*(2), 148–154. http://dx.doi.org/10.1080/09084282.2013.780173

Meyers, J. E., Miller, R. M., Thompson, L. M., Scalese, A. M., Allred, B. C., Rupp, Z. W., et al. (2014). Using likelihood ratios to detect invalid performance with performance validity measures. *Archives of Clinical Neuropsychology*, *29*(3), 224–235. http://dx.doi.org/10.1093/arclin/acu001

Meyers, J. E., Millis, S. R., & Volkert, K. (2002). A validity index for the MMPI-2. *Archives of Clinical Neuropsychology*, *17*(2), 157–169. http://dx.doi.org/10.1016/S0887-6177(00)00107-4

Meyers, J. E., Volbrecht, M., Axelrod, B. N., & Reinsch-Boothby, L. (2011). Embedded symptom validity tests and overall neuropsychological test performance. *Archives of Clinical Neuropsychology*, *26(1)*, 8–15. http://dx.doi.org/10.1093/arclin/acq083

Miele, A. S., Gunner, J. H., Lynch, J. K., & McCaffrey, R. J. (2011). Are embedded validity indices equivalent to free-standing symptom validity tests? *Archives of Clinical Neuropsychology*, *27*(1), 10–22. http://dx.doi.org/10.1093/arclin/acr084

Miller, A. K., Rufino, K. A., Boccaccini, M. T., Jackson, R. L., & Murrie, D. C. (2011). On individual differences in person perception: Raters' personality traits relate to their Psychopathy Checklist-Revised scoring tendencies. *Assessment*, *18*(2), 253–260.

Miller, H. A. (2001). *M-Fast: Miller Forensic Assessment of Symptoms Test professional manual.* Odessa, FL: Psychological Assessment Resources.

Miller, H. A. (2004). Examining the use of the M-FAST with criminal defendants incompetent to stand trial. *International Journal of Offender Therapy and Comparative Criminology*, *48*(3), 268–280. http://dx.doi.org/10.1177/0306624X03259167

Miller, H. A. (2005). The Miller-Forensic Assessment of Symptoms Test (M-Fast): Test generalizability and utility across race literacy, and clinical opinion. *Criminal Justice and Behavior*, *32*(6), 591–611. http://dx.doi.org/10.1177/0093854805278805

Miller, R. D. (2003). *People v. Palmer*: Amnesia and competency to proceed revisited. *Journal of Psychiatry and Law*, *31*(2), 165–185. http://dx.doi.org/10.1177/009318530303100203

Millis, S. R. (2009). What clinicians really need to know about symptom exaggeration, insufficient effort, and malingering: Statistical and measurement matters. In J. Morgan & J. Sweet (Eds.), *Neuropsychology of malingering casebook* (pp. 488–493). New York, NY: Psychology Press.

Millon, T., Millon, C., Davis, R. D., & Grossman, S. (1997). *Millon Clinical Multiaxial Inventory–III (MCMI-III): Manual* (2nd ed.). Pearson/PsychCorp. Minneapolis, MN: National Computer Systems.

Mittenberg, W., Patton, C., Canyock, E. M., & Condit, D. C. (2002). Base rates of malingering and symptom exaggerating. *Journal of Experimental and Clinical Neuropsychology*, *24*(8), 1094–1102. http://dx.doi.org/10.1076/jcen.24.8.1094.8379

Mogge, N. L., Lepage, J. S., Bell, T., & Ragatz, L. (2010). The Negative Distortion Scale: A new PAI validity scale. *Journal of Forensic Psychiatry and Psychology*, *21*(1), 77–90. http://dx.doi.org/10.1080/14789940903174253

Morel, K. R. (1998). *Manual for the Morel Emotional Numbing Test for Post-Traumatic Stress Disorder* (MENT). Printed in USA.

Morey, L. C. (1991). *Personality Assessment Inventory* (PAI). Lutz, FL: Psychological Assessment Resources.

Morey, L. (2007). *Personality Assessment Inventory-Adolescent* (PAI-A). Lutz, FL: Psychological Assessment Resources.

Moss, A., Jones, C., Fokias, D., & Quinn, D. (2003). The mediating effects of effort upon the relationship between head injury severity and cognitive functioning. *Brain Injury, 17*(5), 377–387. http://dx.doi.org/10.1080/0269905031000070125

Mossman, D. (2000). The meaning of malingering data: Further applications of Bayes theorem. *Behavioral Sciences and the Law, 18*(6), 761–779. http://dx.doi.org/10.1002/bsl.419

Mossman, D., & Berger, J. O. (2001). Intervals for posttest probabilities: A comparison of 5 methods. *Medical Decision Making, 21*(6), 498–507.

Mossman, D., Miller, W. G., Lee, E. R., Gervais, R. O., Hart, K. J., & Wygant, D. B. (2015). A Bayesian approach to Mixed Group Validation of performance validity tests. *Psychological Assessment, 27*(3), 763–776. http://dx.doi.org/10.1037/pas0000085

Mossman, D., Noffsinger, S. G., Ash, P., Frierson, R. L., Gerbasi, J., Hackett, M., . . . & Wall, B. W. (2007). AAPL practice guideline for the forensic psychiatric evaluation of competence to stand trial. *Journal of the American Academy of Psychiatry and the Law Online, 35*(Supplement 4), S3–S72.

Mossman, D., Wygant, D. B., & Gervais, R. O. (2012). Estimating the accuracy of neurocognitive effort measures in the absence of a "gold standard." *Psychological Assessment, 24*(4), 815–822. http://dx.doi.org/10.1037/a0028195

Mossman, D., Wygant, D. B., Gervais, R. O., & Hart, K. J. (in press). Trial 1 vs. Trial 2 of the Test of Memory Malingering: Evaluating accuracy without a "gold standard." *Psychological Assessment.*

Murrie, D. C., & Boccaccini, M. T. (2015). Adversarial allegiance among expert witnesses. *Annual Review of Law and Social Science, 11*, 37–55. http://dx.doi.org/10.1146/annurev-lawsocsci-120814-121714

Murrie, D. C., Boccaccini, M. T., Zapf, P. A., Warren, J. I., & Henderson, C. E. (2008). Clinician variation in findings of competence to stand trial. *Psychology, Public Policy, and Law, 14*, 177–193. http://dx.doi.org/10.1037/a0013578

Musick, J. E., & Otto, R. K. (2010). *Inventory of Legal Knowledge professional manual.* Lutz, FL: Psychological Assessment Resources.

Myers, B. A. (1987). The Mini Mental State in those with developmental disabilities. *Journal of Nervous and Mental Disease, 175*(2), 85–89.

Myers, W. C., Hall, R. C., & Tolou-Shams, M. (2013). Prevalence and assessment of malingering in homicide defendants using the Mini-Mental State Examination and the Rey 15-Item memory test. *Homicide Studies, 17*(3), 314–328. http://dx.doi.org/10.1177/1088767912465609.

Nathan, D. (2011). *Sybil exposed: The extraordinary story behind the famous multiple personality case.* Glencoe, IL: Free Press.

National Research Council, Committee on Identifying the Needs of the Forensic Science Community. (2009). *Strengthening forensic science in the United States: A path forward.* Washington, DC: The National Academies Press. Retrieved from https://www.ncjrs.gov/pdffiles1/nij/grants/228091.pdf

Nayani, T. H., & David, A. S. (1996). The auditory hallucination: A phenomenological survey. *Psychological Medicine, 26*(1), 177–189. http://dx.doi.org/10.1017/S003329170003381X

Neal, T. M., & Grisso, T. (2014a, September 25). Assessment practices and expert judgment methods in forensic psychology and psychiatry: An international snapshot. *Criminal Justice and Behavior*. Published online. doi:10.1177/0093854814548449

Neal, T., & Grisso, T. (2014b). The cognitive underpinnings of bias in forensic mental health evaluations. *Psychology, Public Policy, Law, 20*(2), 200–211. http://dx.doi.org/10.1037/a0035824

Nelson, N. W., Hoelzle, J. B., Sweet, J. J., Arbisi, P. A., & Demakis, G. J. (2010). Updated meta-analysis of the MMPI-2 Symptom Validity Scale (FBS): Verified utility in forensic practice. *Clinical Neuropsychologist, 24*(4), 701–724. http://dx.doi.org/10.1080/13854040903482863

Nelson, N. W., Sweet, J. J., Berry, D. T., Bryant, F. B., & Granacher, R. P. (2007). Response validity in forensic neuropsychology: Exploratory factor analytic evidence of distinct cognitive and psychological constructs. *Journal of the International Neuropsychological Society, 13*(3), 440–449. http://dx.doi.org/10.1017/S1355617707070373

Ney v. City of Troy, 3 N.Y. Suppl. 679 (1888).

Niesten, I. J., Nentjes, L., Merckelbach, H., & Bernstein, D. P. (2015). Antisocial features and "faking bad": A critical note. *International Journal of Law and Psychiatry, 41*, 34–42.

Nørbech, P. C. B., Fodstad, L., Kuisma, I., Lunde, K. B., & Hartmann, E. (2016). Incarcerated violent offenders' ability to avoid revealing their potential for violence on the Rorschach and the MMPI-2. *Journal of Personality Assessment, 98*(4), 419–429.

Norris, M. P., & May, M. C. (1998). Screening for malingering in a correctional setting. *Law and Human Behavior, 22*(3), 315–323. http://dx.doi.org/10.1023/A:1025706606774

Norton, K. A., & Ryba, N. L. (2010). An investigation of the ECST-R as a measure of competence and feigning. *Journal of Forensic Psychology Practice, 10*(2), 91–106. http://dx.doi.org/10.1080/15228930903446625

O'Bryant, S. E., Engel, L. R., Kleiner, J. S., Vasterling, J. J., & Black, F. W. (2007). Test of Memory Malingering (TOMM) Trial 1 as a screening measure for insufficient effort. *Clinical Neuropsychologist, 21*(3), 511–521.

O'Bryant, S. E., Gavett, B. E., McCaffrey, R. J., O'Jile, J. R., Huerkamp, J. K., Smitherman, T. A., & Humphreys, J. D. (2008). Clinical utility of Trial 1 of the Test of Memory Malingering (TOMM). *Applied Neuropsychology, 15*(2), 113–116.

Odland, A. P., Lammy, A. B., Martin, P. K., Grote, C. L., & Mittenberg, W. (2015). Advanced administration and interpretation of multiple validity tests. *Psychological Injury and Law, 8*(1), 46–63. http://dx.doi.org/10.1007/s12207-015-9216-4

Ohayon, M. M., Mahowald, M. W., Dauvilliers Y., Krystal, A. D., & Leger, D. (2012). Prevalence and comorbidity of nocturnal wandering in the US adult general population. *Neurology, 78*(20), 1583–1589. http://dx.doi.org/10.1212/WNL.0b013e3182563be5

Ohlemacher, S. (2013). *Judges: Social Security pushes approval of claims*. Washington, DC: Associated Press.

Ornish, S. A. (2001). A blizzard of lies: Bogus psychiatric defenses. *American Journal of Forensic Psychiatry, 22*(1), 19–30.

Otto, R. K., DeMier, R., & Boccaccini, M. (2014). *Forensic reports and testimony: A guide to effective communication for psychologists and psychiatrists*. Hoboken, NJ: Wiley.

Otto, R. K., Musick, J. E., & Sherrod, C. B. (2010). *Inventory of Legal Knowledge professional manual*. Lutz, FL: Psychological Assessment Resources.

Otto, R. K., Musick, J. E., & Sherrod, C. (2011). Convergent validity of a screening measure designed to identify defendants feigning knowledge deficits related to competence to stand trial. *Assessment, 18*(1), 60–62.

Otto, R. K., Slobogin, C., & Greenberg, S. A. (2007). Legal and ethical issues in accessing and utilizing third-party information. In A. Goldstein (Ed.), *Forensic psychology: Emerging topics and expanding roles* (pp. 190–205). New York, NY: Wiley.

Parwatikar, S. D., Holcomb, W. R., & Menninger, K. A. (1985). The detection of malingered amnesia in accused murderers. *Bulletin of the American Academy of Psychiatry and the Law*, 13(1), 97–103.

Perper, J. A., Twerski, A., & Wienand, J. W. (1986). Tolerance at high blood alcohol concentrations: A study of 110 cases and review of the literature. *Journal of Forensic Sciences, 31*(1), 212–221. http://dx.doi.org/10.1520/JFS11873J

Perry, P. J., Argo, T. R., Barnett, M. J., Liesveld, J. L., Liskow, B., Hernan, J. M., . . . & Brabson, M. A. (2006). The association of alcohol-induced blackouts and grayouts to blood alcohol concentrations. *Journal of Forensic Sciences, 51*(4), 896–899. http://dx.doi.org10.1111/j.1556-4029.2006.00161.x/

Peters, M. J., van Oorsouw, K. I., Jelicic, M., & Merckelbach, H. (2013). Let's use those tests! Evaluations of crime-related amnesia claims. *Memory, 21*(5), 599–607. http://dx.doi.org/10.1080/09658211.2013.771672

Philipsborn, J. T. (2015). Keynote address to the American Psychology Law Society. Available at: https://www.youtube.com/watch?v=p60UiuuHM1k

Piper, A., & Merskey, H. (2004). The persistence of folly: Critical examination of dissociative identity disorder. Part II. The defence and decline of multiple personality or dissociative identity disorder. *Canadian Journal of Psychiatry, 49*(10), 678–683.

Pirelli, G., Gottdiener, W. H., & Zapf, P. A. (2011). A meta-analytic review of competency to stand trial research. *Psychology, Public Policy, Law, 17*(1), 1–53. http://dx.doi.org/10.1037/a0021713

Pirelli, G., Otto, R. K., & Estoup, A. (2016). Using Internet and social media data as collateral sources of information in forensic evaluations. *Professional Psychology: Research and Practice, 47*(1), 12–17. http://dx.doi.org/10.1037/pro0000061.

Pirelli, G., Zapf, P. A., & Gottdiener, W. H. (2011). Competency to stand trial research: Guidelines and future directions. *Journal of Forensic Psychiatry and Psychology, 22*(3), 340–370. http://dx.doi.org/10.1080/14789949.2011.552622

Pivovarova, E., Rosenfeld, B., Dole, T., Green, D., & Zapf, P. (2009). Are measures of cognitive effort and motivation useful in differentiating feigned from genuine psychiatric symptoms? *International Journal of Forensic Mental Health, 8*(4), 271–278. http://dx.doi.org/10.1080/14999011003635514

Pollock, P. H. (1997). A cautionary note on the determination of malingering in offenders. *Psychology, Crime and Law, 3*(2), 97–110. http://dx.doi.org/10.1080/10683169608409798

Pollock, P. (1998). Feigning auditory hallucinations. *Journal of Forensic Psychiatry, 9*(2), 305–327. http://dx.doi.org/10.1080/09585189808402199

Porter, S., & Woodworth, M. (2007). I'm sorry I did it . . . but he started it: A comparison of the official and self-reported homicide descriptions of psychopath and non-psychopaths. *Law and Human Behavior, 31*(1), 91–107. http://dx.doi.org/10.1007/s10979-006-9033-0

Porter, S., Woodworth, M., & Doucette, N. (2007). Memory for murder. In S. A. Christianson (Ed.), *Offenders' memories of violent crimes* (pp. 115–134). Mauldin, MA: Wiley.

Powell, M. R., Gfeller, J. D., Hendricks, B. L., & Sharland, M. (2004). Detecting symptom- and test-coached simulators with the Test of Memory Malingering. *Archives of Clinical Neuropsychology, 19*(5), 693–702. http://dx.doi.org/10.1016/j.acn.2004.04.001

Poyner, G. (2010). Psychological evaluations of veterans claiming PTSD disability with the Department of Veterans Affairs: A clinician's viewpoint. *Psychological Injury and Law, 3*(2), 130–132. http://dx.doi.org/10.1007/s12207-010-9076-x

Poythress, N. G., Edens, J. F., & Watkins, M. M. (2001). The relationship between psychopathic personality features and malingering symptoms of major mental illness. *Law and Human Behavior, 25*(6), 567–582. http://dx.doi.org/10.1023/A:1012702223004

Poythress, N. G., & Feld, D. B. (2002). "Competence restored": What forensic hospital reports should (and should not) say when returning defendants to court. *Journal of Forensic Psychology Practice, 2*(4), 51–58.

Poythress, N., Nicholson, R., Otto, R. K., Edens, J. F., Bonnie, R. J., Monahan, J., et al. (1999). *The MacArthur Competence Assessment Tool–Criminal Adjudication: Professional manual.* Odessa, FL: Psychological Assessment Resources.

Pressman, M. R., & Caudill, D. S. (2013). Alcohol-induced blackout as a criminal defense or mitigating factor: An evidence-based review and admissibility as scientific evidence. *Journal of Forensic Sciences, 58*(4), 932–940. http://dx.doi.org/10.1111/1556-4029.12134

Pressman, M. R., Mahowald, M. W., Schenck, C. H., & Cramer Bornemann, M. (2007). Alcohol-induced sleepwalking or confusional arousal as a defense to criminal behavior: A review of scientific evidence, methods, and forensic considerations. *Journal of Sleep Research, 16*(2), 198–212. http://dx.doi.org/10.1111/j.1365-2869.2007.00586.x

Proto, D. A. (2008). *The detection of malingered mental retardation in high- and low-cognitive ability individuals* (Unpublished master's thesis). Baton Rouge: Louisiana State University.

Proto, D. A., Pastorek, N. J., Miller, B. I., Romesser, J. M., Sim, A. H., & Linck, J. F. (2014). The dangers of failing one or more performance validity tests in individuals claiming mild traumatic brain injury–related postconcussive symptoms. *Archives of Clinical Neuropsychology, 29*(7), 614–624. http://dx.doi.org/10.1093/arclin/acu044

Purdon, S. E., Purser, S. M., & Goddard, K. M. (2011). MMPI-2 Restructured Form overreporting scales in first-episode psychosis. *Clinical Neuropsychologist, 25*(5), 829–842. http://dx.doi.org/10.1080/13854046.2011.585141

Pyszora, N. M., Barker, A. F., & Kopelman, M. D. (2003). Amnesia for criminal offences: A study of life sentence prisoners. *Journal of Forensic Psychiatry, 14*(3), 475–490. http://dx.doi.org/10.1080/1478994031000 1599785

Pyszora, N. M., Fahy, T., & Kopelman, M. D. (2014). Amnesia for violent offenses: Factors underlying memory loss and recovery. *Journal of the American Academy of Psychiatry and the Law Online, 42*(2), 202–213.

Raffard, S., Capdevielle, D., Boulenger, J. P., Gely-Nargeot, M. C., & Bayard, S. (2014). Can individuals with schizophrenia be instructed to deliberately feign memory deficits? *Cognitive Neuropsychiatry, 19*(5), 414–426. http://dx.doi.org/10.1080/13546805.2014.896251

Ray, C. L. (2009). The importance of using malingering screeners in forensic practice. *Journal of Forensic Psychology Practice*, *9*(2), 138–146. http://dx.doi.org/10.1080/15228930802575508

Ray, C. L. (2012). Assessment of feigned cognitive impairment: A cautious approach to the use of the Test of Memory Malingering for individuals with intellectual disability. *Open Access Journal of Forensic Psychology*, *4*, 24–50.

Ray, J. V., Hall, J., Rivera-Hudson, N., Poythress, N. G., Lilienfeld, S. O., & Morano, M. (2013). The relation between self-reported psychopathic traits and distorted response styles: A meta-analytic review. *Personality Disorders: Theory, Research, and Treatment*, *4*(1), 1–14. http://dx.doi.org/10.1037/a0026482

Rees, L. M., Tombaugh, T. N., & Boulay, L. (2001). Depression and the Test of Memory Malingering. *Archives of Clinical Neuropsychology*, *16*(5), 501–506. http://dx.doi.org/10.1016/S0887-6177(00)00064-0

Resnick, P. J. (1984). The detection of malingered mental illness. *Behavioral Sciences and the Law*, *2*(1), 21–38. http://dx.doi.org/10.1002/bsl.2370020104

Resnick, P. J., & Knoll, J. (2008). Malingered psychosis. In Rogers, R. (Ed.), *Clinical assessment of malingering and deception* (pp. 51–68). New York: Guilford.

Reuber, M., & Mackay, R. D. (2008). Epileptic automatisms in the criminal courts: 13 cases tried in England and Wales between 1975 and 2001. *Epilepsia*, *49*(1), 138–145. http://dx.doi.org/10.1111/j.1528-1167.2007.01269.x

Rey, A. (1941). L'examen psychologia dans las cas d'enchaphalopathie traumatique. *Archives de Psychologie*, *28*, 286–340.

Rey, A. (1958). *L'examen clinique en psychologie* [The psychological examination]. Paris: Presses Universitaires de France.

Reznek, L. (2005). The Rey 15-Item Memory Test for malingering: A meta-analysis. *Brain Injury*, *19*(7), 539–543. http://dx.doi.org/10.1080/02699050400005242

Rienstra, A., Groot, P. F., Spaan, P. E., Majoie, C. B., Nederveen, A. J., Walstra, G. J., . . . & Schmand, B. (2013). Symptom validity testing in memory clinics: Hippocampal-memory associations and relevance for diagnosing mild cognitive impairment. *Journal of Clinical and Experimental Neuropsychology*, *35*(1), 59–70. http://dx.doi.org/10.1080/13803395.2012.751361

Rienstra, A., Spaan, P. E. J., & Schmand, B. (2010). Validation of symptom validity tests using a "child-model" of adult cognitive impairments. *Archives of Clinical Neuropsychology*, *25*(5), 371–382. http://dx.doi.org/10.1093/arclin/acq035

Rios, J., & Morey, L. C. (2013). Detecting feigned ADHD in later adolescence: An examination of three PAI-A negative distortion indicators. *Journal of Personality Assessment*, *95*(6), 594–599. http://dx.doi.org/10.1080/00223891.2013.821071

Roberts, J. R., & Dollard, D. (2010). Alcohol levels do not accurately predict physical or mental impairment in ethanol-tolerant subjects: Relevance to emergency medicine and dram shop laws. *Journal of Medical Toxicology*, *6*(4), 438–442. http://dx.doi.org/10.1007/s13181-010-0048-z

Robinson, R., & Acklin, M. W. (2010). Fitness in paradise: Quality of forensic reports submitted to the Hawaii judiciary. *International Journal of Law and Psychiatry*, *33*(3), 131–137. http://dx.doi.org/10.1016/j.ijlp.2010.03.001

Roesch, R., Zapf, P. A., & Eaves, D. (2006). *Fitness Interview Test—Revised: A structured interview for assessing competency to stand trial.* Sarasota, FL: Professional Resource Press.

Roesch, R., Zapf, P. A., Eaves, D., & Webster, C. D. (1998). *Fitness Interview Test* (Rev. ed.). Burnaby, BC: Simon Fraser University, Mental Health, Law and Policy Institute

Rogers, R. (1984). Towards an empirical model of malingering and deception. *Behavioral Sciences and the Law, 2*, 93–112.

Rogers, R. (1997). Researching dissimulation. In R. Rogers (Ed.), *Clinical assessment of malingering and deception* (2nd ed., pp. 398–426). New York, NY: Guilford.

Rogers, R. (2008a). An introduction to response styles. In R. Rogers (Ed.), *Clinical assessment of malingering and deception* (3rd ed., pp. 3–13). New York, NY: Guilford.

Rogers, R. (2008b). Detection strategies for malingering and defensiveness. In R. Rogers (Ed.), *Clinical assessment of malingering and deception* (3rd ed., pp. 14–35). New York, NY: Guilford.

Rogers, R. (2008c). Researching response styles. In R. Rogers (Ed.), *Clinical assessment of malingering and deception* (3rd ed., pp. 411–434). New York, NY: Guilford.

Rogers, R. (2008d). Current status of clinical methods. In R. Rogers (Ed.), *Clinical assessment of malingering and deception* (3rd ed., pp. 391–410). New York, NY: Guilford.

Rogers, R., Bagby, R. M., & Dickens, S. E. (1992). *Structured Interview of Reported Symptoms (SIRS) and professional manual.* Lutz, FL: Psychological Assessment Resources.

Rogers, R., & Bender, S. D. (2003). Evaluation of malingering and deception. In A. M. Goldstein and I. B. Weiner (Eds.), *Handbook of psychology: Forensic psychology* (Vol. 11, pp. 109–129). New York, NY: Wiley.

Rogers, R., Bender, S. D., & Johnson, S. F. (2011). A critical analysis of the MND criteria for feigned cognitive impairment: Implications for forensic practice and research. *Psychological Injury and Law, 4*(2), 147–156. http://dx.doi.org/10.1007/s12207-011-9107-2

Rogers, R., & Correa, A. A. (2008). Determinations of malingering: Evolution from case-based methods to detection strategies. *Psychiatry, Psychology, and Law, 15*, 213–223. http://dx.doi.org/10.1080/13218710802014501

Rogers, R., Gillard, N. D., Berry, D. T., & Granacher, R. P. (2011). Effectiveness of the MMPI-2-RF validity scales for feigned mental disorders and cognitive impairment: A known-groups study. *Journal of Psychopathology and Behavioral Assessment, 33*(3), 355–367.

Rogers, R., Gillard, N. D., Wooley, C. N., & Kelsey, K. R. (2013). Cross-validation of the PAI Negative Distortion Scale for feigned mental disorders: A research report. *Assessment, 20*(1), 36–42. http://dx.doi.org/10.1177/1073191112451493

Rogers, R., Gillard, N. D., Wooley, C. N., & Ross, C. A. (2012). The detection of feigned disabilities: The effectiveness of the Personality Assessment Inventory in a traumatized inpatient sample. *Assessment, 19*(1), 77–88. http://dx.doi.org/10.1177/1073191111422031

Rogers, R., Hinds, J. D., & Sewell, K. W. (1996). Feigning psychopathology among adolescent offenders: Validation of the SIRS, MMPI-A, and SIMS. *Journal of Personality Assessment, 67*(2), 244–257.

Rogers, R., Jackson, R. L., Sewell, K. W., & Harrison, K. S. (2004). An examination of the ECST-R as a screen for feigned incompetency to stand trial. *Psychological Assessment, 16*(2), 139–145. http://dx.doi.org/10.1037/1040-3590.16.2.139

Rogers, R., Kropp, P. R., Bagby, R. M., & Dickens, S.E. (1992). Faking specific disorders: A study of the Structured Interview of Reported Symptoms (SIRS). *Journal of Clinical Psychology, 48*(5), 643–648.

Rogers, R., Payne, J. W., Berry, D. T., & Granacher, R. P., Jr. (2009). Use of the SIRS in compensation cases: An examination of its validity and generalizability. *Law and Human Behavior, 33*(3), 213–224. http://dx.doi.org/10.1007/s10979-008-9145-9

Rogers, R., Payne, J. W., Correa, A. A., Gillard, N. D., & Ross, C. A. (2009). A study of the SIRS with severely traumatized patients. *Journal of Personality Assessment, 91*(5), 429–438. http://dx.doi.org/10.1080/00223890903087745

Rogers, R., Robinson, E. V., & Gillard, N. D. (2014). The SIMS screen for feigned mental disorders: The development of detection-based scales. *Behavioral Sciences and the Law, 32*(4), 455–466. http://dx.doi.org/10.1002/bsl.2131

Rogers, R., Robinson, E. V., & Henry, S. A. (2017). Feigned adjudicative incompetence: Testing effectiveness of the ILK and SAMA with jail detainees. *Assessment, 24*(2), 173–182. http://dx.doi.org/073191115605613.

Rogers, R., Salekin, R. T., Sewell, K. W., Goldstein, A., & Leonard, K. (1998). A comparison of forensic and nonforensic malingerers: A prototypical analysis of explanatory models. *Law and Human Behavior, 22*(4), 353–367. http://dx.doi.org/10.1023/A:1025714808591

Rogers, R., Sewell, K. W., Cruise, K. R., Wang, E. W., & Ustad, K. L. (1998). The PAI and feigning: A cautionary note on its use in forensic-correctional settings. *Assessment, 5*(4), 399–405.

Rogers, R., Sewell, K. W., & Gilliard, N. (2010). *Structured Interview of Reported Symptoms–2 and professional manual.* Odessa, FL: Psychological Assessment Resources.

Rogers, R., Sewell, K. W., Grandjean, N. R., & Vitacco, M. J. (2002). The detection of feigned mental disorders on specific competency measures. *Psychological Assessment, 14*(2), 177–183. http://dx.doi.org/10.1037/1040-3590.14.2.177

Rogers, R., Sewell, K. W., Martin, M. A., & Vitacco, M. J. (2003). Detection of feigned mental disorders: A meta-analysis of the MMPI-2 and malingering. *Assessment, 10*(2), 160–177. http://dx.doi.org/10.1177/1073191103010002007

Rogers, R., Sewell, K. W., Morey, L. C., & Ulstad, K. L. (1996). Detection of feigned mental disorders on the Personality Assessment Inventory: A discriminant analysis. *Journal of Personality Assessment, 67*(3), 629–640. http://dx.doi.org/10.1207/s15327752jpa6703_15

Rogers, R., Tillbrook, C. E., & Sewell, K. W. (2004). *Evaluation of Competency to Stand Trial–Revised (ECST-R).* Odessa, FL: Psychological Assessment Resources.

Rohling, M. L. (2013, May). When are your trial data real? Poster presented at the 53rd annual conference of the American Society for Clinical Psychopharmacology, Hollywood, FL.

Rohling, M. L., & Demakis, G. J. (2010). Bowden, Shores, & Mathias (2006): Failure to replicate or just failure to notice. Does effort still account for more variance in neuropsychological test scores than TBI severity? *Clinical Neuropsychologist, 24*(1), 119–136. http://dx.doi.org/10.1080/13854040903307243

Rosenfeld, B., Green, D., Pivovarova, E., Dole, T., & Zapf, P. (2010). What to do with contradictory data? Approaches to the integration of multiple malingering measures.

International Journal of Forensic Mental Health, 9(2), 63–73. http://dx.doi.org/10.1080/14999013.2010.499559

Ross, S. R., & Adams, K. M. (1999). Test review: One more test of malingering? *Clinical Neuropsychologist, 13*(1), 112–116. http://dx.doi.org/10.1076/clin.13.1.112.1973

Rubenzer, S. J. (2009). Posttraumatic stress disorder: Assessing response style and malingering. *Psychological Injury and Law, 2*(2), 114–142. http://dx.doi.org/10.1007/s12207-009-9045-4.

Rubenzer, S. J. (2010). Review of the Structured Interview of Reported Symptoms–2. *Open Access Journal of Forensic Psychology, 2*, 273–286.

Rubenzer, S. J. (2011a). Review of the Inventory of Legal Knowledge. *Open Access Journal of Forensic Psychology, 3*, 70–81.

Rubenzer, S. J. (2011b). Judging intoxication. *Behavioral Sciences & the Law, 29*(1), 116–137. http://dx.doi.org/10.1002/bsl.935

Rubenzer, S. J. (2018). A survey of competency to stand trial examiners. In *Assessing negative response style in competency to stand trial evaluations* (pp. 169–188). New York, NY: Oxford University Press.

Rudman, N., Oyebode, J. R., Jones, C. A., & Bentham, P. (2011). An investigation into the validity of effort tests in a working age dementia population. *Aging and Mental Health, 15*(1), 47–57. http://dx.doi.org/10.1080/13607863.2010.508770

Ruff, R. M., Iverson, G. L., Barth, J. T., Bush, S. S., & Broshek, D. K. (2009). Recommendations for diagnosing a mild traumatic brain injury: A National Academy of Neuropsychology education paper. *Archives of Clinical Neuropsychology, 24*(1), 3–10. http://dx.doi.org/10.1093/arclin/acp006

Ruff, R. M., Klopfer, J., & Blank, J. (2016). Homogenous base rates for malingering in neuropsychological examination of litigants. *Psychological Injury and Law, 9*(2), 143–153. http://dx.doi.org/10.1007/s12207-016-9259-1.

Ruocco, A. C., Swirsky-Sacchetti, T., Chute, D. L., Mandel, S., Platek, S. M., & Zilmer, E. A. (2008). Distinguishing between neuropsychological malingering and exaggerated psychiatric symptoms in a neuropsychological setting. *Clinical Neuropsychologist, 22*(3), 547–564. http://dx.doi.org/10.1080/13854040701336444

Russo, A. C. (2014). Assessing veteran symptom validity. *Psychological Injury and Law, 7*(2), 178–190. http://dx.doi.org/10.1007/s12207-014-9190-2

Ryba, N. L., Cooper, V. G., & Zapf, P. A. (2003). Juvenile competence to stand trial evaluations: A survey of current practices and test usage among psychologists. *Professional Psychology: Research and Practice, 34*(5), 499–507. http://dx.doi.org/10.1037/0735-7028.34.5.499

Salekin, K. L., & Doane, B. M. (2009). Malingering intellectual disability: The value of available measures and methods. *Applied Neuropsychology, 16*(2), 105–113. http://dx.doi.org/10.1080/09084280902864485

Schagen, S., Schmand, B., de Sterke, S., & Lindeboom, J. (1997). Amsterdam Short-Term Memory Test: A new procedure for the detection of feigned memory deficits. *Journal of Clinical and Experimental Neuropsychology, 19*(1), 43–51. http://dx.doi.org/10.1080/01688639708403835

Schreiber, F. R. (1973). *Sybil*. New York, NY: Warner Books.

Schretlen, D., & Arkowitz, H. (1990). A psychological test battery to detect prison inmates who fake insanity or mental retardation. *Behavioral Sciences and the Law, 8*(1), 75–84. http://dx.doi.org/10.1002/bsl.2370080109

Schretlen, D., Brandt, J., Krafft, L., & Van Gorp, W. (1991). Some caveats in using the Rey 15-Item Memory Test to detect malingered amnesia. *Psychological Assessment: A Journal of Consulting and Clinical Psychology, 3*(4), 667–672. http://dx.doi.org/10.1037/1040-3590.3.4.667

Schretlen, D., Wilkins, S. S., Van Gorp, W. G., & Bobholz, J. H. (1992). Cross-validation of a psychological test battery to detect faked insanity. *Psychological Assessment, 4*(1), 77–83. http://dx.doi.org/10.1037/1040-3590.4.1.77

Schroeder, R. W., Baade, L. E., Peck, C. P., VonDran, E. J., Brockman, C. J., Webster, B. K., & Heinrichs, R. J. (2012). Validation of MMPI-2-RF validity scales in criterion group neuropsychological samples. *Clinical Neuropsychologist, 26*(1), 129–146. http://dx.doi.org/10.1080/13854046.2011.639314

Schroeder, R. W., Buddin, W. H., Hargrave, D. D., VonDran, E. J., Campbell, E. B., Brockman, C. J., . . . & Baade, L. E. (2013). Efficacy of Test of Memory Malingering Trial 1, Trial 2, the Retention Trial, and the Albany Consistency Index in a criterion group forensic neuropsychological sample. *Archives of Clinical Neuropsychology, 28*(1), 21–29. http://dx.doi.org/10.1093/arclin/acs094

Schroeder, R. W., & Marshall, P. S. (2011). Evaluation of the appropriateness of multiple symptom validity indices in psychotic and non-psychotic psychiatric populations. *Clinical Neuropsychologist, 25*(3), 437–453. http://dx.doi.org/10.1080/13854046.2011.556668

Schroeder, R. W., Twumasi-Ankrah, P., Baade, L. E., & Marshall, P. S. (2012). Reliable Digit Span: A systematic review and cross-validation study. *Assessment, 19*(1), 21–30. doi:10.1177/1073191111428764

Shuman, D. W., Whitaker, E., & Champagne, A. (1994). An empirical examination of the use of expert witnesses in the courts—Part II: A three city study. *Jurimetrics, 34*, 193–208.

Schutte, C., Millis, S., Axelrod, B., & VanDyke, S. (2011). Derivation of a composite measure of embedded symptom validity indices. *The Clinical Neuropsychologist, 25*(3), 454–462. https://doi.org/10.1080/13854046.2010.550635

Sellbom, M., & Bagby, M. (2008). Response styles on multiscale inventories. In R. Rogers (Ed.), *Clinical assessment of malingering and deception* (3rd ed. pp. 182–206). New York, NY: Guilford.

Sellbom, M., & Bagby, R. M. (2010). *Psychological Assessment, 22*(4), 757–767. http://dx.doi.org/10.1037/a0020825

Sellbom, M., Toomey, J. A., Wygant, D. B., Kucharski, L. T., & Duncan, S. (2010). Utility of the MMPI–2-RF (Restructured Form) validity scales in detecting malingering in a criminal forensic setting: A known-groups design. *Psychological Assessment, 22*(1), 22–31. http://dx.doi.org/10.1037/a0018222

Sellers, S., Byrne, M. K., & Golus, P. (2006). The detection of malingered psychopathology and cognitive deficits: Employing the Fake Bad Scale and the Raven's Standard Progressive Matrices. *Psychiatry, Psychology and Law, 13*(1), 91–99. http://dx.doi.org/10.1375/pplt.13.1.91

Shandera, A. L., Berry, D. T., Clark, J. A., Schipper, L. J., Graue, L. O., & Harp, J. P. (2010). Detection of malingered mental retardation. *Psychological Assessment, 22*(1), 50–56. http://dx.doi.org/10.1037/a0016585

Sharland, M. J., & Gfeller, J. D. (2007). A survey of neuropsychologists' beliefs and practices with respect to the assessment of effort. *Archives of Clinical Neuropsychology, 22*(2), 213–223. http://dx.doi.org/10.1016/j.acn.2006.12.004

Shaw, D. J., Vrij, A., Mann, S., Leal, S., & Hillman, J. (2014). The guilty adjustment: Response trends on the symptom validity test. *Legal and Criminological Psychology, 19*(2), 240–254. http://dx.doi.org/10.1111/j.2044-8333.2012.02070.x

Siclari, F., Khatami, R., Urbaniok, F., Nobili, L., Mahowald, M. W., Schenck, C. H., . . . & Bassetti, C. L. (2010). Violence in sleep. *Brain, 133*(12), 3494–3509. http://dx.doi.org/10.1093/brain/awq296

Sigelman, C. K., Winer, J. L., & Schoenrock, C. J. (1982). The responsiveness of mentally retarded persons to questions. *Education and Training of the Mentally Retarded, 17*(2), 120–124.

Silk-Eglit, G. M., Stenclik, J. H., Miele, A. S., Lynch, J. K., & McCaffrey, R. J. (2015). Rates of false-positive classification resulting from the analysis of additional embedded performance validity measures. *Applied Neuropsychology: Adult, 22*(5), 1–13. http://dx.doi.org/10.1080/23279095.2014.938809

Simon, M. J. (2007). Performance of mentally retarded forensic patients on the Test of Memory Malingering. *Journal of Clinical Psychology, 63*(4), 339–344. http://dx.doi.org/10.1002/jclp.20351

Singhal, A., Green, P., Ashaye, K., Shankar, K., & Gill, D. (2009). High specificity of the Medical Symptom Validity Test in patients with very severe memory impairment. *Archives of Clinical Neuropsychology, 24*(8), 721–728. http://dx.doi.org/10.1093/arclin/acp074

Skeem, J. L., Golding, S. L., Cohn, N. B., & Berge, G. (1998). Logic and reliability of evaluations of competence to stand trial. *Law and Human Behavior, 22*(5), 519–547. http://dx.doi.org/10.1023/A:1025787429972

Slick, D. J., & Sherman, E. M. S. (2012). Differential diagnosis of malingering and related clinical presentations. In E. M. S. Sherman & B. L. Brooks (Eds.), *Pediatric forensic neuropsychology* (pp. 113–135). New York, NY: Oxford University Press.

Slick, D. J., & Sherman, E. M. S. (2013). Differential diagnosis of malingering. In D. Carone & S. Bush (Eds.), *Mild traumatic brain injury: Symptom validity assessment and malingering* (pp. 57–72). New York, NY: Springer.

Slick, D. J., Sherman, E. M. S., & Iverson, G. L. (1999). Diagnostic criteria for malingered neurocognitive dysfunction: Proposed standards for clinical practice and research. *Clinical Neuropsychologist, 13*(4), 545–561. http://dx.doi.org/10.1076/1385-4046(199911)13:04;1-Y;FT545

Smith, D., & Resnick, P. (2007). Amnesia and competence to stand trial. *Journal of the American Academy of Psychiatry and the Law Online, 35*(4), 541–543.

Smith, G. P. (2008). Brief screening measures for the detection of feigned psychopathology. In R. Rogers (Ed.), *Clinical assessment of malingering and deception* (3rd ed., pp. 323–342). New York, NY: Guilford.

Smith, G. P., & Burger, G. K. (1997). Detection of malingering: Validation of the Structured Inventory of Malingered Symptomatology (SIMS). *Journal of the American Academy of Psychiatry and the Law Online, 25*(2), 183–189.

Smith, K., Boone, K., Victor, T., Miora, D., Cottingham, M., Ziegler, E., . . . & Wright, M. (2014). Comparison of credible patients of very low intelligence and non-credible patients on neurocognitive performance validity indicators. *Clinical*

Neuropsychologist, *28*(6), 1048–1070. http://dx.doi.org/10.1080/13854046.2014.931465

Smith, S. A., & Donmoyer, S. (n.d.). *Competency to stand trial and intelligence: Defendants with mental retardation*. Unpublished manuscript.

Social Security Administration Program Operations Manual System. (2013). DI 22510.006 When not to purchase a consultative examination (CE). Retrieved from https://secure.ssa.gov/apps10/poms.nsf/lnx/0422510006, April 16, 2015

Soliman, S., & Resnick, P. J. (2010). Feigning in adjudicative competence evaluations. *Behavioral Sciences and the Law*, *28*(5), 614–629. http://dx.doi.org/10.1002/bsl.950

Sollman, M. J., & Berry, D. T. (2011). Detection of inadequate effort on neuropsychological testing: A meta-analytic update and extension. *Archives of Clinical Neuropsychology*, *26*(8), 774–789. http://dx.doi.org/10.1093/arclin/acr066

Sollman, M. J., Ranseen, J. D., & Berry, D. T. (2010). Detection of feigned ADHD in college students. *Psychological Assessment*, *22*(2), 325–335. http://dx.doi.org/10.1037/a0018857

Sopko, K. (2012). *Detecting feigned reading learning disability and attention deficit hyperactivity disorder: The effects of coaching* (Unpublished doctoral dissertation, St. Louis University).

Spanos, N. P. (1996). *Multiple identities and false memories: A sociocognitive perspective*. Washington, DC: American Psychological Association.

Spiegel, H., & Spiegel, D. (1978). *Trance and treatment: Clinical uses of hypnosis*. Washington, DC: American Psychiatric Press.

Springman, R. E., & Vandenberg, B. R. (2009). The effects of test-strategy coaching on measures of competency to stand trial. *Journal of Forensic Psychology Practice*, *9*(3), 179–198. http://dx.doi.org/10.1080/15228930902809856

State of Louisiana v. Brooks, 648 So. 2d 366 (La. 1995).

State v. Demesmin, 159 N.H. 595; 992 A.2d 569; 2010 N.H. LEXIS 7 7.

Steadman, H. J. (1979). *Beating a rap? Defendants found incompetent to stand trial*. Chicago, IL: University of Chicago Press.

Steffan, J. S., & Morgan, R. D. (2008). Diagnostic accuracy of the MMPI-2 Malingering Discriminant Function Index in the detection of malingering among inmates. *Journal of Personality Assessment*, *90*(4), 392–398. http://dx.doi.org/10.1080/00223890802108204

Steffan, J. S., Morgan, R. D., Lee, J., & Sellbom, M. (2010). A comparative analysis of MMPI-2 malingering detection models among inmates. *Assessment*, *17*(2), 185–196. http://dx.doi.org/10.1177/1073191109359382

Stein, L. A. R., Graham, J. R., & Williams, C. R. (1995). Detecting fake-bad MMPI-A profiles. *Journal of Personality Assessment*, *65*(3), 415–427. http://dx.doi.org/10.1207/s15327752jpa6503_3

Steinberg, M. (1993). *Structured clinical interview for DSM-IV dissociative disorders (SCID-D)*. Washington, DC: American Psychiatric Press.

Stenclik, J. H., Miele, A. S., Silk-Eglit, G., Lynch, J. K., & McCaffrey, R. J. (2013). Can the sensitivity and specificity of the TOMM be increased with differential cutoff scores? *Applied Neuropsychology: Adult*, *20*(4), 243–248. http://dx.doi.org/10.1080/09084282.2012.704603

Stevens, A., Friedel, E., Mehren, G., & Merten, T. (2008). Malingering and uncooperativeness in psychiatric and psychological assessment: Prevalence and effects in a

German sample of claimants. *Psychiatry Research, 157*(1), 191–200. http://dx.doi.org/10.1016/j.psychres.2007.01.003

Stevens, A., Schneider, K., Liske, B., Hermle, L., Huber, H., & Hetzel, G. (2014). Is subnormal cognitive performance in schizophrenia due to lack of effort or to cognitive impairment? *German Journal of Psychiatry, 17*(1), 1–9.

Stimmel, M., Green, D., Belfi, B., & Klaver, J. (2012). Exploring the accuracy and utility of the Rey Fifteen Item Test (RMT) with recognition trial in a forensic psychiatric population. *International Journal of Forensic Mental Health, 11*(1), 51–58. http://dx.doi.org/10.1080/14999013.2012.676148

Stredney, R. V., Torres, A. N., & Wolber, G. J. (2009). "Parallel assessment" of competence to stand trial. *American Journal of Forensic Psychology, 27*(4), 5–22.

Suen, H. K. (1990). *Principles of test theories.* Hillsdale, NJ: Lawrence Erlbaum Associates.

Suesse, M., Wong, V. W., Stamper, L. L., Carpenter, K. N., & Scott, R. B. (2015). Evaluating the clinical utility of the Medical Symptom Validity Test (MSVT): A clinical series. *Clinical Neuropsychologist,* (ahead-of-print), 1–18. http://dx.doi.org/10.1080/13854046.2015.1022226

Sullivan, J. B., Hauptman, M., & Bronstein, A. C. (1987). Lack of observable intoxication in humans with high plasma alcohol concentrations. *Journal of Forensic Sciences, 32*(6), 1660–1665. http://dx.doi.org/10.1520/JFS11224J.

Sweet, J., & Giuffre Meyer, D. (2011). Well-documented, serious brain dysfunction followed by malingering. In J. E. Morgan, I. S. Baron, & J. H. Ricker (Eds.), *Casebook of clinical neuropsychology* (pp. 200–212). New York, NY: Oxford University Press.

Swihart, G., Yuille, J., & Porter, S. (1999). The role of state-dependent memory in "red-outs." *International Journal of Law and Psychiatry, 22*(3), 199–212.

Tan, J. E., Slick, D. J., Strauss, E., & Hultsch, D. F. (2002). How'd they do it? Malingering strategies on symptom validity tests. *Clinical Neuropsychologist, 16*(4), 495–505. http://dx.doi.org/10.1076/clin.16.4.495.13909

Tarescavage, A. M., & Glassmire, D. M. (2016, April 14). Differences between Structured Interview of Reported Symptoms (SIRS) and SIRS-2 sensitivity estimates among forensic inpatients: A criterion groups comparison. *Law and Human Behavior.* Advance online publication. http://dx.doi.org/10.1037/lhb0000191

Tarescavage, A. M., Wygant, D. B., Gervais, R. O., & Ben-Porath, Y. S. (2013). Association between the MMPI-2 Restructured Form (MMPI-2-RF) and malingered neurocognitive dysfunction among non–head injury disability claimants. *Clinical Neuropsychologist, 27*(2), 313–335. http://dx.doi.org/10.1080/13854046.2012.744099

Taylor, P. J., & Kopelman, M. D. (1984). Amnesia for criminal offences. *Psychological Medicine, 14*(3), 581–588. http://dx.doi.org/10.1017/S003329170001518X

Teichner, G., & Wagner, M. T. (2004). The Test of Memory Malingering (TOMM): Normative data from cognitively intact, cognitively impaired, and elderly patients with dementia. *Archives of Clinical Neuropsychology, 19*(3), 455–464. http://dx.doi.org/10.1016/S0887-6177(03)00078-7

Tellegen, A., & Ben-Porath, Y. S. (2008). *Minnesota Multiphasic Personality Inventory-2-RF technical manual.* Minneapolis: University of Minnesota Press.

Texas Health and Human Services Commission, Department of State Health Services, State Hospital Section. 2016. Management Plan, 3rd Quarter FY 2016 Report. https://www.dshs.texas.gov/mhreports/PIMHpub.shtm

Thigpen, C. H., & Cleckley, H. M. (1957). *The three faces of Eve*. New York, NY: McGraw Hill.

Thigpen, C. H., & Cleckley, H. M. (1984). On the incidence of multiple personality disorder: A brief communication. *International Journal of Clinical and Experimental Hypnosis*, *32*(2), 63–66.

Thomas, A. (2001). Factitious and malingered dissociative identity disorder. *Journal of Trauma and Dissociation*, *2*(4), 59–77. doi:10.1300/J229v02n04_04

Thomas, A., Donnell, A. J., & Young, T. R. (2004). Factor structure and differential validity of the Expanded Brief Psychiatric Rating Scale. *Assessment*, *11*(2), 177–187. doi: 10.1177/1073191103262893.

Thomas, K. M., Hopwood, C. J., Orlando, M. J., Weathers, F. W., & McDevitt-Murphy, M. E. (2012). Detecting feigned PTSD using the Personality Assessment Inventory. *Psychological Injury and Law*, *5*(3–4), 192–201. http://dx.doi.org/10.1007/s12207-011-9111-6

Tolin, D. F., Steenkamp, M. M., Marx, B. P., & Litz, B. T. (2010). Detecting symptom exaggeration in combat veterans using the MMPI-2 symptom validity scales: A mixed group validation. *Psychological Assessment*, *22*(4), 729–736. http://dx.doi.org/10.1037/a0020973

Tombaugh, T. N. (1996). *Test of Memory Malingering*. North Tonawonda, NY: Multi-Health Systems. http://dx.doi.org/10.1007/978-0-387-79948-3_216

Toomey, J. A., Kucharski, L. T., & Duncan, S. (2009). The utility of the MMPI-2 malingering discriminate function index in the detection of malingering: A study of criminal defendants. *Assessment*, *16*(1), 115–121. http://dx.doi.org/10.1177/1073191108319713

Tsushima, W. T., Geling, O., & Fabrigas, J. (2011). Comparison of MMPI-2 validity scale scores of personal injury litigants and disability claimants. *Clinical Neuropsychologist*, *25*(8), 1403–1414. http://dx.doi.org/10.1080/13854046.2011.613854

Tsushima, W. T., Geling, O., & Woo, A. (2013). Comparison of four MMPI-2 validity scales in identifying invalid neurocognitive dysfunction in traumatic brain injury litigants. *Applied Neuropsychology: Adult*, *20*(4), 263–271. http://dx.doi.org/10.1080/09084282.2012.701679

Tyner, E. A. (2009). Validating the SIRS with MGV using the MMPI-2 validity scales as estimators of base rate. In R. Frederick (Chair), Validating tests without criterion groups. Symposium conducted at the American Psychology Law Society meeting, San Antonio, TX.

Tyner, E. A., & Frederick, R. I. (2013). Rates of computational errors for scoring the SIRS primary scales. *Psychological Assessment*, *25*(4), 1367–1369. http://dx.doi.org/10.1037/a0033696

Tysse, J. E. (2005). Note: The right to an imperfect trial—Amnesia, malingering, and competency to stand trial. *William Mitchell Law Review*, *32*, 353–387.

Urso, T., Gavaler, J. S., & Van Thiel, D. H. (1981). Blood ethanol levels in sober alcohol users seen in an emergency room. *Life Sciences*, *28*(9), 1053–1056. http://dx.doi.org/10.1016/0024-3205(81)90752-9

United States v. Batista, 483 F.3d 193 (3d Cir. 2007).

United States v. Binion, 132 F. App'x 89 (8th Cir. 2005).*United States v. Tucker*, 489 S.W.3d 731 (2016).

United States v. Denny-Shaffer, 2 F.3d 999, 1006 (10th Cir. 1993).

United States v. Deruiter, 2015 U.S. Dist. LEXIS 176591. Retrieved from www.lexisnexis.com/hottopics/lnacademic

United States v. Gigante, 982 F. Supp. 140 (E.D.N.Y. 1997).

United States v. Greer, 158 F.3d 228, 238–239 (5th Cir. 1998).

United States v. Kokoski, 865 F. Supp. 325, 329–336 (S.D. W. Va. 1994).

United States v. Merriweather, 921 F Supp. 2d 1265 (ND Ala, 2013).

United States v. Rothman, Case no. 08-20895-CR Unagaro/Simonton, US District Court for the Southwestern District of Florida (2010).

United States v. Tucker, 2010 U.S. Dist. LEXIS 91754, *3, (E.D. Pa., Sept. 3, 2010).

Vallabhajosula, B., & Van Gorp, W. G. (2001). Post-Daubert admissibility of scientific evidence on malingering of cognitive deficits. *Journal of the American Academy of Psychiatry and the Law Online, 29*(2), 207–215.

Van Dyke, S. A., Millis, S. R., Axelrod, B. N., & Hanks, R. A. (2013). Assessing effort: Differentiating performance and symptom validity. *The Clinical Neuropsychologist, 27*(8), 1234–1246. https://doi.org/10.1080/13854046.2013.835447

Van Egmond, J. J., & Kummeling, I. (2002). A blind spot for secondary gain affecting treatment outcome. *European Psychiatry, 17*(1), 46–54. http://dx.doi.org/10.1016/S0924-9338(02)00622-3

Van Egmond, J., Kummeling, I., & Balkom, T. (2005). Secondary gain as hidden motive for getting psychiatric treatment. *European Psychiatry, 20*(5–6), 416–421. http://dx.doi.org/10.1016/j.eurpsy.2004.11.012

van Impelen, A., Merckelbach, H., Jelicic, M., & Merten, T. (2014). The Structured Inventory of Malingered Symptomatology (SIMS): A systematic review and meta-analysis. *Clinical Neuropsychologist, 28*(8), 1336–1365. http://dx.doi.org/10.1080/13854046.2014.984763

Van Oorsouw, K., & Merckelbach, H. (2010). Detecting malingered memory problems in the civil and criminal arena. *Legal and Criminological Psychology, 15*(1), 97–114. doi:10.1348/135532509X451304

Veazey, C. H., Wagner, A. L., Hays, J. R., & Miller, H. A. (2005). Validity of the Miller Forensic Assessment of Symptoms Test in psychiatric patients. *Psychological Reports, 96*(3), 771–774. http://dx.doi.org/10.2466/pr0.96.3.771-774

Verschuere, B., Meijer, E., & Crombez, G. (2008). Symptom validity testing for the detection of simulated amnesia: Not robust to coaching. *Psychology, Crime and Law, 14*(6), 523–528. http://dx.doi.org/10.1080/10683160801955183

Vickery, C. D., Berry, D. T., Inman, T. H., Harris, M. J., & Orey, S. A. (2001). Detection of inadequate effort on neuropsychological testing: A meta-analytic review of selected procedures. *Archives of Clinical Neuropsychology, 16*(1), 45–73. http://dx.doi.org/10.1016/S0887-6177(99)00058-X

Victor, T. L., & Boone, K. B. (2007). Identification of feigned mental retardation. In K. B. Boone (Ed.), *Assessment of feigned cognitive impairment: A neuropsychological perspective* (pp. 310–345). New York, NY: Guilford.

Victor, T. L., Boone, K. B., Serpa, J. G., Buehler, J., & Ziegler, E. A. (2009). Interpreting the meaning of multiple symptom validity test failure. *Clinical Neuropsychologist, 23*(2), 297–313. http://dx.doi.org/10.1080/13854040802232682

Victor, T. L., Kulick, A. D., & Boone, K. B. (2013). Assessing noncredible attention, processing speed, language, and visuospatial/perceptual function in mild traumatic brain injury cases. In D. Carone & S. Bush (Eds.), *Mild traumatic brain injury: Symptom validity assessment and malingering* (pp. 231–267). Hoboken, NJ: Springer.

Vissia, E. M., Giesen, M. E., Chalavi, S., Nijenhuis, E. R. S., Draijer, N., Brand, B. L., & Reinders, A. A. (2016). Is it trauma- or fantasy-based? Comparing dissociative identity disorder, post-traumatic stress disorder, simulators, and controls. *Acta Psychiatrica Scandinavica, 134*(2), 111–128. http://dx.doi.org/10.1111/acps.12590

Vitacco, M. J., Jackson, R. L., Rogers, R., Neumann, C. S., Miller, H. A., & Gabel, J. (2008). Detection strategies for malingering with the Miller Forensic Assessment of Symptoms Test: A confirmatory factor analysis of its underlying dimensions. *Assessment, 15*(1), 97–103. http://dx.doi.org/10.1177/1073191107308085.

Vitacco, M., Rogers, R., & Gabel, J. (2007). An evaluation of malingering screens with competency to stand trial patients: A known-groups comparison. *Law and Human Behavior, 31*(3), 249–260. http://dx.doi.org/10.1007/s10979-006-9062-8

Vitacco, M. J., Rogers, R., & Gabel, J. (2009). An investigation of the ECST-R in male pretrial patients evaluating the effects of feigning on competency evaluations. *Assessment, 16*(3), 249–257. http://dx.doi.org/10.1177/1073191108325057

Wager, J. G., & Howe, L. L. (2010). Nonverbal Medical Symptom Validity Test: Try faking now! *Applied Neuropsychology, 17*(4), 305–309. http://dx.doi.org/10.1080/09084282.2010.525093

Wall, B. W., & Christopher, P. P. (2012). A training program for defendants with intellectual disabilities who are found incompetent to stand trial. *Journal of the American Academy of Psychiatry and the Law Online, 40*(3), 366–373.

Wall, T. D., Wygant, D. B., & Gallagher, R. W. (2015). Identifying overreporting in a correctional setting: Utility of the MMPI-2 Restructured Form validity scales. *Criminal Justice and Behavior, 42*(6), 610–622. doi:10.1177/0093854814556881

Walters, G. D., White, T. W., & Greene, R. L. (1988). Use of the MMPI to identify malingering and exaggeration of psychiatric symptomatology in male prison inmates. *Journal of Consulting and Clinical Psychology, 56*(1), 111–117.

Watson, M. E., & Kivisto, A. J. (2017). The Inventory of Legal Knowledge (ILK) and adults with intellectual disabilities. *Journal of Intellectual Disabilities and Offending Behaviour, 8*(2), 83–89. https://doi.org/10.1108/JIDOB-10-2016-0018

Warren, J. I., DuVal, J., Komarovskaya, I., Chauhan, P., Buffington-Vollum, J., & Ryan, E. (2009). Developing a forensic service delivery system for juveniles adjudicated incompetent to stand trial. *International Journal of Forensic Mental Health, 8*(4), 245–262.

Washington v. State of Florida, No. 4D13-1213. District Court of Appeal of Florida, Fourth District (2015).

Wasyliw, O. E., Benn, A. F., Grossman, L. S., & Haywood, T. W. (1998). Detection of minimization of psychopathology on the Rorschach in cleric and noncleric alleged sex offenders. *Assessment, 5*(4), 389–397.

Webb, J. W., Batchelor, J., Meares, S., Taylor, A., & Marsh, N. V. (2012). Effort test failure: Toward a predictive model. *The Clinical Neuropsychologist, 26*(8), 1377–1396.

Wechsler, D. (1981). Wechsler Adult Intelligence Scale (Rev. ed.). San Antonio, TX: Psychological Corporation.

Wechsler, D. (1997). Wechsler Adult Intelligence Scale (3rd ed.). San Antonio, TX: Psychological Corporation.

Wechsler, D. (2008). Wechsler Adult Intelligence Scale (4th ed.). San Antonio, TX: Psychological Corporation.

Wechsler, D. (2009). *WASI: Wechsler abbreviated scale of intelligence.* Psychological Corporation.

Weinborn, M., Orr, T., Woods, S. P., Conover, E., & Feix, J. (2003). A validation of the Test of Memory Malingering in a forensic psychiatric setting. *Journal of Clinical and Experimental Neuropsychology*, *25*(7), 979–990. http://dx.doi.org/10.1076/jcen.25.7.979.16481

Weinborn, M., Woods, S. P., Nulsen, C., & Leighton, A. (2012). The effects of coaching on the Verbal and Nonverbal Medical Symptom Validity Tests. *Clinical Neuropsychologist*, *26*(5), 832–849. http://dx.doi.org/10.1080/13854046.2012.686630

Weiss, R. A., Rosenfeld, B., & Farkas, M. R. (2011). The utility of the Structured Interview of Reported Symptoms in a sample of individuals with intellectual disabilities. *Assessment*, *18*(3), 284–290. http://dx.doi.org/1073191111408230

Welburn, K. R., Fraser, G. A., Jordan, S. A., Cameron, C., Webb, L. M., & Raine, D. (2003). Discriminating dissociative identity disorder from schizophrenia and feigned dissociation on psychological tests and structured interview. *Journal of Trauma and Dissociation*, *4*(2), 109–130.

White, A. M. (2003). What happened? Alcohol, memory blackouts, and the brain. *Alcohol Research and Health*, *27*(2), 186–196.

Whiteside, D. M., Dunbar-Mayer, P., & Waters, D. P. (2009). Relationship between TOMM performance and PAI validity scales in a mixed clinical sample. *Clinical Neuropsychologist*, *23*(3), 523–533. http://dx.doi.org/10.1080/13854040802389169

Whiteside, D. M., Galbreath, J., Brown, M., & Turnbull, J. (2012). Differential response patterns on the Personality Assessment Inventory (PAI) in compensation-seeking and non-compensation-seeking mild traumatic brain injury patients. *Journal of Clinical and Experimental Neuropsychology*, *34*(2), 172–182. http://dx.doi.org/10.1080/13803395.2011.630648

Whitney, K. A. (2013). Predicting Test of Memory Malingering and Medical Symptom Validity Test failure within a Veterans Affairs Medical Center: Use of the Response Bias Scale and the Henry–Heilbronner Index. *Archives of Clinical Neuropsychology*, *28*(3), 222–235. http://dx.doi.org/10.1093/arclin/act012

Whitney, K. A., Davis, J. J., Shepard, P. H., & Herman, S. M. (2008). Utility of the Response Bias Scale (RBS) and other MMPI-2 validity scales in predicting TOMM performance. *Archives of Clinical Neuropsychology*, *23*(7), 777–786. http://dx.doi.org/10.1016/j.acn.2008.09.001

Whitney, K. A., Shepard, P. H., & Davis, J. J. (2013). WAIS-IV Digit Span variables: Are they valuable for use in predicting TOMM and MSVT failure?. *Applied Neuropsychology: Adult*, *20*(2), 83–94. https://doi.org/10.1080/09084282.2012.670167

Widows, M. R., & Smith, G. P. (2005). *SIMS: Structured Inventory of Malingered Symptomatology: Professional manual*. Lutz, FL: Psychological Assessment Resources.

Wiggins, C. W., Wygant, D. B., Hoelzle, J. B., & Gervais, R. O. (2012). The more you say the less it means: Overreporting and attenuated criterion validity in a forensic disability sample. *Psychological Injury and Law*, *5*(3–4), 162–173. http://dx.doi.org/10.1007/s12207-012-9137-4

Williams, C. (1992). *The Minnesota Multiphasic Personality Inventory-Adolescent*. Minneapolis, MN: Pearson Assessments.

Williams, C. L., Butcher, J. N., Gass, C. S., Cumella, E., & Kally, Z. (2009). Inaccuracies about the MMPI-2 fake bad scale in the reply by Ben-Porath, Greve, Bianchini, and Kaufman (2009). *Psychological Injury and Law*, *2*(2), 182–197. http://dx.doi.org/10.1007/s12207-009-9046-3

Williams, J. M. (2011). The malingering factor. *Archives of Clinical Neuropsychology*, *26*(3), 280–285. http://dx.doi.org/10.1093/arclin/acr009

Williamson, D. J., Holsman, M., Chaytor, N., Miller, J. W., & Drane, D. L. (2012). Abuse, not financial incentive, predicts non-credible cognitive performance in patients with psychogenic non-epileptic seizures. *Clinical Neuropsychologist*, *26*(4), 588–598. http://dx.doi.org/10.1080/13854046.2012.670266

Wilson v. United States, 391 F.2d 460 (1968).

Wisdom, N. M., Callahan, J. L., & Shaw, T. G. (2010). Diagnostic utility of the structured inventory of malingered symptomatology to detect malingering in a forensic sample. *Archives of Clinical Neuropsychology*, *25*(2), 118–125. doi:10.1093/arclin/acp110

Wisdom, N. M., Brown, W. L., Chen, D. K., & Collins, R. L. (2012). The use of all three Test of Memory Malingering trials in establishing the level of effort. *Archives of Clinical Neuropsychology*, *27*(2), 208–212. http://dx.doi.org/10.1093/arclin/acr107

Wise, E. A. (2009). Selected MMPI-2 scores of forensic offenders in a community setting. *Journal of Forensic Psychology Practice*, *9*(4), 299–309. doi:10.1080/15228930902936048

Wise, S. L., & Smith, L. F. (2011). A model of examinee test-taking effort. In J. A. Bovlard, K. F. Geisinger, & C. W. Buckendahl (Eds.), *High-stakes testing in education: Science and practice in K–12 settings* (pp. 139–153). Washington, DC: American Psychological Association. http://dx.doi.org/10.1037/12330-009

Witt, P. H. (2010). Forensic report checklist. *Open Access Journal of Forensic Psychology*, *2*, 233–240.

Woodworth, M., Porter, S., ten Brinke, L., Doucette, N. L., Peace, K., & Campbell, M. A. (2009). A comparison of memory for homicide, non-homicidal violence, and positive life experiences. *International Journal of Law and Psychiatry*, *32*(5), 329–334. http://dx.doi.org/10.1016/j.ijlp.2009.06.008

Wooley, C., & Rogers, R. (2015). The effectiveness of the Personality Assessment Inventory with feigned PTSD: An initial investigation of Resnick's model of malingering. *Assessment*, *22*(4), 449–458. http://dx.doi.org/10.1177/1073191114552076

Worthen, M. D., & Moering, R. G. (2011). A practical guide to conducting VA compensation and pension exams for PTSD and other mental disorders. *Psychological Injury and Law*, *4*(3–4), 187–216. http://dx.doi.org/10.1007/s12207-011-9115-2

Wygant, D. B., Anderson, J. L., Sellbom, M., Rapier, J. L., Allgeier, L. M., & Granacher, R. P. (2011). Association of the MMPI-2 restructured form (MMPI-2-RF) validity scales with structured malingering criteria. *Psychological Injury and Law*, *4*(1), 13–23. http://dx.doi.org/10.1007/s12207-011-9098-z

Wygant, D. B., Ben-Porath, Y. S., Arbisi, P. A., Berry, D. T. R., Freeman, D. B., & Heilbronner, R. L. (2009). Examination of the MMPI-2 restructured form (MMPI-2-RF) validity scales in civil forensic settings: Findings from simulation and known group samples. *Archives of Clinical Neuropsychology*, *24*(7), 671–680. http://dx.doi.org/10.1093/arclin/acp073.

Wygant, D. B., Sellbom, M., Ben-Porath, Y. S., Stafford, K. P., Freeman, D. B., & Heilbronner, R. L. (2007). The relation between symptom validity testing and MMPI-2 scores as a function of forensic evaluation context. *Archives of Clinical Neuropsychology*, *22*(4), 489–499. http://dx.doi.org/10.1016/j.acn.2007.01.027

Wygant, D. B., Sellbom, M., Gervais, R. O., Ben-Porath, Y. S., Stafford, K. P., Freeman, D. B., & Heilbronner, R. L. (2010). Further validation of the MMPI-2 and MMPI-2-RF Response Bias Scale: Findings from disability and criminal forensic settings. *Psychological Assessment*, *22*(4), 745–756. http://dx.doi.org/10.1037/a0020042

Wymer, J. H. (2006). Validation of the Barkemeyer-Callon-Jones Malingering Detection Scale. *American Journal of Forensic Psychiatry, 24*(1), 1–11.

Wynkoop, T. F., & Denney, R. L. (2005). Test review: Green's Word Memory Test (WMT) for Windows. *Journal of Forensic Neuropsychology, 4*(3), 101–105.

Yanez, Y. T., Fremouw, W., Tennat, J., Strunk, J., & Coker, K. (2006). Effects of severe depression on TOMM performance among disability-seeking outpatients. *Archives of Clinical Neuropsychology, 21*(2), 161–165. http://dx.doi.org/10.1016/j.acn.2005.07.009

Young, G. (2014). *Malingering, feigning, and response bias in psychiatric/psychological injury*. Heidelberg: Springer Dordrecht. http://dx.doi.org/10.1007/978-94-007-7899-3

Young, J. C., Kearns, L. A., & Roper, B. L. (2011). Validation of the MMPI-2 Response Bias Scale and Henry Heilbronner Index in a U.S. veteran population. *Archives of Clinical Neuropsychology, 26*(3), 194–204. http://dx.doi.org 10.1093/arclin/acr015

Youngjohn, J. R., Wershba, R., Stevenson, M., Sturgeon, J., & Thomas, M. L. (2011). Independent validation of the MMPI-2-RF somatic/cognitive and validity scales in TBI litigants tested for effort. *Clinical Neuropsychologist, 25*(3), 463–476. http://dx.doi.org/10.1080/13854046.2010.550635

Zapf, P. A., & Dror, I. E. (2017). Understanding and mitigating bias in forensic evaluation: Lessons from forensic science. *International Journal of Forensic Mental Health*, 1–12.

Zapf, P. A., Kukucka, J., Kassin, S., & Dror, I. (in press). Cognitive bias in forensic mental health evaluation: A survey of evaluators. *Psychology, Public Practice, and the Law.*

Zapf, P. A., & Roesch, R. (2009). *Best practices in forensic mental health assessment: Evaluation of competence to stand trial.* New York, NY: Oxford University Press.

Zavodny, D. (2016, December 15). Feigning in CST exams for juveniles. Message posted to PSYLAW-L@LISTSERV.UNL.EDU electronic mail archived at http://listserv.unl.edu/cgi-bin/wa?A0=psylaw-l

INDEX

Tables, figures, and boxes are indicated by an italic *t, f,* and *b* following the page number.

www.ingramcontent.com/pod-product-compliance
Lightning Source LLC
Chambersburg PA
CBHW062141140826
49870CB00032B/848